Gregory J. del Zoppo Etsuro Mori
Werner Hacke (Eds.)

Thrombolytic Therapy in Acute Ischemic Stroke II

With 60 Figures and 41 Tables

Springer-Verlag
Berlin Heidelberg New York
London Paris Tokyo
Hong Kong Barcelona
Budapest

Gregory J. del Zoppo, M.D.
Department of Molecular and Experimental Medicine,
The Scripps Research Institute
and Division of Hematology/Medical Oncology,
Scripps Clinic and Research Foundation,
10666 North Torrey Pines Road, La Jolla, CA 92037, USA

Etsuro Mori, M.D.
Neurology Service, Hyogo Brain and Heart Center at Himeji
520 Saisho-ko, Himeji, 670, Japan

Prof. Dr. Werner Hacke
Neurologische Klinik, Ruprecht-Karls-Universität Heidelberg
Im Neuenheimer Feld 400, W-6900 Heidelberg 1, FRG

Publication of this volume was substantially underwritten by
The Roon Foundation, Inc., of La Jolla, California, USA.

ISBN-13: 978-3-540-56442-3 e-ISBN-13: 978-3-642-78061-5
DOI: 10.1007/ 978-3-642-78061-5

Library of Congress Cataloging-in-Publication Data. Thrombolytic therapy in acute ischemic stroke II/Gregory J. del Zoppo, Etsuro Mori, Werner Hacke (eds.). p. cm. Includes bibliographical references and index. 1. Cerebrovascular disease – Chemotherapy – Congresses. 2. Thrombolytic therapy – Congresses. 3. Tissue plasminogen activator – Therapeutic use – Congresses. 4. Fibrinolysis – Congresses. 5. Thrombolytic Therapy – congresses. I. Del Zoppo, Gregory J. II. Mori, Etsuro, 1951– . III. Hacke, W, (Werner), 1948– . [DNLM: 1. Cerebral Ischemia – drug therapy – congresses. 2. Fibrinolysis – congresses. 3. Fibrinolytic Agents – therapeutic use – congresses. WL 355 T5314 1993] RC388.5.T4773 1993 616.8'10651–dc20

Typesetting: K+V Fotosatz GmbH, Beerfelden
25/3130-5 4 3 2 1 0 – Printed on acid-free paper

Preface

With the demonstration that cerebral arterial recanalization is feasible, there has been a more active pursuit of thrombolysis as a therapeutic option for patients in the acute stages of ischemic stroke. Since the inaugural symposium held in Heidelberg in May 1990, plans for prospective controlled trials of both fibrin-selective thrombolytic agents and fibrinogenolytic agents have matured. Several recently completed prospective trials give insights into the profile of hemorrhagic transformation and its risk, and limited information about clinical benefit. The possibility of early recanalization suggests an adjunctive role for possible neuronal protectants, new antithrombotics, and other novel agents and marries two major investigational directions. These and related topics provided the content for the Second International Symposium on Thrombolysis in Acute Ischemic Stroke, held in La Jolla 1–2 May 1992. This volume contains selected papers from that meeting, and a summary of the discussions which accompanied the papers.

The editors wish to express their gratitude for the extraordinary support of this symposium by a number of sponsors, including the Roon Foundation, Abbott Laboratories, Genentech Inc., Knoll Pharmaceuticals, Sumitomo Pharmaceuticals Co., Ltd., Dr. Karl Thomae GmbH (Boehringer Ingelheim Deutschland), and the Upjohn Company. Preparation of the manuscripts was facilitated by Ms. J. Koehler and her team and Ms. S. Larsen at the Scripps Research Institute. We wish to again thank Springer-Verlag, Heidelberg, for its generous assistance in the preparation and publication of this volume. Of course, this effort would not have been possible without the provocative contributions of a growing number of investigators to this exciting area.

La Jolla

Gregory J. del Zoppo
Etsuro Mori
Werner Hacke

Contents

Insights into the Pathogenesis of Cerebral Ischemia Relevant to Fibrinolysis

Diagnosis and Assessment of Outcomes in Acute Cerebral Ischemia

Open Communications

Clinical Trial Development

List of Contributors

Addresses are given at the beginning of the respective contribution.

Background to Thrombolytic Therapy in Acute Ischemic Stroke

Therapy for Acute Ischemic Stroke: Clinical Needs and Statistical Burdens

L. R. Caplan[1] and M. Gent[2]

Acute Stroke Treatment: Clinical Needs

Although brain ischemia involves very complex cellular and biochemical events, the issues in treating patients with brain ischemia can be viewed rather simply. Supplying blood and energy to the brain through the cardiovascular system can be compared to watering a lawn through a series of hoses. If water is not getting to a part of the lawn, there is either something wrong with the pump system (inadequate pressure or water volume) or the hose supplying that part of the lawn is blocked. Since this meeting concerns mostly thrombolysis, let us look at the situation of a blocked hose.

A number of options are available to keep the lawn green: 1) The most obvious and direct approach is to unblock the hose. This could be done by cutting open the hose and repairing it (surgery), if accessible. Alternatively, using a tool (angioplasty) or chemical substance (thrombolysis) might work. 2) If the hose could not be unblocked, one could try increasing flow by increasing the pressure and water volume. This might increase flow through a partially blocked hose or, more likely, increase flow through the other unblocked hoses (collateral circulation). Flow could be directed into the blocked hose beyond the obstruction by mechanically connecting the region with one of the other hoses (vascular shunt). Chemical installation into the system might be able to dilate some of the hoses and so augment flow into the desired region of the lawn (targeted vasodilatation). 3) Perhaps changing the fuel or water might help. The present water might be too thick (reduce viscosity) or carry too little energy. Increasing the oxygen content or energy-carrying capability might compensate for the reduced flow. 4) If the flow could not be improved, perhaps something could be placed on the grass to make it more resistant to damage.

[1] Department of Neurology, Tufts-New England Medical Center, Boston, MA, USA
[2] McMaster University and The Hamilton Civic Hospitals Research Centre, Henderson General Hospital, Hamilton, Ontario, Canada

G. J. del Zoppo, E. Mori, W. Hacke (Eds.)
Thrombolytic Therapy in Acute Ischemic Stroke II

Table 1. Factors related to the blocked artery

1. Size and location of the artery involved.
2. Time duration of the occlusion.
3. Occlusion mechanism: Embolic (thrombus arising proximally) vs thrombotic (thrombus arising in situ).
4. If embolic, nature of material blocking the artery: Red fibrin-dependent thrombus, white platelet plug, calcific particle, cholesterol plaque.
5. If thrombotic, the nature and severity of the underlying stenosis: Is it mostly fibromuscular or cholesterol-rich plaque? Is the blockage all plaque, all thrombus, or various intermediate mixes of plaque and thrombus?
6. Is thrombus loose and free or organized and adherent?
7. Length of the thrombus: Length is somewhat related to vascular anatomy and size of the artery. The internal carotid, middle cerebral and basilar arteries are likely all different.

Table 2. Ischemic brain and blood flow factors

1. Reversibility of ischemia: Is brain normal, irreversibly damaged, or stunned (diminished function but reversible).
2. Size of ischemic/infarcted regions.
3. Duration of ischemia.
4. Vascular damage by ischemia, foci or hemorrhage, or vasogenic edema within the infarct.
5. Blood pressure, especially presence and severity of hypertension.
6. Prior hypertension or other vascular injury.
7. Blood composition: Cellular constituents, coagulability, viscosity, and other hemorrheological factors.

Evaluation of Treatments – Trials

Any of these strategies potentially could be systematically studied in a therapeutic trial. The researcher could try one strategy and keep all other variables constant, then simply look at the grass to determine if the strategy worked. Alas, in human brains and arteries, the situation is far more complex and daunting. Limiting the discussion to one strategy, thrombolysis, there are still many diverse factors that probably influence the success or failure of the treatment. These include: factors related to the blocked artery (Table 1), factors related to the ischemic brain and its fine blood flow (Table 2), and factors related to the delivery of the thrombolytic agent (Table 3).

To make things even more complex, it might not be so easy to document or quantify the success of the treatment (Table 4). Since brain ischemia involves different brain regions, each of which has very different functions, comparison between functions is difficult. How will a hemianopia to be compared against stupor, weakness, numbness, ataxia, aphasia, etc.? Should the presence and size of the resulting infarct be used instead? How can small brain stem or spinal cord infarcts, in which a half centimeter lesion can be devastating, be compared to a similar sized small lesion in a cerebral lobe or the cerebellum where no, or very slight, deficit might result? Should we instead use sophisticated

Table 3. Delivery of thrombolytic agent

1. Agent used
2. Dose
3. Means of delivery: Intravenous or intra-arterial by catheter
4. Rate of delivery
5. Duration of delivery
6. Time delivery started and finished in relation to time thrombus formed and brain ischemia began
7. Use of other drugs, e.g., aspirin and heparin, before, during and after thrombolytic drug

Table 4. Evaluation of efficacy

1. Functional outcome: How to compare different deficits? How to compare grapes and grapefruits?
2. Size of infarct determined by neuroimaging or necropsy: How to compare different loci – brain stem *vs* cerebral lobes *vs* cerebellum?
3. Opening of the blocked artery: How and when will reperfusion be determined and measured?

neurophysiological or biochemical data to assess dysfunction? Alternatively, should the outcome measured be the presence and extent of vascular reopening? Vascular opening was the parameter measured in some early thrombolytic studies; however, what good is opening of the artery if the brain and patient are not better off, or possibly even worse, after reperfusion?

Statistical Analysis and Theoretical Problems with Trials

Trials will also, of course, have to include measures of complications. Reperfusion might cause bleeding or edema in the reperfused zone [1]. The treatment could also lead to systemic bleeding. Other complications might relate to drug delivery by catheters and the use of concomitant treatments. Drugs might have to be given after thrombolysis to maintain perfusion. So far, I have mentioned only the variability and complexity of factors involved and the factors to be evaluated. What about analysis of the results and statistical issues? All now agree that randomized, placebo-controlled therapeutic trials are potentially very important in making therapeutic progress. Many now view these trials in the same class as motherhood – unassailable and beyond reproach or question. There are, however, problems in the design, planning, performance, analysis and applicability of individual trials.

The main theoretical limitation of trials is summed up in the issue of numbers *vs* specificity. For the results of trials to have sufficient power to be statistically valid and important, the trial must include lots of patients – numbers. In order to include enough patients, the condition to be studied must be very common. To achieve numbers, a lumping strategy is usually needed rather than a "splitting" one. For example, to get enough patients for a thrombolytic trial, all blocked arteries and mechanisms of blockage would probably be needed. However, for the results of a trial to be useful for a practicing physician applying the data to care for an individual patient, the sample would need to include enough patients with features matching the patient to be treated. The more a trial lumps diverse subgroups, the more general are the results and the applicability to specific patients' declines. Subgroups can be managed by prospective stratification, that is, by randomizing patients using predetermined variables (e.g., artery, stroke mechanism, time since symptom onset, etc.) to ensure that subgroups will be relatively equally represented in the different treatment groups. Alternatively, the treatment results can be retrospectively analyzed by subgroup determinants. Some have raised issues about subgroup analysis [3].

Practical Issues in Trials

Besides the theoretical issues, there are very practical problems which are enumerated in Table 5. The first problem is money-funding. Trials are big operations. They require multiple centers, personnel, hardware and software, and equipment. Designing and writing grants takes time and great effort. The next hurdle is institutional review boards (IRBs) at each center. In my experience, these IRBs are usually administered by inflexible people who insist on dotting every "i" and crossing every "t". They are obsessed with consent forms that spell out every possible disaster and include, and even emphasize, that the study will not compensate the patient for complications. Few of us would sign these consent forms if we actually read them.

The next problem is inclusion and exclusion criteria. In some studies nearly every concurrent illness excludes the patient. Many patients usually have to be screened to find one that fits the inclusion/exclusion criteria. Estimates of eligible patients are nearly always exaggerated so that pilot trial runs are usually needed to create reasonable estimates of recruitment during the trial. Once the

Table 5. Some practical problems in trials

1. Funding
2. Time, personnel and experience for grant writing
3. Consent forms
4. Institutional review boards
5. Entry inclusions and exclusions
6. Forms
7. Uniformity of patient evaluations
8. Uniformity of evaluation of investigations (e.g., CT, MRI, angiography)
9. Uniformity of data entry onto forms
10. Recruitment
11. Ensuring continuation and follow-up in the trial
12. Compliance
13. Unblinded observers
14. Patient safety
15. Statistical analysis

funds are generated, the criteria and evaluation chosen, the consent forms written, and the IRB passed, then the next hurdle is actually recruiting patients into the trial. Many individuals conceive of trials as something good for everyone else. They do not want to be the "guinea pigs." If they are told that the doctors treating them do not know which is the best treatment for a condition, some will choose other doctors that seem to know already what is best. Considerable experience, patience, time and skill are needed for successful recruitment. Often relatives, friends and significant others must also be dealt with before consent is reached. Even then, some potential recruits change their minds or drop out very early in the study.

Forms must be designed. If forms are too long and laborious to fill out, many data items will be ignored. If too brief, they will omit key data. Who will fill out the forms? Often the most junior individual who is the least familiar with the subject is "elected" making the validity of the data suspect. Sometimes a clerk or nurse fill out the forms. It is very difficult to get senior clinicians to spend the time filling out or reviewing carefully the forms. Will the patient evaluations and form filling out be uniform and comparable across centers? Validity checks may be needed.

The next practical challenge is ensuring that patients stay in the trial, do not change treatment groups, and remain available for follow-up. In large urban centers, such as New York, Chicago and Los Angeles, some groups of patients are very difficult to trace after hospital discharge. Some will not return to the hospital or clinic. Some neighborhoods are dangerous to visit. Compliance is another important problem. How will the trialist know if patients got their treatments as prescribed? Will there be clues from one treatment that practically unblind the observers so that they might lose their objectivity? Safety, of course, is a critical issue. None of us would want to harm our patients. How can we be sure that patient safety is watched and preserved? Usually, an independent safety monitoring committee is needed.

Lastly, how will the results be analyzed statistically? You are all aware of the well known characterization – "lies, damn lies, and statistics." Statistics, like "creative accounting," can be used by some analysts to prove any of a series of hypotheses. Dr. Gent, in the remainder of this introductory chapter, will consider how best to deal with some of these theoretical and practical limitations. After all, we need trials to work and to give us the maximal useful data.

Acute Stroke Treatment: Statistical Requirements

I am unclear of the intent of Dr. Caplan's introduction. Was he suggesting that I am conniving and manipulative, or was he likening me to that great statesman Disraeli to whom the phrase "lies, damn lies, and statistics" is most often credited? I will assume it was the latter!

The concept of the randomized, controlled clinical trial was first promoted by Bradford Hill in the late 1940s and has now become established as the basic

Table 6. Methodological standards

1. Study objectives	6. Follow-up schedule
2. Population studied	7. Outcome events
3. Study treatments	8. Feasibility
4. Treatment allocation	9. Statistical analysis
5. Blinding	10. Organization

research strategy for the sound evaluation of therapeutic and prophylactic regimens. Since that time, various components of the methodology and organization have been refined and there is now general acceptance of the broad methodological requirements for good quality, large-scale intervention studies.

The methodological standards which are generally accepted today relate to some of the key components of the study protocol and execution which are listed in Table 6 and discussed below.

Study Objectives

The primary objective of a study should be the test of a stated hypothesis relating to the possible benefits of some defined treatment. For this objective to be clear and unambiguous, specific details need to be given about the treatment to be evaluated, about the patient population to which the findings of the trial would be applicable, and about the assessment of benefit in terms of which outcome events will be expected to be modified and in what time frame.

A prerequisite, of course, is that there be a sound rationale for the study based on the biology and pathogenesis of the clinical disorder being investigated and on the mechanism of action of the study treatment.

Population Studied

Specific inclusion criteria, together with criteria for exclusion, should be defined to describe the patients potentially eligible for consideration for the study. These are required for validation of appropriate patient selection relative to the research objectives, for consistency between collaborating clinical centers, and for replication by other investigators and by practitioners. Those patients satisfying the inclusion criteria would need to pass a screen of exclusion criteria which might include associated comorbid conditions; the presence of life-limiting diseases (e.g., cancer); contraindications to the test treatment; and any geographic inaccessibility that might present difficulty in following the patient carefully during the study.

One needs a careful balance between increased heterogeneity of the defined patient population in order to maximize the patient base for generalization, and a more selected group which may be more consistent with the rationale behind the test intervention and at high risk for the targeted outcome measures.

Study Treatments

The treatment regimen to be evaluated must be described in sufficient detail that it could be replicated exactly by another investigator or by a clinician who wanted to implement the results of the clinical trial in practice. With a drug intervention, therefore, it would be necessary to describe who did what to whom and with what formulation and dose; administered where and under what circumstances; with what dose adjustments and titrations; when it was initiated, for how long it was continued, and what the criteria were for deciding that the doses should be increased, tapered or terminated. The treatment should be consistent with current understanding of human structure and function, pharmacology, and clinical practice. The doses, durations, and dose-settings should conform to current understanding and convention or be justified if they do not.

Treatment Allocation

When assessing the possible benefit of a new treatment, it is necessary to compare the outcomes for a group of patients to whom the intervention has been applied to those of a corresponding control group. In these circumstances, one should ensure that these two groups of patients are similar at baseline in all relevant respects and that their subsequent management is similar, except in the test treatments received. This implies that satisfactory controls should be concurrent in time and place. The control group should receive the best treatment currently available and may need to receive, in addition, a placebo which is identical in appearance to the experimental treatment.

The only valid way to allocate patients to their respective treatment groups, i.e., to avoid bias, is according to some prescribed randomized arrangement. Randomization is also a prerequisite for the valid application of statistical tests in the assessment of differences in outcome between the respective treatment groups. To be appropriate, the method of randomization should be based on generated random numbers.

Before randomization, the patients can be stratified with respect to some of the important prognostic factors in order to maximize the initial comparability of the two treatment groups. Such stratification also facilitates the evaluation of treatment within defined patient subgroups, which might show that the magnitude of the benefit of the intervention was related to one or more identified risk factors. There are practical limitations to the number of factors on which one can stratify for any given study, but adjustments for additional prognostic factors can be made post hoc by applying appropriate statistical methods in the analysis of the data.

Blinding

An advantage of the use of an identical-appearing placebo treatment in the control group is that the study can be made double-blind wherein neither the attending physician nor the patient knows which treatment is being administered and, as such, the ascertainment and evaluation of outcomes are likely to be made free from bias. This is particularly important when there may be a subjective element in the assessment of important clinical outcomes.

It is sometimes not possible to maintain blindness – for example, because of characteristic side effects which clearly identifies the test treatment or because it is simply not feasible or ethical. In these circumstances, every effort should be made to have the outcome assessments made by someone who is unaware of the treatment a particular patient is receiving.

Follow-up Schedule

For patients entered into the study there must be a baseline assessment which documents the required demographic, laboratory, and clinical data. There must also be a schedule of clinic follow-up visits at times appropriate to monitoring and maintaining protocol adherence, as well as the detection of outcomes relating to both efficacy and safety.

Outcome Events

The outcome events or measures should be feasible and most relevant to the objectives of the study. In patients with cerebrovascular disease, for example, ischemic stroke, myocardial infarction and vascular death are significant outcomes which one would expect to be preventable by antiplatelet drugs. Furthermore, the use of the composite outcome of ischemic stroke, myocardial infarction, or vascular death provides a clinically sensible cluster which increases the expected incidence of outcomes in the control group and thus impacts favorably on sample size requirements. There should be specific criteria for such outcome events.

Feasibility

The estimated number of patients required in a clinical trial depends upon four parameters: 1) the rate at which the principal outcome events can be expected to occur in the control group (π); 2) the postulated benefit of the test treatment, measured by the relative risk reduction (Δ) in the expected rate at which the principal outcome events occur when given the experimental treatment; 3) the risk of concluding the treatment is of benefit when it is not [Type I error (α); the level of statistical significance]; and 4) the risk of concluding the test treatment is of no benefit when it is really of the magnitude specified in 2) above [Type II error (β); 1-β is the power of the test].

Table 7. Sample size

		Expected rate of outcomes in control group (%)		
		10	20	30
Expected Rate of outcomes in experimental group (%)	15		1028	144
	10		237	77
	5	513	95	46

$\alpha = 0.05$ (one sided)
$\beta = 0.10$

The risks α and β are virtually fixed by convention and are usually chosen to be 0.05 and 0.10, respectively. The required sample size is therefore essentially a function of only two parameters we can influence, namely π and Δ; the greater π and/or Δ, the smaller the sample size required, as shown in Table 7. These two parameters which relate to risk and response can be maximized by the appropriate selection of patients and choice of outcome events.

Efficiency can also be increased by the use of factorial designs in which patients are allocated to both of two experimental interventions, to one or other of the interventions, or to neither. This strategy worked well in the Canadian Cooperative Study [4] which evaluated aspirin and sulfinpyrazone and in ISIS-2 [2] which evaluated aspirin and streptokinase.

Statistical Analysis

The statistical methods used in the analysis should be described clearly. In carrying out the analysis, a demonstration of the comparability of the two groups at baseline with respect to important prognostic factors is necessary; attention should be paid to complications caused by incomplete follow-up; mortality from all causes as well as that due to the target clinical condition should be reported. The analysis should include the entire group of patients in the study as well as appropriate predefined subgroups.

Organization

The organization of large-scale, multicentered trials should include, in addition to the clinical centers, a coordinating and methods center, a clinical monitoring center, and appropriate policy, validation, and monitoring committees. A Steering Committee, which has overall responsibility for the design and execution of the study, should meet at least every six months to address and resolve policy issues encountered during the course of the study and to ensure the prompt and accurate completion of study documentation. A Central Validation Committee should be responsible for validating the outcome events reported by the investigators, using previously established criteria. An independent External Safety and Efficacy Monitoring Committee, a group with necessary expertise, should be responsible for ongoing unblinded monitoring of safety and efficacy. This monitoring should be based on quarterly summaries it receives from an independent interim analysis group which receives the necessary data from the coordinating and methods center. Only the independent safety committee and interim analysis group should be aware of the randomization code during the study.

Summary

Some considerations in the design, execution, and organization of large- scale clinical trials have been reviewed and attention has been drawn to the basic methodological requirements for the sound evaluation of new interventions.

References

1. Caplan LR (1991) Reperfusion of ischemic brain: Why and why not. In: Hacke W, del Zoppo GJ, Hirschberg M (eds) Thrombolytic therapy in acute ischemic stroke. Springer-Verlag, Berlin Heidelberg New York, p 36
2. ISIS-2 (Second International Study of Infarct Survival) Collaborative Group (1988) Randomised trial of intravenous streptokinase, oral aspirin, both, or neither among 17, 187 cases of suspected acute myocardial infarction: ISIS-2. Lancet 13 August:349–360
3. Oxman AD, Guyatt GH (1992) A consumer's guide to subgroup analyses. Ann Intern Med 116:78–84
4. The Canadian Cooperative Study Group (1978) A randomized trial of aspirin and sulfinpyrazone in threatened stroke. N Engl J Med 299:53–59

Clinical Outcome of Acute Ischemic Stroke: Prospective Angiographic Studies

C. Fieschi, M. L. Sacchetti, C. Argentino, M. Fiorelli, D. Toni, C. Gori, S. Bastianello, and G. Sette

Studies of supratentorial ischemic stroke have shown that the sooner an angiography is performed, the easier it is to detect the middle cerebral artery (MCA) trunk or branch occlusion [2, 3, 6]. Early angiography has demonstrated that up to 70% of strokes are due to complete occlusion of an arterial vessel downstream from the circle of Willis. This finding is confirmed by noninvasive transcranial doppler ultrasonography [8, 9]. The occlusions are embolic in the vast majority of our series. The emboli frequently disappear or move further downstream in the days following the acute event [1, 3, 5]. Unfortunately, in most patients this spontaneous thrombolysis takes place too late to be of clinical benefit. These considerations provide a rationale for early therapeutic thrombolysis in acute ischemic supratentorial strokes.

Angiographic and SPECT studies performed within the presumed "therapeutic window" have proven that, in almost 50% of cases, the brain region supplied by the occluded vessels already has a significant residual or collateral blood flow in the first hours following the ischemic event [3, 4].

This favorable recovery of collateral flow, which is probably sufficient to ensure tissue survival for the time window of up to 6 h, suggests that humans are more treatable than most animal models of focal brain ischemia, where ischemia is severe enough to prevent recovery beyond 3–4 h. In fact, pathophysiological studies [7] suggest that, when cerebral perfusion is persistently below the ischemic threshold of 8 ml/100 g/min, the chances of recovering function are very scarce even if reperfusion occurs as early as 4–6 h (i.e., the "therapeutic window"). Under these circumstances, the risks of reperfusion may exceed the benefits.

In order to examine the relationships between the level of perfusional deficit at 5 h and clinical outcome, we have analyzed 30-day neurological outcome in a series of 80 consecutive MCA strokes, by means of the Canadian Neurological Scale (C. N. S.) and the Barthel Index (B. I.). One subgroup of these patients (Group A) reached good recovery and functional ability (CNS $\geqslant$7.5, 33% of the patients), while the second subgroup (Group B) showed poor recovery (CNS$<$7.5; 67%; Table 1).

Department of Neurological Sciences, University of Rome, "La Sapienza," Rome, Italy

G. J. del Zoppo, E. Mori, W. Hacke (Eds.)
Thrombolytic Therapy in Acute Ischemic Stroke II

Table 1. Clinical outcome at day 30 after stroke

	Group A (Good outcome)	Group B (Poor outcome)
CNS Score	33%	67%
B.I. Score	32%	68%

The number of patients is expressed as percent of total series. Strikingly similar percent values for the two groups (A and B) were obtained using the Barthel index value of 60 as break point between good and poor outcome groups.

Table 2. Early vascular filling by angiography

	Present %	Absent %
Group A, good outcome ($n = 26$)	85	15
Group B, poor outcome ($n = 54$)	54	46

The two outcome groups (A and B) are as defined for Table 1.

SPECT scans, obtained in 32 of these patients within 5 h from stroke, were analyzed in a blinded fashion. The data analysis showed that all but one of the group A patients had good collateral perfusion downstream of the MCA, while group B showed either very severe CBF reduction or good perfusion in the same proportion of patients [4]. Similar observations were obtained from the angiograms (Table 2).

It may be presumed that, in Group B patients who presented good vascular filling within 5 h, the collateral circulation was either re-established too late to prevent tissue damage or that it was insufficient to restore CBF values over the ischemic threshold.

These two groups of patients (A and B) with different outcomes may represent two potentially different indications for thrombolytics, in that the greatest improvement is expected in the group with severe deficits and poor outcome (group B). However, if the target of reperfusion is dead tissue, deterioration with high risk of hemorrhagic and/or massive edema complications can be expected.

On the other hand, in the group with moderate-to-good spontaneous recovery (Group A), one might expect fewer risks except that in some of these patients the therapeutic thrombolysis might add little to the already favorable outcome. Consequently, in randomized trials these subgroups should be analyzed separately.

We have treated, with almost complete recovery, two such patients, within 4 h from clinical onset, with intravenous urokinase and rt-PA, respectively. Our experience suggests the "safe" administration of the drug, at least in cases with mild initial perfusional deficit, despite an MCA embolic occlusion.

Table 3. CT scan abnormalities (early hypodensity and/or ventricular shift and/or effacement of subarachnoid spaces) with 5 h of stroke

	Positive (%)	Negative (%)
Group A, good outcome ($n = 18$)	44	56
Group B, poor outcome ($n = 34$)	53	47

The two outcome groups (A and B) are defined as for Table 1.

Table 4. Clinical outcome according to the site of arterial occlusion at angiography 5 h after stroke

	Good (%)	Poor (%)
ICA occlusion ($n = 25$)	12	88
MCA occlusion ($n = 36$)	39	61
Absence of occlusion ($n = 19$)	47	53

Clinically, in patients it is difficult to distinguish between good and poor residual perfusion. Angiography and/or SPECT are, in fact, not always available and they are time-consuming. For this reason, these investigations cannot be included in a multicenter pragmatic trial and in day-to-day protocols.

How, then, can a proper thrombolytic treatment design be made on pathophysiological bases?

In order to answer this question, we analyzed the very early CT scan data of our series, and a larger series of 800 patients is currently being examined. Patients with poor residual/collateral flow have shown a high incidence of early CT scan abnormalities, suggestive of irreversible ischemic damage. However, the information obtained with CT scan is not clinically satisfactory. Almost half of our patients with normal early CT scans ended up with very severe neurological deficits, while 44% with a subsequent good outcome had a positive early CT scan (Table 3). Functional images are, in this early phase, more sensible than the morphological ones [4], including MRI (Fiorelli et al., 1991 unpublished data). Angiography also showed an unexpected correlation with outcome; i.e., an occlusion of the cervical internal carotid artery (ICA) predicted a much poorer outcome than an isolated MCA occlusion (Table 4). This suggests that a carotid artery Doppler scan must be performed in all randomized reperfusional studies in order to stratify patients at least for a posthoc analysis.

Considering these limitations, we should refine the clinical investigation itself and match whatever predictive information can be obtained from other techniques. We could better separate two prognostic groups of patients by using the initial C. N. S. score rather than by the early CT scan [3]. Furthermore,

Table 5. Changes in neurological score in the acute phase (6–24 h) in 80 patients

22% Progressing (65% poor outcome)	27% Improving (75% good outcome)

Those patients (65%) with progressing neurological deficits in this early phase, were included in the poor outcome group as determined at the 30-day neurological evaluation. In contrast, 75% of patients who showed improving neurological deficits in the 6- to 24-hour interval were included in the good outcome group.

the clinical course might represent an unexploited source of information.

Repeated neurological evaluations within the first 24 h have shown that the neurological score changes in about 50% of patients (Table 5). This appears to be highly predictive of outcome (Table 5).

Neurological scales could be repeated between "time 0," when the patient is first seen, and the "time 0+90 min," before any possible effect of treatment. Supposing that this apparently too short interval is in fact related to the underlying pathophysiological conditions, what are the disadvantages of testing this hypothesis by repeating a semi-quantitative neurological scale at these two time points?

Finally, we believe that the clinical neurologist plays the most important role in the course and evaluation of clinical trials in acute cerebral ischaemia. The application of neurological scales requires both motivation and accuracy, which should be part of the training of all physicians dealing with acute stroke management, while the roles of investigational techniques should not be overemphasized in the clinical setting of efficacy trials.

References

1. Dalal PM, Shah PM, Seth SC, Deshpande CK (1965) Cerebral embolism angiographic observations on spontaneous clot lysis. Lancet i:61–64
2. del Zoppo GJ, Poeck K, Pessin MS, 16 co-authors of the rt-PA Acute Stroke Study Group (1992) Recombinant tissue plasminogen activator in acute thrombotic and embolic stroke. Ann Neurol 32:78–86
3. Fieschi C, Argentino C, Lenzi GL, Sacchetti ML, Toni D, Bozzao L (1989) Clinical and instrumental evaluation of patients with ischemic stroke within the first six hours. J Neurol Sci 91:311–321
4. Giubilei F, Lenzi GL, Di Piero V, et al (1990) Predictive value of brain perfusion single-photon emission computed tomography in acute ischemic stroke. Stroke 21:895–900
5. Hakim AM, Pokrupa RP, Villanueva J, et al (1987) The effect of spontaneous reperfusion on metabolic function in early human cerebral infarcts. Ann Neurol 21:279–289
6. Horowitz SH, Zito JL, Donnarumma R, Patel M, Arvil J (1991) Computed tomographic-angiographic findings within the first five hours of cerebral infarction. Stroke 22:1245–1253
7. Pulsinelli W (1992) Pathophysiology of acute stroke. Lancet 369:533–536
8. Ringelstein B (1992) Transcranial doppler ultrasonography in acute stroke management. 2nd International Symposium on Thrombolytic Therapy in Acute Ischemic Stroke, La Jolla, CA, USA
9. Zanette EM, Fieschi C, Bozzao L, et al (1989) Comparison of cerebral angiography and transcranial doppler sonography in acute stroke. Stroke 20:899–903

The Ischemic Penumbra: Usefulness of PET*

W. J. Powers

Studies in experimental animals have provided a detailed description of the changes in cerebral blood flow (CBF) and metabolism that occur during and after transient focal cerebral ischemia [2, 8, 9, 13, 15]. When a vessel is occluded, a central core of severe ischemia is produced that is surrounded by zone with less reduction in blood flow where perfusion is maintained by collateral circulation. No changes in brain metabolism or function occur as long as CBF is above approximately 20 ml 100 g^{-1} min^{-1}. Below this level, brain electrical activity fails and neurological deficits appear. Normal cellular biochemistry is disrupted as energy supply becomes insufficient due to inadequate supply of oxygen. Depletion of high energy phosphate stores (ATP, phosphocreatine [PCr]) occurs. Anaerobic metabolism of the small amount of residual glucose from intracellular stores and remaining blood flow results in lactic acidosis. With more severe reduction in CBF to approximately 10–12 ml 100 g^{-1} min^{-1}, integrity of cell membranes is lost with leakage of intracellular K^{+} into extracellular spaces and influx of extracellular Ca^{++} into cells. Cell death will follow if reperfusion does not occur. Following reperfusion, biochemical and ionic perturbations resolve to variable degrees depending on the severity of the ischemic insult. However, further cell damage may occur due to generation of free radicals and prostanoids and to the influx of blood-borne leukocytes.

The ability of neurons to survive a period of transient cerebral ischemia depends on both the severity and duration. Other factors such as age, species, temperature, glucose availability and the different sensitivity of different neuronal populations also affect ischemic tolerance. The pathophysiologic state that occurs in acute ischemia in which neurons are nonfunctional but alive and salvageable by reperfusion has been called the ischemic penumbra [2]. In experimental animals, this pathophysiologic state is unstable and, even without further reduction in CBF, neurons usually go on to die within hours. The extent and duration of this ischemic penumbra in human stroke is unknown.

* Supported by Grants NS06833, NS 28700, and NS 28947 of the National Institutes of Health, the Lillian Strauss Institute for Neuroscience and the Jewish Hospital of St. Louis.

Department of Neurology, The Jewish Hospital of St. Louis, Washington University Medical Center, St. Louis, MO, USA

G. J. del Zoppo, E. Mori, W. Hacke (Eds.)
Thrombolytic Therapy in Acute Ischemic Stroke II

CBF thresholds for brain function and cell death similar to those found in animals have been demonstrated in humans. In patients undergoing carotid endarterectomy, EEG slowing and flattening occur when hemispheric CBF falls below approximately 18 ml 100 g^{-1} min^{-1} [14, 16]. In patients with carotid artery disease, positron emission tomography (PET) has shown that CBF as low as 19 ml 100 g^{-1} min^{-1} and cerebral metabolic rate of oxygen ($CMRO_2$) of 60 μM 100 g^{-1} min^{-1} (1.3 ml 100 g^{-1} min^{-1}) may occur without neurological dysfunction. $CMRO_2$ below 60 μM 100 g^{-1} min^{-1} is found only in infarcted tissue. CBF in infarcted tissue is variable depending on the state of reperfusion, but values below 12 ml 100 g^{-1} min^{-1} have only been observed in infarcts (except for newborn infants). All of these PET studies were performed on patients who were neurologically stable. In three patients with acute ischemic neurological deficits that subsequently reversed, CBF was 13–16 ml 100 g^{-1} min^{-1} and $CMRO_2$ was $\geqslant$60 μ*M* 100 g^{-1} min^{-1} [1, 4, 11, 12].

In acute ischemic stroke, a focal reduction in CBF is accompanied by a reduction in $CMRO_2$. In patients studied within the first 48 h, this reduction in CBF is often proportionately greater than the reduction in $CMRO_2$ corresponding to an increase in oxygen extraction fraction (OEF) [3, 4, 17]. The closer to the ictus, the more likely is there to be an increase in OEF. Patients with elevated OEF usually have CBF below 20 ml 100 g^{-1} min^{-1} whereas those with lower OEF have flows above this value [6]. Hakim and colleagues reported CBF above 20 ml 100 g^{-1} min^{-1} in 5 of 12 patients with early cerebral infarcts who were studied within 48 h, indicating the occurrence of early spontaneous reperfusion without tissue recovery. The initial period of increased OEF has been interpreted as indicating a state of "critical perfusion" in still viable tissue during which restoration of flow should restore both metabolism and function, i.e., the ischemic penumbra. The increased OEF is also consistent with changes in CBF and $CMRO_2$ that occur during post-ischemic hypoperfusion in animals.

PET studies of patients with acute ischemic strokes performed within 48 h have demonstrated a dense core of ischemia with CBF and $CMRO_2$ values similar to those seen in later studies of areas of fully developed infarction [3, 5, 7]. Surrounding this dense core is a region consistent with a region of ischemic penumbra in which $CMRO_2$ is above 60 μM 100 g^{-1} min^{-1} and CBF is 10–20 ml 100 g^{-1} min^{-1}. When these patients are re- studied 1–2 weeks later, this peri-infarct region has undergone metabolic deterioration with further reduction in $CMRO_2$, even though CBF has increased [7, 10]. Recent studies in baboons subjected to middle cerebral artery occlusion have indicated that this metabolic deterioration may take place very early. Between 50±3 min and 2.5±0.6 h postocclusion, $CMRO_2$ showed a further decline of 15%–20%, even though CBF did not change appreciably [10].

In one patient with persistently increased OEF on day 4, Wise and coworkers raised systemic blood pressure by angiotensin infusion, resulting in increased blood flow to the infarcted region. Regional OEF decreased but $rCMRO_2$ did not change, and there was no neurological improvement. Thus, they were unable to confirm an association between increased OEF and the ischemic penumbra [17]. This patient was unusual in that the OEF elevation persisted for so long. Nevertheless, this case demonstrates that an increase in OEF is not sufficient as a marker for the ischemic penumbra.

The potential application of PET measurements of CBF and $CMRO_2$ to the detection of a small penumbral region of nonfunctional but viable neurons around an area of infarcted tissue is subject to methodologic restraints that may greatly reduce its accuracy. Due to partial volume averaging, PET measurements of regional CBF and $CMRO_2$ at the edge of an infarct will be influenced both by values within the infarct and those in the surrounding brain tissue. We have investigated the effect of partial volume averaging on the detection of an ischemic penumbra by performing computer simulations of cerebral infarcts with and without an ischemic penumbra [12]. These simulations were based on a digitized image of an actual brain slice with a gray–white ratio of 80:20 for CBF and 5:1.25 for $CMRO_2$. In the right Sylvian region of this image, a circular infarcted area 18.9 mm in diameter was created with CBF of 5 and $CMRO_2$ of 0.2. Surrounding this infarct, penumbral rings 2.7 or 5.4 mm wide were created with CBF of 15 and $CMRO_2$ of either 2.5 or 1.5 (corresponding to oxygen extraction fractions of 1.0 and 0.6, respectively). These original digitized images with and without penumbras were subjected to simulated scanning and reconstruction procedures based on the design and performance characteristics of the PETT VI tomograph to produce a final image with resolution of 18 mm FWHM.

In the case of infarction without penumbra we have assumed that there is an abrupt decrease in CBF and $CMRO_2$ levels from normal to those found in infarcted tissue. Due to partial volume averaging, this abrupt decrease will be imaged by PET as a gradual transition. Regional values for CBF and $CMRO_2$ within the penumbral range will be detected in this transition zone even when no actual regions with these values exist in the brain. When a penumbral region surrounds the infarct, PET measurements will again show this transition zone. There is little difference between the two scans except the apparent area of infarction looks larger in the infarct with penumbra because the total area of abnormal tissue is larger.

Fortunately, the situation for OEF is not the same. OEF is increased in the penumbra as compared to both normal tissue or infarct. Thus, partial volume averaging which tends to blur differences in spatially contiguous regions can cause a true increase in OEF to be of smaller magnitude, but it cannot produce an artifactual zone of increase where it is not really present. Thus, an area of increased OEF associated with CBF of 10–20 ml 100 g^{-1} min^{-1} and $CMRO_2 > 1.3$ ml 100 g^{-1} min^{-1} may indicate viable, nonfunctioning tissue in some patients. There may also be an interaction between the time since the stroke occurred and the level of CBF and $CMRO_2$ which indicate normal viability on reperfusion. The metabolism of glial cells which make up approximately 50% of the brain and are more resistant than neurons to ischemia may further complicate the issue. Proof of the value of PET in identifying the ischemic penumbra rests on studying patients during periods of acute cerebral ischemia, documenting that tissue reoxygenation occurs with therapeutic intervention, and then correlating the subsequent clinical course with the initial PET measurements. To date, such studies have not been performed and this clinical application of PET, although attractive, remains theoretical. Even if such studies do demonstrate the accuracy of PET for identifying reversible ischemia, the time required to make the necessary PET measurements may be an obstacle to routine clinical application. Under the very best of circumstances, PET measurements of CBF and $CMRO_2$ take an hour. In acute stroke, where the time interval between the onset of ischemia and the institution of therapy is likely to have direct bearing on outcome, the additional time necessary to perform PET may be critical. The data obtained would need to have crucial bearing on therapeutic decisions in order to be worth the delay. Merely predicting who would and who would not respond to a given therapy may not be enough, unless the therapy itself were very expensive or carried significant morbidity and mortality. If the data derived from PET could be used to minimize these complications, then PET might be worthwhile.

References

1. Altman DI, Powers WJ, Perlman JM, et al (1988) Cerebral blood requirements for brain viability in newborn infants is lower than in adults. Ann Neurol 24:218–226
2. Astrup J, Siesjo BK, Symon L (1981) Thresholds in cerebral ischemia – the ischemic penumbra. Stroke 12:723–725
3. Baron JC, Rougemont D, Bousser MG, Lebrum-Grandie P, Iba-Zizen MT, Chivas JC (1983) Local CBF, oxygen extraction fraction and $CMRO_2$: Prognostic value in recent supratentorial infarction. J Cereb Blood Flow Metab 3(Suppl 1):S1–S2
4. Baron JC, Rougemont D, Lebrun-Grandie P, et al (1983) Measurement of local blood flow and oxygen consumption in evolving irreversible cerebral infarction: An in vivo study in man. In: Meyer JS, Lechner H, Reivich M, Ott EO (eds) Cerebral vascular disease 4. Excerpta Medica, Princeton, p 205
5. Hakim AM, Evans AC, Berger L, et al (1989) The effect of nimodipine on the evolution of human cerebral infarction studied by PET. J Cereb Blood Flow Metab 9:523–534
6. Hakim AM, Pokrupa RP, Villanueva J, et al (1987) The effect of spontaneous reperfusion on metabolic function in early human cerebral infarcts. Ann Neurol 21:279–289
7. Heiss W-D, Huber M, Fink GR et al (1992) Progressive derangement of peri-infarct viable tissue in ischemic stroke. J Cereb Blood Flow Metab 12:193–203
8. Heiss WD, Rosner G (1983) Functional recovery of cortical neurons as related to degree and duration of ischemia. Ann Neurol 14:294–301
9. Hossman K-A (1988) Pathophysiology of cerebral infarction. In: Vinken PJ, Bruyn GW, Klawans HL, Toole JF (eds) Handbook of clinical neurology, Vol. 53. Elsevier Science Publishing Co., New York, p 107
10. Pappata S, Fiorelli A, Hartmann A, et al (1991) PET study of local brain hemodynamics and oxygen metabolism in primate-model of acute middle cerebral artery occlusion (MCAO). J Cereb Blood Flow Metab 11(Suppl 2):S655
11. Powers WJ, Grubb RL, Jr., Darriet D, Raichle ME (1985) Cerebral blood flow and cerebral metabolic rate of oxygen requirements for cerebral function and viability in man. J Cereb Blood Flow Metab 5:600–608
12. Powers WJ, Mintun MA (1987) The role of positron emission tomography in identification of the ischemic penumbra. In: Powers WJ, Raichle WE (eds) Cerebrovascular diseases. Fifteenth Research (Princeton) Conference. Raven Press, New York

13. Siesjo BK (1984) Cerebral circulation and metabolism. J Neurosurg 60:883–908
14. Sundt T, Sharbrough F, Anderson R, Michenfelder J (1974) Cerebral blood flow measurements and electroencephalograms during carotid endarterectomy. J Neurosurg 41:310–320
15. Symon L, Pasztor E, Branston NJM (1974) The distribution and density of reduced cerebral blood flow following acute middle cerebral artery occlusion: An experimental study by the technique of hydrogen clearance in baboons. Stroke 5:355–364
16. Trojaborg W, Boysen G (1973) Relation between EEG, regional cerebral blood flow and internal carotid artery pressure during carotid endarterectomy. Electroencephalogr Clin Neurophysiol 34:61–69
17. Wise RJS, Bernardi S, Frackowiak RSJ, et al (1983) Serial observations on the pathophysiology of actue stroke. Brain 106:197–222

Thrombolytic Agents: Lessons for Their Use in Acute Stroke from Myocardial Infarction Experience

M. Verstraete

As for patients with acute myocardial infarction, thrombolytic treatment of acute stroke is not a recent proposal. This is not surprising, as both conditions are most often caused by a common etiology, a thrombotic occlusion of a coronary or cerebral atherosclerotic artery, respectively. Initial clinical studies with streptokinase in acute myocardial infarction and in acute stroke patients suffered from many technical problems and clinical limitations. Since thrombolysis of acute myocardial infarction came of age in the last decade, there has been a concomitant resurgence of interest in the thrombolytic treatment of ischemic stroke. Advances in clinical and radiological diagnostic techniques, the use of superselective arterial catheters and the availability of a new generation of more fibrin- specific thrombolytic agents are also responsible for the renewed interest in this difficult area of neurological investigations.

The presence of an acute arterial occlusion precipitates a myocardial infarction and ischemic stroke, which calls for the same thrombolytic treatment. However, there are important differences between the two clinical conditions which may have a bearing on investigational therapeutic approaches.

Myocardial Stunning and the "No-Reflow" Phenomenon Versus Cerebral Reperfusion Injury

Much skepticism has surrounded coronary thrombolysis in the early 1980s, as the potential of risks was widespread [8]. The possibility that coronary vasospasm, calcium overload accompanying suffusion of jeopardized myocardium with blood from recanalized arteries and the "no-reflow" phenomenon (microvascular compromise secondary to platelet and leukocyte plugging, endothelial swelling, or vasoconstriction) were seriously entertained. The myth of reperfusion injury was rampant but did not materialize in the vast majority of patients with myocardial infarction treated with thrombolytic drugs. The same holds for reperfusion arrhythmias. Myocardial stunning defined as a

Center for Thrombosis and Vascular Research, Katholieke Universiteit Leuven, Leuven, Belgium

G. J. del Zoppo, E. Mori, W. Hacke (Eds.)
Thrombolytic Therapy in Acute Ischemic Stroke II

postischemic transient dysfunction of viable myocardium appears, however, to be of clinical relevance in patients [5, 31].

There is the hypothesis that within certain limits, brain damage after experimental global brain ischemia is not only determined during the ischemic insult but also by the postischemic changes initiated by the ischemia which add to the ultimate degree of neurologic deficit sustained. The no-reflow phenomenon described in the brain by Ames and co-workers [2] may result from neuronal, glial, and capillary endothelial edema, red cell aggregation and lysosomal enzyme activation resulting from cytolysis and infarction [13]. Intracranial pressure due to ischemic brain swelling may in this regard be a much more important factor than for the myocardium which is not confined in a closed box [19].

Incidence of Coronary Thrombosis and Cerebral Embolism

Coronary thrombosis on an underlying atherosclerotic plaque is now accepted as the factor which precipitates acute myocardial infarction in the vast majority of patients, fibrin emboli and platelet aggregates in the coronary circulation being rarely the cause of a transmural infarction.

In contrast, the cause of an ischemic stroke in the cortical middle cerebral artery territory is considered to be in 44% due to carotid artery atherosclerosis with distal embolization, whereas in 40% cardiogenic embolism was the suspected mechanism [4]. Small embolic fragments only 3–4 mm in diameter can occlude the middle cerebral artery and cause devastating stroke. In general, about 15% of all ischemic strokes are due to a cardiogenic embolism [10]. Ulcerated plaques in the aortic arch are highly suspected as a cause of cerebral embolism [1].

The frequency of embolism in causing ischemic stroke is striking when compared with myocardial infarction. Cerebral emboli result in a more severe neurologic deficit in patients without atherosclerosis and thus without developed collaterals in the brain circulation which may narrow the time window for effective treatment.

Coronary Stenosis Versus Narrowing of Extracranial Arteries

In the heart there seems to be a direct relation between the magnitude of collateral development and the severity of coronary artery stenosis. The increased flow capacity of collateral coronary arteries has important implications for the preservation of myocardial function [27]. Myocardial damage, profound left ventricular dysfunction, and probably sudden death are more likely to occur after sudden occlusion of a coronary artery with underlying mild atherosclerotic narrowing, rather than after an occlusion of a vessel with a more severe stenosis.

While an atherosclerotic carotid stenosis of 75% or greater of the luminal diameter increases sharply the risk for the development of ischemic symptoms, there is much less evidence that a stenosis in extracranial arteries develops collateral circulation in the intracranial circulation as does progressive coronary stenosis in nearby coronary arteries. As noted above, this is of major importance if the ischemic stroke is due to an embolus detached from an atherosclerotic plaque in the aortic arch and its cervical branches.

Stuttering Myocardial Infarction and Abrupt Stroke

A novel concept is that myocardial infarction is often a stuttering event, a dynamic process evolving over hours rather than a few minutes. It may be difficult to define with acceptable accuracy the time of onset of myocardial infarction as chest pain, electrocardiographic ST segment and T-wave changes, arrhythmias and other clinical criteria are notoriously unreliable for this purpose. This explains the controversy on the relative benefit of thrombolytic treatment when the interval between the onset of infarction and the start of thrombolytic treatment increases over 6 h [16, 18, 20, 33].

Most often the symptoms of a stroke are sudden and its beginning can be more sharply defined than in patients having a myocardial infarction. This may shorten the critical time interval required for effective thrombolytic treatment in patients with acute stroke in a still more remarkable manner as has been witnessed in the last years for patients with myocardial infarction [9, 11, 12].

Is the Therapeutic Time Window Larger in Acute Myocardial Infarction than in Ischemic Stroke?

The time course of development of irreversible myocardial damage after coronary occlusion was studied by Schaper [29] in various animal species. In rats and rabbits the infarct appeared to be completed after approximately 1 hour occlusion, such that subsequent reperfusion in these species did not salvage any myocardial tissue. On the other hand, reperfusion of the ischemic myocardium in cats and dogs after 1–3 h of occlusion resulted in salvage of approximately half of the myocardium at risk, while in guinea pigs coronary occlusion did not result in myocardial necrosis at all. Other groups confirmed that after experimentally induced myocardial infarction in dogs with no collaterals, the infarction process usually is completed within 6 h after coronary occlusion [21]. The results of recent clinical trials called this theory of a limited time window into question. Although the benefits of thrombolysis lessen as the interval between the appearance of symptoms and treatment increases, some benefits are still apparent up to 24 h after symptom onset.

After ischemic stroke, the level of residual blood flow is a major variable in determining the speed at which the ischemic process evolves towards an irreversible stage and therefore in determining the time interval until irreversible damage has occurred. For instance, it is commonly thought that electrically silent ischemic brain tissue (the ischemic penumbra described by Astrup and colleagues [3]) surrounding the main infarction area remains potentially viable for a few hours provided a residual "critical" perfusion is maintained [14, 23–25]. It is still an open question whether thrombolytic treatment in patients begun 6–8 h after the clinical symptoms of an ischemic brain infarction will be effective, as some data in experimental animal models suggest [34–36]. Opening up of a cerebral artery might help if patients are at the critical stage of cerebrovascular reserve exhaustion but still before the ischemic process has started. Late spontaneous restoration of blood flow [15] is not associated with clinical benefit.

Incidence of Drug-Induced Cerebral Bleeding Versus Myocardial Hemorrhage

Spontaneous hemorrhage in the myocardium only occurs as a rare complication of antithrombotic or thrombolytic treatment [17]. In contrast, a number of vascular pathologies may produce a hemorrhagic stroke which accounts for about 15% of all strokes. Subarachnoid bleeding occurs when an arterial aneurysm ruptures, while spontaneous primary intracerebral hemorrhage is most often associated with changes in small vessels. The latter condition is mainly related to age and hypertension, but has no direct link with atherosclerosis.

The risk of cerebral bleeding in patients treated with thrombolytic drugs is circa 0.6% [22]. Why the brain is more susceptible to bleeding than, for instance, the retina where a minute hemorrhage also has devastating consequences is an unsolved question. Still unidentified local cerebrovascular factors such as prior head trauma, silent cerebral emboli, and concomitant angiopathies may play an additional role to the hypocoagulable state in causing intracranial hemorrhage [22].

Local Versus Intravenous Administration of Thrombolytic Drugs in Acute Myocardial Infarction and Ischemic Stroke

When cardiologists eventually became interested in the thrombolytic treatment of acute myocardial infarction, they preferred the intracoronary administration of thrombolytic drugs. The direct delivery of a thrombolytic agent at the intended site and the immediate visual angiographic control of clot lysis convinced even skeptical cardiologists. However, in order to offer the benefit of thrombolytic treatment to a greater proportion of patients as soon as possible after their myocardial infarction, short and simple therapeutic schemes must be developed [32]. The logistics are, of course, in favor of the intravenous use of thrombolytic drugs which are the only realistic therapeutic approach as well in acute myocardial infarction as in ischemic stroke.

Relative Importance of Adjunctive Treatment to Thrombolysis for the Improvement of Myocardial Infarction or Cerebral Function

A modest but significant improvement in regional left ventricular function has been obtained with all thrombolytic agents in patients when coronary recanalization was successful, with no change evident in patients in whom persistent recanalization had not been induced [30]. This benefit was obtained regardless of adjunctive treatment with β-adrenergic blockers, calcium antagonists, nitrates and other agents which may retard cell death in ischemic myocardial tissue [6, 7].

It is an unresolved matter whether the ischemic brain would need additional protection therapy before blood flow is restored. Possible candidates are *N*-methyl-D-aspartate (NMDA) receptor blockers, calcium ion channel blockers, calcium overload blockers, glycerol and free radical scavengers (e.g., 21-aminosteroids) [13]. The fact that these agents used alone were not convincingly shown to be valuable in patients [28] does not exclude the possibility that in conjunction with thrombolytic treatment some neuroprotective drugs administered timely and for days prevent ischemia- related abnormalities in brain cells. It is indeed possible that even a small increase in blood flow may optimize the volume of moderately ischemic brain that is responsive to neuroprotective agents [26].

References

1. Amarenco P, Duyckaerts C, Tzourio C, Hénin D, Bousser MG, Hauw JJ (1992) The prevalence of ulcerated plaques in the aortic arch in patients with stroke. N Engl J Med 326:221–225
2. Ames A,III, Wright RL, Kowada M, Thurston JM, Majno G (1968) Cerebral ischemia. II. The no-reflow phenomenon. Am J Pathol 52:437–453
3. Astrup J, Siesjoe BK, Symon L (1981) Thresholds in cerebral ischemia – the ischemic penumbra. Stroke 12(6):723–725
4. Bogousslavsky J, Van Melle G, Rigli F (1989) Middle cerebral artery pial territory infarcts: A study of the Lausanne stroke registry. Ann Neurol 25:555–560
5. Bolli R, Triana JF, Jeroudi MO (1990) Prolonged impairment of coronary vasodilatation after reversible ischemia: Evidence for microvascular "stunning". Circ Res 67:322–343
6. Braunwald E (1985) The aggressive treatment of acute myocardial infarction. Circulation 71:1087–1092

7. Braunwald E (1987) The path to myocardial salvage by thrombolytic therapy. Circulation 76(Suppl II):II2–II7
8. Bresnahan GF, Roberts R, Shell WE, Ross J, Jr., Sobel BE (1974) Deleterious effects due to hemorrhage after myocardial reperfusion. Am J Cardiol 33:82–86
9. Brott T, Haley C, Levy D, et al (1990) Safety and potential efficacy of tissue plasminogen activator (t-PA) for stroke. Stroke 21:181 (Abstract)
10. Chesebro JH, Fuster V, Halperin JL (1990) Atrial fibrillation – Risk marker for stroke. N Engl J Med 323:1556–1558
11. del Zoppo GJ, Ferbert A, Otis S, et al (1988) Local intra-arterial fibrinolytic therapy in acute carotid territory stroke. A pilot study. Stroke 19:307–313
12. del Zoppo GJ, Poeck K, Pessin MS, and 16 coauthors of the rt-PA Acute Stroke Study Group (1992) Recombinant tissue plasminogen activator in acute thrombotic and embolic stroke. Ann Neurol 32:78–86
13. Editorial (1991) Treatment for stroke? Lancet 337:1129–1130
14. Fieschi C, Argentino C, Lenzi GL, et al (1988) Therapeutic window for pharmacological treatment in acute focal cerebral ischemia. Ann NY Acad Sci 522:662–666
15. Fieschi C, Argentino C, Lenzi GL, Sacchetti ML, Toni D, Bozzao L (1989) Clinical and instrumental evaluation of patients with ischemic stroke within the first six hours. J Neurol Sci 91:311–321
16. Fox KAA, Saffitz JE, Corr PB (1987) Pathophysiology of myocardial perfusion. In: Sobel BE (ed) Cardiology clinics: Thrombolysis and the heart. WB Saunders, Philadelphia, p 31
17. Fujiwara H, Onodera T, Tanaka M, et al (1986) A clinicopathologic study of patients with hemorrhagic myocardial infarction treated with selective coronary thrombolysis with urokinase. Circulation 73:749–757
18. Grip L, Ryden L (1991) Late streptokinase infusion and antithrombotic treatment in myocardial infarction reduce subsequent myocardial ischemia. Am Heart J 121:737–747
19. Hossmann KA, Zimmerman V (1974) Resuscitation of the monkey brain after 1 h complete ischemia. I. Physiological and morphological observations. Brain Res 81:59–74
20. ISIS-2 (Second International Study of Infarct Survival) Collaborative Group (1988) Randomized trial of intravenous streptokinase, oral aspirin, both, or neither among 17, 187 cases of suspected acute myocardial infarction: ISIS-2. Lancet 13 August:349–360
21. Jenning RB, Reimer KA, Lowe JE, et al (1977) The "wavefront phenomenon" of myocardial infarction cell death. I. Myocardial infarct size vs duration of coronary occlusion in dogs. Circulation 56:786–794
22. Kase CS, Pessin MS, Zivin JA, et al (1992) Intracranial hemorrhage after coronary thrombolysis with tissue plasminogen activator. Am J Med 92:384–390
23. Meyer FB, Sundt TM, Yanagihara T, Anderson RE (1987) Focal cerebral ischemia: Pathophysiologic mechanisms and rational for future avenues of treatment. Mayo Clin Proc 62:35–55
24. Olsen TS (1986) Regional cerebral blood flow after occlusion of the middle cerebral artery. Acta Neurol Scand 73:321–337
25. Olsen TS, Larsen B, Herning M, et al (1983) Blood flow and vascular reactivity in collaterally perfused brain tissue. Evidence of an ischemic penumbra in patients with acute stroke. Stroke 14(3):332–341
26. Pulsinelli W (1992) Pathophysiology of acute ischaemic stroke. Lancet 339:533–536
27. Rentrop KP, Thornton CJ, Feit F, Van Buskirk M (1988) Determinants and protective potential of coronary collaterals as assessed by an angioplasty model. Am J Cardiol 61:677–684
28. Sandercock P, Willems H (1992) Medical treatment of acute ischaemic stroke. Lancet 339:537–539
29. Schaper W (1983) Natural defense mechanisms to ischemia. Eur Heart J 4(Suppl D):73–78
30. Sobel BE (1992) Thrombolysis in the treatment of acute myocardial infarction. In: Fuster V, Verstraete M (eds) Thrombosis in cardiovascular disorders. WB Saunders, Philadelphia, p 289
31. Trevi GP, Shuban I (1992) Chronic ischaemic ("hibernating") and post-ischemic ("stunned") dysfunctional but viable myocardium. Eur Heart J 12(Suppl G):20–26
32. Verstraete M (1985) Intravenous administration of a thrombolytic agent is the only realistic therapeutic approach in evolving myocardial infarction. Eur Heart J 6:586–593

33. Verstraete M (1992) Unresolved issues in the thrombolytic treatment of myocardial infarction. J Myocardial Ischemia 4:72–84
34. Zivin JA, et al (1986) Delayed therapy of embolic stroke with tissue plasminogen activator. Ann Neurol 20:154
35. Zivin JA, Fisher M, DeGirolami U, Hemenway CC, Stashak JA (1985) Tissue plasminogen activator reduced neurological damage after cerebral embolism. Science 230:1289–1292
36. Zivin JA, Lyden PD, De Girolami U, et al (1988) Tissue plasminogen activator reduction of neurologic damage after experimental embolic stroke. Arch Neurol 45:387–391

Pathogenesis of Secondary Brain Hemorrhage After Ischemia: Lessons from Animal Models ... and a few from man: too!

G.F. Molinari

Both open label and controlled clinical trials of thrombolytic therapy for acute stroke are careful to define and distinguish between hemorrhagic infarctions and intracerebral hematomas in addressing possible complications of treatment. Since the major and potentially unacceptable risk of this type of treatment is brain hemorrhage [16, 17] and because certain types of stroke are apt to produce some hemorrhagic complications as part of the untreated natural history [22, 23], it has become very important to stratify and quantitate secondary brain hemorrhages at least into two strata, acceptable and unacceptable.

Hemorrhagic infarction is defined in classical neuropathological terms as diapedesis of red blood cells into a relatively preserved background matrix of tissue characterized by irreparable nerve cell damage, but with preservation of many of the glial and vascular components. Clinical caveats, known only since the advent of transcranial imaging of lesions in man, have been added to the descriptive definition: hemorrhagic complications may be delayed and progressive over days, and there may be no clinical change correlating with that slow hemorrhagic change. Often, the CT scan may look worse while the patient is getting better. Hemorrhagic transformation usually begins 12 h or more after onset of ischemia and is related to infarct size. Hematomas, on the other hand, even when complicating an infarct, caused by presumed excessive anticoagulation or surgical reperfusion not only wipe out any necrotic matrix that may have been present, but produce a confluent blood clot that distorts the surrounding tissues due to associated pressure gradients. Clinically, that type of hemorrhage is almost always signalled by dramatic clinical deterioration [3, 15, 22–25, 27].

It has been suggested that a complication rate of less than 15% "significant hemorrhages" may be acceptable. The criteria for "significance" are not precisely defined but presumed to include clinical deterioration. Three significant hemorrhages out of 20 patients treated would stop one study and perhaps the treatment modality. The implications of how the incidence of less significant hemorrhagic infarction may influence the future of an intervention study and the treatment rationale is less clear. By the proposed methodology of data

Department of Neurology, George Washington University Medical Center, Washington, DC, USA

G.J. del Zoppo, E. Mori, W. Hacke (Eds.)
Thrombolytic Therapy in Acute Ischemic Stroke II

analysis, it seems to make sense to treat hemorrhagic infarctions which may have little to no clinical significance and cerebral hematomas, which cause clinical decline, as separate clinical as well as pathological entities.

Historically and perhaps even currently, there are those who might argue that the distinction is not quite so clear, both from the perspectives of experimental neuropathology and from some human clinicopathological correlations as well.

Experimental Neuropathology

In 1953, in the same volume of the journal that carried his obituary, Joseph Globus, along with his associate Joseph Epstein, published the last in a series of reports of animal experiments that led them to the conclusion that there is a continuous spectrum of neuropathological entities that begin with ischemic or bland infarction and end with fatal, destructive expanding mass lesions resembling the spontaneous intracerebral hematomas seen in man [11, 12]. Those authors concluded that, at least in animal models, not only hemorrhagic infarctions, but hematomas, could be induced under certain time-dependent conditions. Acute hypertension induced by neosynephrine several days to a week after irreversible intracranial arterial ligation caused hemorrhagic staining of the ischemic vascular territory; in areas of ischemic softening, reperfusion of injured but viable small arteries, traversing early porencephalic cavities, weakened unsupported arterial walls. Arterial rupture with bleeding into cystic cavities without opposing pressure formed massive hematomas. Their hand-drawn schematic illustrations resemble a combined form of acutely acquired Charcot-Bouchard aneurysms and "etat lacunaire" described in modern neuropathology texts [28]. Their work at the time was criticized by many as artificial, not related to anything seen in man at the autopsy table. Some who looked at their pathological materials interpreted the experimental lesions as merely variations in the intensity of hemorrhagic infarction. The semantics were impeccable. After all, the experimental lesions were originally infarctions and later became hemorrhages.

Furthermore, there was a reported variation in the incidence of hemorrhagic complications of experimentally produced infarcts according to the species of animal used. Hemorrhage was a relatively common complication in dogs and cats, but uncommon in monkeys [13]. Globus attributed that variation to some unmeasured difference in either the degree or pattern of collateralization among species [11].

In an apparently obscure, seldom quoted paper in the same journal many years later, Laurent and colleagues [18] reported experiments duplicating some of Globus' work, using a nonmigrating embolism model in monkeys. Those authors confirmed that both hemorrhagic infarctions and hematomas could be induced by manipulating collateral circulation in the early recovery period after ischemic stroke. They used modern vasopressor drugs and vasodilatation by hypercapnia and were able to overcome the native resistance of the species to hemorrhagic transformation. Critical to the induction of either complication, just as in Globus' methodology, was a latency of 5 to 10 days between infarction and vasomotor alteration of the ischemic and collateral vascular beds.

Throughout most of that interval, the ischemic and adjacent vascular beds are dysautoregulatory, and, as reported by Globus and his coworkers, tissue necrosis also progresses and early pseudocysts form around relatively spared blood vessel walls.

In human pathological material, McCormick and Schochet describe "cracking," an artifact occurring within 36–48 h of onset, as a curvilear plane of cleavage, separating necrotic tissue from relatively intact adjacent tissue [19]. Their Figure 164 shows a "crack" contiguous with a blood clot penetrating the lateral ventricle in the proximal distribution of a very bloody hemorrhagic infarct from a marantic embolism. Dissection of clotted blood along a similar path from a deep homogeneous blood clot to the ipsilateral ventricle was a common observation in some of our early unpublished dog specimens, and in the Laurent primate series [18].

The experimentally induced hemorrhagic transformations in the latter series [18] consistently displayed either of two patterns, both seen in man. One pattern was that of cortical staining with extravasated blood, evident by light microscopy to surround structurally identifiable elements of the capillaries and reactive microvasculature. Topographically, those lesions were distal to the nonmigratory embolism and contiguous with the brain surface but no matter how large, never approached the ventricular system. The second type, however, was one of confluent hematoma, occurring in deep structures within the distribution of the lateral striate penetrating arteries, also distal to the in situ occlusive particle, contiguous with the zone of "cracking" observed in nonhemorrhagic control specimens of similar age, and in human pathological specimens, and always isolated from the brain surface by an intact strip of cortex and capsula extrema. They were usually accompanied by mass effect and dissection into the ipsilateral ventricle.

Current literature of experimental pathology continues to support the principle that selective vulnerability of the component tissues of the brain parenchyma to ischemia parallels the order of susceptibility to anoxia; irreversible change occurs in nerve cells before glia, and glia succumb before endothelium [1, 8, 9, 21, 29]. Little is known about the tolerance times of smooth muscle and elastica to ischemia before necrosis.

Basic references in anatomy [10], physiology [26], pathology [1, 28], and clinical stroke [20] indicate that the penetrating arterioles of the brain are in many ways different from arteries of similar size in other organs. They originate at right angles to their parent conduit arteries on the surface; there is an abrupt reduction in internal diameter from the large surface vessel to the penetrating branch, an often 10-fold reduction; they are very thin walled; they apparently have no functional precapillary anastomoses. While they have an internal elastic membrane and a defined muscularis media, vessels of this caliber

(50–100 μm) constitute the "resistance" vascular bed in other organs; in the brain, although the vessels at the base are referred to as the resistance vascular bed, the precise segments over which perfusion pressure reduces from arterial to capillary levels is not known. From cerebral blood flow studies, it is inferred that while the large surface conduit arteries of the brain are under sympathetic nervous system control, the penetrating vessels to the interior are primarily regulated by local metabolism [14].

Certainly during the acute dysautoregulatory phase after a stroke, the pressure in such reperfused arteries is proportionate to the systemic blood pressure.

If ischemic injury has affected only or mainly the capillary vascular bed which is not necrotic but rather "leaky," or if the hypoperfusion of the ischemic bed has persisted long enough to permit clotting on the venous side, or if the proliferating capillaries in the subacute reactive phase of ischemia are not quite competent, then hemorrhagic infarction may occur by passive diapedesis of formed blood elements around tiny vessels discernible by the light microscope within the bloody patch: the pattern seen by all who have examined the experimental and clinical neuropathology of "red" infarction.

If, on the other hand, primarily deep, proximal vascular territory infarction has been severe enough and persistent long enough to affect the integrity of the somewhat fragile precapillary arteriolar vessels, hematomas could develop by active bleeding from the arteriolar side, especially in the newly forming pseudocyst, dissecting along the course of least resistance to ipsilateral ventricle.

Hemorrhage into infarcted areas may have histologic characteristics of "hemorrhagic infarction" in some sections, clearly homogeneous clot penetrating the ipsilateral ventricle in other specimens, and in still other sections the same specimen may show the features of "hematomas" and "red infarctions."

Such experiments suggest the distinction between hemorrhagic infarction and intracerebral hematoma to be semantic, arbitrary, artificial and no more than quantitative. The as yet unquantified variable may be the critical tolerance of elastic and smooth muscle tissue to ischemia.

Clinical Neuropathology

By the time of his death in 1952, Globus' idea about the pathogenesis of hemorrhage complicating ischemic infarction had been supplanted by the still popular concept of primary occlusion, secondary distal migration with reperfusion of previously occluded vessels, published in a long abstract by Fisher and Adams in 1951 [6].

Initially, the latter authors had their own detractors. In the published commentary on their paper, presented at the annual meeting of the American Association of Neuropathologists meeting in 1950, Drs. Kubick and Hiller commented that perhaps the observations could be explained by an alternative hypothesis, that distal ischemic fields were hemorrhagic because they were cortical and that is where all the collaterals are [6]!

Drs. Adams and Fisher rejoined that often there was a bland ischemic area, distal to or surrounded by the hemorrhagic component. This they felt to represent further evidence that reperfusion followed distal migration of the embolic occlusive clot, and that distal to the final position of the embolism the infarct remains bland. This idea dominated the standard teaching on the mechanism of hemorrhages complicating ischemia for the next 35 years.

Ironically, the discussion among the authors and their critics at the time of the presentation concluded with the deferral to the experimentalists to resolve the vagaries of pathogenesis of hemorrhagic transformation, a group that had been and still is largely ignored by clinicians.

Clinical Neurology

Not until relatively recently, due to the resurgent interest and emphasis on therapy, have these old concepts resurfaced to haunt us. Ideas developed by classical clinicopathological correlation are being reexamined by in vivo imaging methods that permit more precise distinctions between ischemic and hemorrhagic regions of brain and hopefully the more subtle differences between hemorrhagic infarctions and intracerebral hematomas.

During the last decade, the benefits and the potential risks of anticoagulation with heparin were reexamined and recommendations made in the hope of avoiding disastrous bleeding, complicating otherwise successful prophylactic treatment of subsequent embolism [2, 3, 15, 22, 23, 25, 27].

There is now general consensus that bleeding into ischemic infarcts occurs gradually during the first 24 h after onset of ischemia or may be delayed for days; that infarct size seems more important than hypertension in the pathogenesis of spontaneous hemorrhagic transformation; and that in the case of large infarctions, anticoagulation should be delayed for 5 to 7 days [3]. This recommendation was made despite at least one prospective controlled clinical trial of anticoagulation that showed better outcomes in all categories of lesion size when anticoagulation was provided immediately [2].

One important prospective study of pathogenesis of hemorrhagic transformation [15] identified the most important risk factors as: severity of neurological deficit; disturbance of consciousness; large infarction with mass effect; and early enhancement by contrast medium on CT. The authors also performed lumbar punctures in some of their patients and thought that alteration of the blood/CSF barrier disturbances tended to parallel early contrast enhancement and were therefore predictive. They also felt that early transformations tended to produce hematomas and later transformations, in the second week, were related to less dangerous petechial bleeding in cortical areas of infarction. All of their patients received plasma volume expanders, and 65% were given "low dose" heparin (5000 IU every 12 h), the other 35% aspirin or heparin plus aspirin. Therefore, the control group in that study cannot be considered a proper natural history cohort.

The ubiquitous reference to the Fisher and Adams hypothesis used throughout the clinical and experimental literature on this subject was almost invariably to their "long abstract," published in 1951 [6].

Not until 1987 did the full text of their paper appear in the archival literature complete with illustrations [7]. Their Figure 2.2 in the long paper shows what they call a "hemorrhagic infarction of caudate and lenticular nuclei," which seems to be a glistening homogeneous blood clot dissecting into and contiguous with identical clot in the ipsilateral ventricle. "Pale infarction" is noted in the temporal lobe but less obviously in the frontal and parietal lobes.

Other examples of these phenomena abound, in the clinicopathological literature, in commercially available series of neuropathology teaching slides, and in each of our own clinical experiences. The most important examples include: a) a pattern of hemorrhagic infarction which dominates cortical areas contiguous with the brain's surface, b) hematomas which occur in deep vascular territories and are isolated from the brain surface, c) the architecture of hemorrhagic infarction suggesting passive, lowpressure bleeding, d) hematomas as destructive lesions, associated with mass effects and dissection suggesting active bleeding under pressure, and e) all of these phenomena may occasionally be seen in the same specimen, human or subhuman, in the same vascular territory, at the same time interval following embolism with severe ischemic infarction.

Implications for Fibrinolytic Therapy

It was inevitable that the unsettled issues regarding the natural history of brain hemorrhages complicating ischemia would demand resolution in the era of renaissance of fibrinolytic therapy for strokes [4, 5, 16, 24].

Since the finding of as few as three intracerebral hematomas in a group of 20 treated patients would exceed the predefined safety limits, a single avoidable "significant" hemorrhage could close a doserange cohort or even end a study. There might be an observer bias among investigators to overdiagnose the less ominous hemorrhagic infarction and underdiagnose hematoma.

Hemorrhagic infarctions do not dissect into the ventricular system, whereas hematomas often do. Therefore, blood in the ipsilateral ventricle may prove a useful additional criterion, in conjunction with clinical deterioration and evidence of pressure gradients and mass effects when the radiodensity and distribution of the hemorrhagic tissue is not adequate to distinguish a homogeneous clot from a "very hemorrhagic infarct." Observations in man used to make critical clinical and policy decisions, while exploiting the benefits of high resolution imaging technology in vivo, lack validation by the traditional "gold standard," pathological correlation.

The timing of administration of fibrinolytic agents may be equally critical to safety as it is to efficacy. While "fibrinolysins" may not be indicated in the vasoproliferative and early necrotic stages following the clinically presenting stroke, subclinical, neurologically silent infarcts must be searched for in the screening CT scan and history taking. For this and other reasons controversy still exists as to whether lacunes, always in the territory of the penetrating arteries and usually periventricular in location, should be included in controlled clinical trials of fibrinolytic therapy. The exclusion criterion of all previous strokes by history or CT is a good one and should not be abandoned to improve the patient accession rate. If there is any doubt as to the age or nature of a given lesion shown on CT scan that is apparently unrelated to the presenting stroke, particularly a lacune, it would be best to perform an enhanced scan or MRI prior to administration of fibrinolytic agents to avoid a possible disastrous complication in a patient and a possible fatal blow to the study.

References

1. Brierly JB, Graham DI (1984) Hypoxia and vascular disorders of the central nervous system. In: Adams HJ, Corsellis JAN, Duchen LW (eds) Greenfield's neuropathology. John Wiley and Sons, New York, p 125
2. Cerebral Embolism Study Group (1983) Immediate anticoagulation of embolic stroke: A randomized trial. Stroke 14:668–676
3. Cerebral Embolism Study Group (1984) Immediate anticoagulation of embolic stroke: Brain hemorrhage and management options. Stroke 15:779–789
4. del Zoppo GJ, Copeland BR, Anderchek K, Hacke W, Koziol JA (1990) Hemorrhagic transformation following tissue plasminogen activator in experimental cerebral infarction. Stroke 21:596–601
5. del Zoppo GJ, Zeumer H, Harker LA (1986) Thrombolytic therapy in acute stroke: Possibilities and hazards. Stroke 17:595–607
6. Fisher CM, Adams RD (1951) Observations on brain embolism with special reference to the mechanism of hemorrhagic infarction. J Neuropathol Exp Neurol 10:92–94
7. Fisher CM, Adams RD (1987) Observations on brain embolism with special reference to hemorrhage infarction. In: Furlan AJ (ed) The heart and stroke. Exploring mutual cerebrovascular and cardiovascular issues. Springer-Verlag, Berlin Heidelberg New York, p 17
8. Garcia JH, Lowry SL, Briggs L, et al (1983) Brain capillaries expand and rupture in areas of ischemia and reperfusion. In: Reivich M, Hurtig HI (eds) Cerebrovascular diseases. Raven Press, New York, p 169
9. Garcia JH, Mitchem HL, Briggs L, et al (1983) Transient focal ischemia in subhuman primates: Neuronal injury as a function of local cerebral blood flow. J Neuropathol Exp Neurol 42:44–60
10. Gillilan LA (1968) The arterial and venous blood supplies to the forebrain (including the internal capsule of primates). Neurology 18:653– 670
11. Globus JH, Epstein JA (1953) Massive cerebral hemorrhage: spontaneous and experimentally induced. J Neuropathol Exp Neurol 12:107–133
12. Globus JH, Epstein JA, Green MA, Marics M (1949) Focal cerebral hemorrhage experimentally induced. J Neuropathol Exp Neurol 8:653–670
13. Hain RF, Westhaysen PU, Swank RL (1952) Hemorrhagic cerebral infarction by arterial occlusion. J Neuropathol Exp Neurol 11:34–43
14. Harper AM, Deshmukh VD, Rowan JO, et al (1972) The influence of sympathetic nervous activity on cerebral blood flow. Arch Neurol 27:16
15. Hornig CR, Dorndorf W, Agnoli AL (1986) Hemorrhagic cerebral infarction: A prospective study. Stroke 17:179–185

16. Kase CS (1991) Intracranial hemorrhage after coronary thrombolysis with tissue plasminogen activator. In: Hacke W, del Zoppo GJ, Hirschberg M (eds) Thrombolytic therapy in acute ischemic stroke. Springer-Verlag, Berlin Heidelberg New York, p 75
17. Kase CS, O'Neal AM, Fisher M, Girgis GN, Ordia JI (1990) Intracranial hemorrhage after use of tissue plasminogen activator for coronary thrombolysis. Ann Intern Med 112:17–21
18. Laurent JP, Molinari GF, Oakley JC (1976) Experimental model of intracerebral hematoma. J Neuropathol Exp Neurol 35:560–568
19. McCormick WF, Schochet SS, Jr. (1976) Infarcts: Morphological determination of age of infarcts. In: Atlas of cerebrovascular disease. WB Saunders, Philadelphia London Toronto, p 148
20. Millikan CH, McDowell F, Easton JD (1987) Pathology of primary intracerebral hemorrhage (PIH). In: Stroke. Lea and Febiger, Philadelphia, p 53
21. Molinari GF (1986) Experimental models of ischemic stroke. In: Barnett HJ, Morh JP, Stein BM, Yatsu FM (eds) Stroke: Pathophysiology, diagnosis, management. Churchill Livingstone, New York, p 57
22. Okada Y, Yamaguchi T, Minematsu K, et al (1989) Hemorrhagic transformation in cerebral embolism. Stroke 20:598–603
23. Ott BR, Zamani A, Kleefield J, Funkenstein HH (1986) The clinical spectrum of hemorrhagic infarction. Stroke 17:630–637
24. Papadopoulos SM, Chandler WF, Salamat MS, Topol EJ, Sackellares JC (1987) Recombinant human tissuetype plasminogen activator therapy in acute thromboembolic stroke. J Neurosurg 67:394–398
25. Pessin MS (1991) Hemorrhagic transformation in the natural history of acute embolic stroke. In: Hacke W, del Zoppo GJ, Hirschberg M (eds) Thrombolytic therapy in acute ischemic stroke. Springer-Verlag, Berlin Heidelberg New York, p 67
26. Purves MJ (1972) Some aspects of the anatomy of the cerebral blood vessels. In: The physiology of the cerebral circulation. Cambridge University Press, Cambridge, p 1
27. Shields RW, Laureno R, Lachman T, Victor M (1984) Anticoagulantrelated hemorrhage in acute cerebral embolism. Stroke 15:426–437
28. Weller RO (1984) Spontaneous intracranial hemorrhage. In: Adams HJ, Corsellis JAN, Duchen LW (eds) Greenfield's neuropathology. John Wiley and Sons, New York, p 125
29. Yashida Y, Dereski MO, Garcia JH, Hetzel FW, Chopp M (1992) Photoactivated photofrin II: Astrocytic swelling precedes endothelial injury in rat brain. J Neuropathol Exp Neurol 51:91–100.111

Clinical Trials of Fibrinolytic Agents in Carotid Territory Cerebral Ischemia

Symptom-Based Trials of Intravenous rt-PA in Acute Stroke*

T. Brott

As thrombolytic therapy developed as a potential intervention for acute ischemic stroke during the 1980s, early clinical investigation depended upon pretreatment cerebral arteriography [5]. The pathologic cerebral anatomy was first defined, and then thrombolytic therapy could be administered selectively to the site of thrombosis via the intra-arterial route [3, 6, 11]. These intra-arterial thrombolytic interventions, carried out with the benefit of computed tomographic (CT) scanning to exclude hemorrhagic stroke, demonstrated the feasibility of cerebral arterial clot lysis. Several thrombolytic agents administered in a variety of doses [3–6, 11–13] were shown to accomplish partial or complete arterial recanalization in the setting of acute cerebral embolism or thrombosis.

In the mid- and late 1980s, symptom-based delivery of thrombolytic therapy for acute ischemic stroke emerged as a complementary strategy. It was hoped that delivery of agents very early after the onset of symptoms [1], prior to the performance of cerebral arteriography, could offset the disadvantages of treatment without knowledge of arterial anatomy. Potential benefits were neuronal protection, enhanced clot lysis, and lowered risk for thrombolysis-related intracerebral hematoma. The symptom-based approach was not original to stroke investigators. Symptom-based delivery of thrombolytic therapy for myocardial infarction [9] had already come to supersede angiographically mediated delivery, both clinically and in large clinical trials.

At the First International Symposium on Thrombolytic Therapy in Acute Ischemic Stroke, held in Heidelberg, the results from a symptom-based trial sponsored by the National Institutes of Health (NIH) were presented [10]. This pilot dose-escalation study of intravenous recombinant tissue plasminogen activator (rt-PA; alteplase) demonstrated the feasibility of urgent treatment (within 90 [2] and 91–180 min [7] of symptom onset) and also suggested acceptable safety for doses up to 0.95 mg/kg.

Following completion of the NIH pilot study, three other trials proceeded, each with a double-blind, placebo-controlled design. These trials are described

* This work was supported in part by the National Institute of Neurological Disorders and Stroke.

Department of Neurology, University of Cincinnati College of Medicine, Cincinnati, OH, USA

G. J. del Zoppo, E. Mori, W. Hacke (Eds.)
Thrombolytic Therapy in Acute Ischemic Stroke II

below. One has been completed, and the other two are scheduled to be completed in 1993 or 1994.

The rt-PA Bridging Study

At the termination of the NIH pilot trial, a pilot-randomized trial of rt-PA [8] was organized at the University of Cincinnati and the University of Virginia, supported by Genentech, Inc. The purpose of the trial was to provide a bridge between the completion of the NIH pilot trial and the beginning of a large NIH-sponsored randomized trial of rt-PA which was anticipated to begin in 1991. The bridging trial was designed to test the feasibility of such a larger trial as well as to identify potential pitfalls in the performance of such a trial. Under a randomized, double-blind, placebo-controlled protocol, patients were entered into two groups, based upon the time of symptom onset. In the first group, randomization occurred within 90 min, and patients were then treated with either 0.85 mg/kg of rt-PA (alteplase) given intravenously over 60 min, or placebo. In the second group, randomization occurred at 91 – 180 min. Neurological outcome was assessed with the NIH Stroke Scale, and volume measurements of the cerebral infarction were determined by CT.

Among the 20 patients randomized within 90 min, 6 of 10 patients treated with rt-PA had a $\geqslant$4 point improvement at 24 h in the NIH Stroke Scale, compared to 1 of 10 patients treated with placebo ($p = 0.03$, Fisher's Exact Test). Among the 7 patients randomized at 91 – 180 min, 2 of the 4 patients treated with rt-PA had a $\geqslant$4 point improvement at 24 h compared to 1 of 3 patients treated with placebo. One fatal intracerebral hemorrhage occurred among all 27 patients, occurring in a patient receiving placebo in the 91- 180 min group. The investigators concluded that a larger randomized trial of rt-PA was feasible. They also hypothesized that rt-PA treatment within 90 min may be associated with early neurological improvement.

NINDS t-PA Stroke Trial

A relatively large multicenter controlled trial of rt-PA as acute therapy for acute ischemic stroke is now underway, also sponsored by NIH and administered by the National Institute for Neurological Disorders and Stroke (NINDS). This trial is being carried out at 8 clinical centers with the Henry Ford Hospital serving as the study Coordinating Center. The study design is that of a double-blind, randomized, controlled trial of very early therapy of intravenous rt-PA (alteplase) for acute ischemic stroke. The primary hypotheses are that there is a difference between the rt-PA- treated group and the placebo group with regard to the proportion showing significant early neurological improvement for a) those enrolled within 90 min of symptom onset, b) those enrolled between 91–180 min from symptom onset, and c) those enrolled within 180 min of symptom onset. Significant early neurological improvement is defined as an improvement in the NIH Stroke Scale of ⩾4 points at 24 h or a complete resolution of the neurological deficit at 24 h. The sample size required to test these hypotheses was derived from the results of the NINDS t-PA pilot trial. It was estimated that 40% of the rt-PA group would show significant early improvement. Accordingly, with 280 patients the power was calculated to be 0.95 to detect an absolute difference of 20% in significant neurological improvement (e.g., 40% in the rt-PA group vs. 20% in the placebo group) at the $p < 0.05$ level of significance. It was also estimated that, with 140 patients in each of the time groups (0–90 min and 91–180 min), the power would be 0.90 to detect an absolute difference of 24% between the rt-PA and placebo-treated patients at the $p < 0.05$ level. Secondary outcomes to be compared in the rt-PA and placebo patients include a ⩾5 point improvement in the NIH Stroke Scale at 7–10 days, the median change in the NIH score at 3 months, the mean infarction volume by CT at 7–10 days and 3 months, and the median Barthel index at 7–10 days and 3 months.

The inclusion criteria for the study are age 18–80 years; ischemic stroke with deficits in language, motor, cognitive, or visual function; time to treatment 0–90 or 91–180 min; and the number of patients at any given clinical center enrolled in the 91- to 180-min group cannot exceed the number enrolled in the 0–90 min group by more than 2 patients. This latter inclusion criterion was added so as to guarantee balanced numbers in the two time groups and to enforce a discipline of time so as to assure urgent treatment. Exclusion criteria for the trial include hemorrhagic stroke by CT scan, rapid neurological improvement, prior ischemic stroke within 3 months, prior intracerebral hemorrhage thought to imply excess risk, seizure at onset of the stroke, blood pressure >185 mm Hg systolic or 110 mm Hg diastolic, pregnancy, platelet count <100000, prothrombin time >15 s, heparin within 48 h of treatment and elevated partial thromboplastin time, oral anticoagulants, major surgery within 14 days, serious head trauma within 3 months, urinary or GI bleeding within 21 days, glucose <50 or >400 mg/dl, acute myocardial infarction, or post-myocardial infarction pericarditis. An independent Safety and Monitoring Committee oversees operation of the trial and supervises interim analyses of efficacy and safety.

Patient enrollment has been encouraging, and 200 patients had been randomized and treated as of 30 April 1992. Barbara Tilley, the Principal Investigator for the Coordinating Center, discusses some of the unique features of study recruitment in a chapter that follows. An important feature of the recruitment independent of specific techniques has been a multi-hospital approach at more than half of the 8 Clinical Centers. Forty hospitals are participating.

Six-Hour Randomized Trial of rt-PA

Shortly after the organization of the NINDS trial, organization of a second very similar trial was begun, under the sponsorship of Genentech, Inc. This multi-center trial is now underway at 12 centers with additional centers planned for participation.

The study design is that of a double-blind, randomized, placebo-controlled clinical trial of intravenous rt-PA (alteplase) as early therapy for acute ischemic stroke. The first primary hypothesis is that there is a significant difference between rt-PA- and placebo-treated groups in clinical improvement. Clinical improvement is defined as a decrease (improvement) of 4 or more points in the NIH Stroke Scale or complete resolution of symptoms from baseline to 24 h, and from baseline to 30 days. The second primary hypothesis is that there is a significant difference between the rt-PA- and placebo-treated groups in the volume of cerebral infarction as measured by CT at 30 days.

Inclusion criteria are age 18–79 years, the clinical diagnosis of ischemic stroke causing measurable neurological deficit, and the onset of symptoms of ischemic stroke within 6 h of the time to initiation of treatment with the study drug. The exclusion criteria include coma, severe obtundation, fixed eye deviation or complete hemiplegia, minor stroke symptoms (<4 points on the NIH Stroke Scale and normal speech and visual fields) or major symptoms that are rapidly improving by the time of randomization, history of stroke within the previous 6 weeks, a known active seizure disorder or a first seizure within 6 h immediately prior to administration of the study drug, a previous known intracranial hemorrhage, neoplasm, subarachnoid hemorrhage, arteriovenous malformation or aneurysm, a clinical presentation that suggests subarachnoid hemorrhage, systolic blood pressure >185 mm/hg or diastolic blood pressure >110 mm/hg or diastolic blood pressure >110 mm/hg on repeated measures prior to study entry or requiring aggressive treatment to reduce blood pressure within these limits, presumed septic embolus, presumed pericarditis or ventricular thrombus or aneurysm related to recent acute myocardial infarction, surgery or biopsy of a parenchymal organ within 30 days, trauma with internal injuries or ulcerative wounds within 30 days, head trauma within 90 days, active or recent hemorrhage within 30 days, known hereditary or acquired hemorrhagic diathesis, pregnancy, glucose <50 or >400 mg/dl, platelet count <100000, hematocrit <25, other serious, advanced, or terminal illness, or any other condition that the investigator feels would pose a significant hazard to the patient. The study also has CT exclusions of a high-density lesion consistent with hemorrhage of any degree, evidence of significant mass effect or midline shift, or subarachnoid hemorrhage.

In the study, patients are randomized to receive either placebo or 0.9 mg/kg of rt-PA intravenously over 60 min with 10% of the drug as a bolus. The NIH Stroke Scale, CT scans, and the Barthel index are performed at 1, 7, 30, and 90 days. As of 1 April 1992, 20 patients have been enrolled in this multicenter, symptom-based trial.

Comment

Symptom-based trials of thrombolytic therapy have the potential advantage of more rapid treatment delivery, greater ease of patient enrollment, and the potential requirement of smaller sample sizes. The latter potential advantage could be realized if early therapy is more effective than later therapy. Differences between the active-treatment and placebo groups would be larger if earlier treatment is more effective, and so the size of the active-treatment and placebo groups required to demonstrate significant differences could be smaller. Symptom-based trials also have the advantage of wider applicability of results. The studies described above are being carried out within a wide range of American hospitals, including small community hospitals and major tertiary medical centers. The treatment techniques used in these studies should be within the capabilities of essentially any hospital with facilities for emergency CT.

Unfortunately, the rate of patient recruitment has been modest in the symptom-based trials, despite the elimination of pretreatment cerebral arteriography. The protocols are cumbersome, with multiple exclusion criteria and exceptionally demanding data collection. More important, the key people – patients, families, pre-hospital care personnel, and hospital-based health professionals – frequently do not behave as if every minute counts. Delays are endemic: delay in stroke recognition, delay in the call for help, delay in ambulance transport, and delay in emergency department evaluation and referral are all too common. Within the same communities, the standard of care for acute trauma or myocardial infarction is entirely different. Those interested in the stroke patient can best persuade others to behave with a trauma-type urgency if safe and effective therapies are available.

Hopefully, positive results will be forthcoming from these and other randomized trials of thrombolytic therapy for stroke.

Acknowledgements. The author wishes to acknowledge investigators from the trials described above, both for their helpful comments and for their willingness to share details from the protocols they designed. This work was supported in part by the National Institute of Neurological Disorders and Stroke.

References

1. Brott T, Haley EC, Levy D, Barsan W, Broderick J, Marler JR (1991) Strategies for early treatment of acute cerebral infarction. In: Hacke W, del Zoppo GJ, Hirschberg M (eds) Thrombolytic therapy in acute ischemic stroke. Springer-Verlag, Berlin Heidelberg New York, p 196
2. Brott TG, Haley EC, Levy DE, et al (1992) Urgent therapy for stroke. Part I. Pilot study of tissue plaminogen activator administered within 90 minutes. Stroke 23:632–640
3. del Zoppo GJ, Ferbert A, Otis S, et al (1988) Local intra-arterial therapy in acute carotid territory stroke: A pilot study. Stroke 19:307– 313
4. del Zoppo GJ, Poeck K, Pessin MS, and 16 coauthors of the rt-PA Acute Stroke Study Group (1992) Recombinant tissue plasminogen activator in acute thrombotic and embolic stroke. Ann Neurol 32:78–87

5. del Zoppo GJ, Zeumer H, Harker LA (1986) Thrombolytic therapy in acute stroke: Possibilities and hazards. Stroke 17:595–607
6. Hacke W, Zeumer H, Ferbert A, Bruckmann H, del Zoppo GJ (1988) Intra- arterial thrombolytic therapy improves outcome in patients with acute vertebrobasilar occlusive disease. Stroke 19:1216–1222
7. Haley EC, Levy DE, Brott TG, et al (1992) Urgent therapy for stroke. Part II. Pilot study of plasminogen administered 91–180 minutes from onset. Stroke 23:641–645
8. Haley EC, TPA Bridging Study Group (1992) Pilot randomized trial of tissue plaminogen activator in acute ischemic stroke (abstract). Neurology 42 (Suppl 3):203
9. Marder VJ, Sherry S (1988) Thrombolytic therapy. Current status. N Engl J Med 388:1512–1520,–1585–1595
10. Marler JR, Brott T, Haley EC, Levy D (1991) Evaluation of tissue plasminogen activator early in the course of acute ischemic stroke. In: Hacke W, del Zoppo GJ, Hirschberg M (eds) Thrombolytic therapy in acute ischemic stroke. Springer-Verlag, Berlin Heidelberg New York, p 152
11. Mori E, Tabuchi M, Yoshida T, Yamadori A (1988) Intracarotid urokinase with thromboembolic occlusion of the middle cerebral artery. Stroke 19:802–812
12. Mori E, Yoneda Y, Tabuchi M, et al (1992) Intravenous recombinant tissue plasminogen activator in acute carotid artery territory stroke. Neurology 42:976–982
13. von Kummer R, Forsting M, Sartor K, Hacke W (1991) Intravenous recombinant tissue plaminogen activator in acute stroke. In: Hacke W, del Zoppo GJ, Hirschberg M (eds) Thrombolytic therapy in acute ischemic stroke. Springer-Verlag, Berlin Heidelberg New York, p 161

A Safety and Efficacy Study of Intravenous rt-PA in Patients with Acute Stroke

M. J. Alberts for The rt-PA Acute Stroke Study Group

Several studies have proven the safety and efficacy of intravenous (IV) thrombolytic therapy in patients with acute myocardial infarction [26, 27]. Past trials of IV thrombolytic therapy in stroke patients have reported limited efficacy and a disturbing incidence of side effects [11, 14, 16]. Some researchers have indicated that these negative findings were due to poor patient selection, late therapy, and heterogenous drug administration techniques [3]. More recent trials of intra-arterial (IA) thrombolytic therapy in highly selected stroke patients have reported improved safety and efficacy [4, 13]. Because the IV administration of thrombolytic agents is logistically preferable and more widely feasible than IA infusions, it is appropriate to re-study the safety and efficacy of IV recombinant tissue plasminogen activator (rt-PA) in a select group of stroke patients.

This report is a further analysis of a study that has been previously published [5]. The complete report contains more detailed information than this manuscript and will be referred to throughout this paper.

Subjects and Methods

All patients, their next-of-kin, or legal guardian had to give informed consent prior to participation in the study. The study was conducted at 16 major medical centers in the United States and Germany. It was stopped in May, 1990 because of the loss of a patent infringement suit brought against the Burroughs-Wellcome Company, which sponsored this study.

Patients had to be over 21 and under 80 years old with no significant prior neurologic impairment. All patients had to have signs and symptoms of a large vessel thrombotic or embolic stroke. rt-PA had to be started within 8 h of stroke onset.

The study design required that all patients have normal coagulation parameters, and a CT scan that was negative for structural lesions, cerebral hemorrhage, and significant mass affect or edema. Cerebral angiography had to dem-

Department of Neurology, Duke University Medical Center, Durham, NC, USA

G. J. del Zoppo, E. Mori, W. Hacke (Eds.)
Thrombolytic Therapy in Acute Ischemic Stroke II

onstrate a complete arterial occlusion that was appropriate for the patient's clinical findings. Patients with arterial stenosis but no occlusion, suspected arterial dissection, aneurysm, vascular malformation, or vasculitis were excluded.

Following arteriography patients received a 1-h intravenous infusion of two-chain rt-PA (duteplase) without a bolus. Doses of rt-PA ranged from 0.12 million international units per kilogram (MIU/kg) to 0.75 MIU/kg. Following the rt-PA infusion, the cerebral angiogram was repeated to determine reperfusion efficacy. Only those patients who received the full dose of rt-PA at that dose tier were included in the efficacy analysis. Recanalization status was determined using criteria established during the TIMI trials [26], with grade 0–1 being classified as no perfusion, grade 2 as partial perfusion, and grade 3 as complete perfusion. Efficacy was defined as any degree of reperfusion (>grade 1) observed in the posttreatment angiogram.

Patients were monitored by serial neurologic evaluations, and head CT scans 24 h and 10–14 days following the rt-PA infusion. A safety endpoint was defined as any central nervous system (CNS) bleeding causing neurologic deterioration that occurred within 24 h of rt-PA infusion. Patients who received any amount of rt-PA were included in the safety analysis.

Internal and External Safety Monitoring Committees reviewed ongoing results of the trial.

Statistical analyses were performed using Fisher's exact test (two-tailed), the Mantel Hansel test, or the signed Rank test, where appropriate. More complete methodological details can be found in another manuscript [5].

Results

A total of 139 patients underwent cerebral angiography, of whom 104 began the rt-PA infusion. Thirty-five patients did not meet angiographic inclusion criteria. Of the 104 patients who began the rt-PA infusion, 93 received the full dose of rt-PA and were analyzed for efficacy. Among the 93 patients who received the complete dose of rt-PA, the distribution of arterial occlusions is outlined in Table 1. The vast majority of treated patients had occlusion in some portion of the middle cerebral artery.

Table 1. Location of angiographic lesion(s) in patients receiving the entire dose of rt-PA

Arterial localization	*n*	(%)
Internal carotid	11	(12)
Internal carotid and middle cerebral	12	(13)
Middle cerebral (any part)	62	(67)
Multiple/other	8	(8)
Total	93	(100)

Table 2. Recanalization at 60 min following rt-PA infusion at each dose-rate

			Recanalization (%)		
Group	Dose (MIU/kg)	*n*	None	Partial	Comp
A	0.12	4	2(50)	2(50)	0
B	0.20	7	5(71)	2(29)	0
C	0.29	7	4(57)	3(43)	0
D	0.37	15	8(53)	7(47)	0
E	0.43	15	10(67)	2(13)	3(20)
F	0.51	9	7(78)	2(22)	0
G	0.59	14	13(93)	1(7)	0
H	0.67	15	8(53)	6(40)	1(7)
I	0.75	7	4(57)	3(43)	0
Totals		93	61(66)	28(30)	4(4)

Table 3. Recanalization rate by vessel type

	Rate		
Vessel type	(*n*)	(%)	
ICA	2/25	8	
MCA stem	12/46	26	
MCA division	14/40	35	$p = 0.018$*
MCA branch	29/73	40	$p = 0.005$*

* Comparing these groups to the ICA group.

The overall recanalization rate was 34% (32 of 93 patients). The vast majority of responders (87%, 28 of 32 patients) had partial recanalization while 13% (4 of 32 patients) had complete recanalization (see Table 2). There was no clear relationship between recanalization frequency and the dose of rt-PA. When recanalization by vessel type was analyzed, a statistically significant trend for increased recanalization frequency was seen in patients with middle cerebral artery division and middle cerebral artery branch occlusions ($p = 0.018$ and $p = 0.005$, respectively; see Table 3) compared to internal carotid artery occlusions.

CNS bleeding of any type was detected in 32 of 104 patients (30.7%). The bleeding was classified as hemorrhagic infarction in 21 patients and parenchymatous hemorrhage in 11 patients. CNS bleeding with neurologic deterioration within 24 h of the rt-PA infusion was seen in 10 of 104 patients (9.6%). There was a significant association between receiving rt-PA $\geqslant 6$ h after symptom onset and the occurrence of hemorrhagic transformation ($p = 0.006$). The overall mortality rate was 12.5% (13 of 104), of which 4 patients (3.8%) died related to CNS bleeding. There was no correlation between rt-PA dose and the occurrence of CNS hemorrhage of any type, nor was there any correlation between CNS hemorrhage and reperfusion status. Serious or life-threatening non-CNS hemorrhages occurred in 4 patients (3.8%). One patient had another stroke during the post-rt-PA angiogram. This stroke occurred in the hemisphere contralateral to the primary stroke. Other results are included in the primary publication [5].

Discussion

This study failed to identify a dose of intravenous rt-PA (duteplase) that effectively lysed cerebral arterial occlusions in the patients who were treated. This is in contrast to prior studies of IA thrombolytic therapy for stroke and IV thrombolytic therapy for myocardial infarction, which were successful in identifying safe and effective doses. Recent studies of IA fibrinolytic therapy in stroke have reported recanalization rates of 60–80% in selected patients [4, 13]. Intravenous rt-PA administered to patients with acute myocardial infarction results in a 75% frequency of recanalization [26, 27].

One contributor to the reperfusion frequency of 34% after rt-PA infusion may be spontaneous clot lysis, since it is well known that many intravascular cerebral clots may lyse without specific therapy [2, 22]. In this regard, it is of note that no dose response effect was seen, which may support the hypothesis that the recanalizations seen were a reflection of the natural history of these clots. A double-blind, placebo-controlled trial of intravenous rt-PA in patients with carotid territory strokes also failed to identify a significantly increased reperfusion rate in treated patients [21]. However, these observations do not exclude the possibility that higher doses of rt-PA, or a different administration technique, might result in higher rates of recanalization.

The increased frequency of reperfusion seen with MCA division or branch occlusions compared to internal carotid artery occlusions might be explained by several factors. Clots in more distal arterial branches are usually smaller than those in larger vessels, and therefore may be more amenable to either spontaneous or therapeutic thrombolysis. Since no control group was included in this study, it is not possible to determine whether the increased reperfusion rates seen for clots in distal arteries were a therapeutic effect or were indicative of the natural history of such clots. However, no dose-effect relationship was observed for lysis of the clots in the MCA division or branch arteries.

Studies of the natural history of embolic strokes have shown hemorrhagic transformation to occur in up to 43% of patients examined [10, 17, 19, 22, 28]. Neurologic deterioration has been reported in 4%–11% of such cases [1, 17, 23], which is consistent with the findings in this study. Comparisons of safety and complication rates using historical controls is limited because the patients in our study were a highly select group. Definitive statements about hemorrhagic complications and safety will require additional controlled trials. The incidence of hemorrhagic transformation noted above is somewhat higher than that often quoted for stroke; but, this is likely due to the population of stroke patients enrolled in this study. The majority of our patients had cardioembolic strokes, which are more likely to undergo hemorrhagic transformation than small vessel lacunar strokes [17, 22, 23].

The finding that patients treated at 6 h or beyond had a higher frequency of hemorrhagic transformation compared to patients treated less than 6 h after symptom onset may reflect irreparable damage to cerebral vessels. When and if these vessels did become patent (either spontaneously or due to the administered rt-PA), damage of the vessel wall could lead to hemorrhagic transformations [9]. Other mechanisms for hemorrhagic transformation have been postulated, although the exact pathophysiology of this event remains unclear [6, 20].

There are several possible explanations for the overall findings in this study. The lack of a clear dose-response relationship might have been due to the study design. It is possible that some of the clots that did not show lyses at the post-rt-PA angiogram did lyse several minutes or hours later. Therefore, a dose–response relationship may exist, but it was not observed due to the timing of the post-rt-PA angiogram.

Another possibility is that the technique used to administer the rt-PA was not optimal. Other studies of IV thrombolytics have employed dosing regimens that begin with a bolus administration, followed by a slow infusion over several hours. Such a slower rate of administration may result in improved clot lysis [12, 25].

Many of the patients in our trial had cardioembolic strokes. Clots originating in the heart may be relatively old, with relatively little entrapped plasminogen. In vitro studies have shown that clots with little entrapped plasminogen may be difficult to lyse with some thrombolytic agents [24]. Whether cardioemboli within cerebral vessels are more difficult to lyse than in situ coronary occlusions by the systemic administration of rt-PA will require further study. Past studies have shown the efficacy of intra-arterial rt-PA and other thrombolytics in lysing such clots. It is possible that local infusion of thrombolytics will be the best technique to rapidly lyse these clots.

With this study, it was not possible to determine whether higher doses of rt-PA would have resulted in greater cerebral arterial reperfusion. Some comparisons with dose–responses from recent trials with duteplase in acute myocardial infarction (MI) are possible, however. Data from the recent Burroughs-Wellcome Study Group trial component of ISIS-3 [18] showed that 0.60 MIU/kg resulted in a coronary artery patency of 69% following a 4-h infusion of duteplase. In a separate study using a mean dose of 0.35 MIU/kg, 59% of acute MI patients (41 of 70) had coronary artery reperfusion 60 min after initiation of therapy (Burroughs-Wellcome Co., data on file). Coronary artery reperfusion at the highest dosing tier (0.43–0.74 MIU/kg) was 61%. By comparison, overall *cerebral* artery reperfusion in the current study was 34%, with 43% reperfusion at the highest dose rate of 0.75 MIU/kg. It appears that cerebral artery reperfusion and patency with duteplase are below those reported for coronary artery occlusions with the same agents. These observations suggest that cerebral arterial occlusions are somewhat less susceptible than coronary artery occlusions to thrombolysis by intravenous infusion.

The use of cerebral angiography in the setting of acute cerebral infarction has been controversial. Older studies documented complication rates of 5%–12% [8]. Recent studies of cerebral angiography in patients with various types of cerebrovascular disease (i.e., asymptomatic carotid bruits, TIAs, stroke) have reported lower complication rates of 0.4%–4% [7, 15]. Our finding of one permanent neurologic complication among 139 patients and 232 angiograms (complication rate = 0.4% per procedure) suggests that acute cerebral angiography can be performed with relative safety in moderately ill stroke patients.

This study was terminated prior to the identification of an IV dose of rt-PA that effectively lysed cerebral clots in the patient cohort under study. Conclusions about the safety of rt-PA in acute stroke will require further controlled trials. Further studies of thrombolytic agents in stroke are warranted, since prior studies have indicated some efficacy and there are no alternative therapies currently available to acutely reverse the effects of a cerebral infarction. Future protocols should consider the findings of this study when considering the optimal study design, drug administration technique, and outcome measures.

Acknowledgements. The principal investigators in the rt-PA Acute Stroke Study Group are as follows (listed in descending order of patient accrual): Klaus Poeck, M.D., Andreas Ferbert, M.D. (Klinikum, Rheinisch Westfalische Technische Hochschule, Aachen, FRG), Mark J. Alberts, M.D. (Duke University Medical Center), Michael S. Pessin, M.D. (Tufts-New England Medical Center), Justin Zivin, M.D. (University of California, San Diego), Lawrence Wechsler, M.D. (University of Pittsburgh), Anthony J. Furlan, M.D. (The Cleveland Clinic, Cleveland), Otto Busse, M.D. (Klinikum I Minden, Minden, FRG), Ralph Greenlee, Jr., M.D. (University of Texas-Southwestern Medical Center), Lawrence Brass, M.D. (Yale University School of Medicine), Jay Mohr, M.D. (Neurological Insitute), Edward Feldman, M.D. (Rhode Island Hospital), Werner Hacke, M.D. (University of Heidelberg, Heidelberg, FRG), Carlos Kase, M.D. (Boston University Medical Center), Jose Biller, M.D. (The University of Iowa College of Medicine), Gregory J. del Zoppo, M.D., Shirley Otis, M.D.(Scripps Clinic and Research Foundation), and Darryl Gress, M.D. (Massachusetts General Hospital).

The Neuroradiology Core Facility: Tufts-New England Medical Center: Samuel M. Wolpert, M.D., Chief, Section of Neuroradiology.

External Review Committee: Henry Barnett, M.D., Bruce Coull, M.D., and Mark Dyken, M.D.

Internal Review Committee: Anthony J. Furlan, M.D., Mark J. Alberts, M.D., Carlos Kase, M.D., and Michael S. Pessin, M.D.

Data Retrieval and Publications Committees: Gregory J. del Zoppo, M.D., Andreas Ferbert, M.D., Anthony J. Furlan, M.D., Werner Hacke, M.D., Michael S. Pessin, M.D., and Samuel Wolpert, M.D.

We are grateful for the involvement of Richard Kent, M.D., Judith Littlejohn, M.D., Rose Snipes, M.D., and Jacqueline Zinn and the support from the Burroughs-Wellcome Company (Research Triangle Park, NC) which made this study possible.

In addition, the rt-PA Acute Stroke Study Group wishes to thank the many investigators, radiologists, nurses, and other personnel who made this study possible.

The author wishes to thank Dr. Justin Zivin for reviewing the manuscript and offering helpful revisions, and Ms. Tina Brantley for assistance in typing and preparing this manuscript.

References

1. Cerebral Embolism Study Group (1984) Immediate anticoagulation of embolic stroke: Brain hemorrhage and management options. Stroke 15:779–789
2. Dalal PM, Shah PM, Aiyar RR (1965) Arteriographic study of cerebral embolism. Lancet 2:358–361
3. del Zoppo GJ, Copeland BR, Harker LA, et al (1986) Experimental acute thrombotic stroke in baboons. Stroke 17:1254–1265
4. del Zoppo GJ, Ferbert A, Otis S, et al (1988) Local intra-arterial fibrinolytic therapy in acute carotid territory stroke: A pilot study. Stroke 19:307–313
5. del Zoppo GJ, Poeck K, Pessin MS, and 16 coauthors of the rt-PA Acute Stroke Study Group (1992) Recombinant tissue plasminogen activator in acute thrombotic and embolic stroke. Ann Neurol 32:78–86
6. del Zoppo GJ, Zeumer H, Harker LA (1986) Thrombolytic therapy in acute stroke: Possibilities and hazards. Stroke 17:595–607
7. Dion JE, Gates PC, Fox AJ, Barnett HJM, Blom RJ (1987) Clinical events following neuroangiographuy: a prospective study. Stroke 18:997–1004
8. Faught E, Trader SD, Hanna GR (1979) Cerebral complications of angiography for transient ischemia and stroke: prediction of risk. Neurology 29:4–15
9. Fisher CM, Adams RD (1951) Observations on brain embolism with special reference to the mechanism of hemorrhagic infarction. J Neuropathol Exp Neurol 10:92–94
10. Fisher M, Zito JL, Siva A, DeGirolami U (1984) Hemorrhagic infarction: A clinical and CT study. Stroke 15:192
11. Fletcher AP, Alkjaersig N, Lewis M, et al (1976) A pilot study of urokinase therapy in cerebral infarction. Stroke 7:135–142
12. Gruppo Italiano per lo Studio della Sopravvivenza nell'Infarto Miocardico (1990) GISSI-2: A factorial randomised trial of alteplace versus streptokinase and heparin versus no heparin among 12, 490 patients with acute myocardial infarction. Lancet 336:65–71
13. Hacke W, Zeumer H, Ferbert A, Bruckmann H, del Zoppo GJ (1988) Intra-arterial thrombolytic therapy improves outcome in patients with acute vertebrobasilar occlusive disease. Stroke 19:1216–1222
14. Hanaway J, Torack R, Fletcher AP, Landau WM (1976) Intracranial bleeding associated with urokinase therapy for acute ischemic hemispheral stroke. Stroke 7:143–146
15. Hankey GJ, Warlow CP, Sellar RJ (1990) Cerebral angiographic risk in mild cerebrovascular disease. Stroke 21:209–222
16. Herndon RM, Nelson JN, Johnson JF, Meyer JS (1961) Thrombolytic treatment in cerebrovascular thrombosis. In: MacMillan RL, Mustard JF (eds) Anticoagulants and fibrinolysins. Lea and Febiger, Philadelphia, p 154
17. Hornig CR, Dorndorf W, Agnoli AL (1986) Hemorrhagic cerebral infarction: A prospective study. Stroke 17:179–185
18. Kalbfleisch J, Kurnik P, Thadeni U, et al. (1992) Myocardial infarct- artery patency and reocclusion rates after treatment with duteplase at the dose used in International Study of Infarct Survival-3. Am J Cardiol
19. Lodder J (1984) CT-detected hemorrhagic infarction; relation with the size of the infarct, and the presence of midline shift. Acta Neurol Scand 70:329–335
20. Lyden PD, Zivin JA, Clark WA, et al (1989) Tissue plasminogen activator-mediated thrombolysis of cerebral emboli and its effect on hemorrhagic infarction in rabbits. Neurology 39:703–708
21. Mori E, Yoneda Y, Tabuchi M, et al (1992) Intravenious recombinant tissue plasminogen activator in acute carotid artery territory stroke. Neurology 42:976–982
22. Okada Y, Yamaguchi T, Minematsu K, et al (1989) Hemorrhagic transformation in cerebral embolism. Stroke 20:598–603
23. Ott BR, Zamani A, Kleefield J, Funkenstein HH (1986) The clinical spectrum of hemorrhagic infarction. Stroke 17:630–637

24. Sabovic M, Lijnen HR, Keber D, Collen D (1989) Effect of retraction on the lysis of human clots with fibrin specific and non-fibrin specific plasminogen activators. Thromb Haemost 62(4):1083–1087
25. Third International Study of Infarct Survival Collaborative Group (1992) ISIS-3: a randomized comparison of streptokinase vs. tissue plasminogen activator vs. anistreplase and of aspirin plus heparin vs. aspirin alone among 41, 299 cases of suspected acute myocardial infarction. Lancet 339:753–770
26. TIMI Study Group (1985) Special Report: The thrombolysis in myocardial infarction (TIMI) trial. N Engl J Med 312:932–936
27. Van de Werf F, Ludbrook PA, Bergman SR, et al (1984) Coronary thrombolysis with tissue-type plasminogen activator in patients with evolving myocardial infarction. N Engl J Med 310:609–613
28. Weisberg LA (1985) Nonseptic cardiogenic cerebral embolic stroke: clinical-CT correlations. Neurology 35:896–899

Recanalization, Infarct Volume, Cerebral Hemorrhage, and Clinical Outcome After Intravenous Recombinant Tissue Plasminogen Activator and Heparin in Acute Carotid Territory Stroke

R. von Kummer[1], M. Forsting[1], W. Hacke[2], and K. Sartor[2]

In patients with thromboembolic occlusion of the intracranial internal carotid artery (ICA) or middle cerebral artery (MCA), clinical outcome is often poor or fatal. In these patients outcome may be affected by the nature and site of occlusion, the collateral circulation, and by spontaneous recanalization [17]. Recent studies show that recanalization can be achieved safely by local intra-arterial infusion of streptokinase or urokinase [6, 13, 14, 18]. Recombinant tissue plasminogen activator (rt-PA) is an endogenous plasminogen activator with relative fibrin specificity. Experimental work [4] and a recent randomized, placebo-controlled clinical study in 31 patients [15] show that intravenous infusion of rt-PA in acute carotid artery territory stroke is associated with recanalization of the occluded arteries and favorable clinical outcome. We studied the effects of single chain rt-PA, alteplase, in combination with heparin anticoagulation in 40 consecutive patients suffering from acute occlusions of the ICA and MCA. Our observations have been published in part previously [19, 20]. The significance of collateral circulation in these patients is reported in an article by Forsting and colleagues [8] elsewhere in this volume.

Subjects and Methods

Forty consecutive patients presenting with signs of severe hemispheric stroke were treated with an intravenous infusion of 70 ($n = 7$) or 100 mg ($n = 33$) rt-PA (alteplase, Karl Thomae, GmbH Biberach, FRG) over 90 min. Inclusion and exclusion criteria have been adopted from the German rt-PA Multicenter Trial [9]. Among them were 1) informed consent given by the patient or his relatives, 2) patient age between 20 and 70 years, 3) the clinical diagnosis of acute stroke occurring within 6 h of treatment, 4) the absence of hematologic disease and hemorrhage as documented by cranial computed tomography (CT), and 5) angiographic demonstration of the appropriate intracranial ICA,

Departments of [1]Neuroradiology and [2]Neurology, University of Heidelberg, Heidelberg, Federal Republic of Germany

G. J. del Zoppo, E. Mori, W. Hacke (Eds.)
Thrombolytic Therapy in Acute Ischemic Stroke II

MCA trunk, or branch occlusion consistent with the patient's clinical presentation.

The rt-PA infusion was begun immediately after the angiographic documentation of arterial occlusion. Alteplase was given as an initial 15 mg bolus, followed by 50 mg over 30 min and then 35 mg over the next 60 min. Simultaneously, a bolus of 5000 IU heparin was injected which was followed by a continuous infusion of heparin at 1000–1500 IU/h with the aim to double the activated partial thromboplastin time (aPTT) in each patient. Heparin was discontinued when the CT revealed parenchymal hemorrhage. Angiography was repeated immediately after completion of the rt-PA infusion, that is, within 8 h after the onset of symptoms. Reperfusion was then graded as 0, no reperfusion; 1, occlusion with minimal reperfusion; 2, partial reperfusion; or 3, complete reperfusion of the MCA or ICA. Grade 0 and 1 were considered as no reperfusion, grade 2 and 3 as effective reperfusion. Reperfusion was reassessed 12–24 h after symptom onset by transcranial Doppler ultrasound (TCD) ($n = 34$) and a third angiogram ($n = 9$). In two patients neither angiography nor TCD could be performed the day after stroke because of their poor clinical state. In these two patients MCA occlusion was confirmed by postmortem examination within 48 h after the stroke.

Patterns of cerebral infarction were assessed by serial CT or magnetic resonance imaging (MRI) before diagnostic angiography and during follow-up. The extent of cerebral infarction was graded as small (e.g., less than 50% of the presumed MCA territory), large (50%–90%), or total (90%–100%). Whether the infarct volume increased from small or large or the first CT measurement to large or total, respectively, in the second CT was registered. The presence of hemorrhage was defined as hemorrhagic infarction or as parenchymal hematoma according to criteria described by Pessin and colleagues [16].

All patients were monitored and treated on the Neurological Critical Care Unit for at least 3 days. Clinical outcome was defined as good when the patients recovered from their initial deficit so that they were able to walk without assistance at discharge from hospital, or poor when no apparent improvement was seen 4 weeks after the stroke, when compared to presenting deficits. Mortality was assessed separately.

Results

Eighteen women and 22 men aged 28–70 years (median = 60 years, mean ± SD = 56 ± 11 years) entered the study. All patients suffered from severe hemiparesis, conjugate ocular deviation, and impaired consciousness when admitted to the hospital. In 32 patients cardiac disease or arrhythmia suggested cardiac embolism, in 8 patients MCA occlusion was associated with arteriosclerotic stenosis of the cervical ICA. One patient had an isolated distal ICA occlusion with an open MCA trunk. In 13 patients intracranial ICA occlusion was associated with an ipsilateral MCA occlusion. An isolated MCA trunk occlusion was documented in 21 patients, while an MCA branch occlusion at the MCA trifurcation was observed in 5 patients.

The first diagnostic CT study was performed 142±61 min (range 61–292 min, median 124 min) after symptom onset showed areas of slight hypodensity in the cerebral parenchyma in 32 (80%) patients. The region of hypodensity was small in 24 (60%) patients, large in 4 patients (10%), and total in 3 (8%) patients, while the striatum was involved in 24 (60%) patients.

Alteplase and heparin were given by 227±64 min (range = 105–360 min, median = 240 min) after symptom onset. The overall frequency of recanalization was 35% (n = 14) when assessed immediately after the alteplase infusion, and 50% (n = 20) at 12–24 h after the stroke. Reocclusion was observed in 1 patient. The effects of different alteplase dosages, the site of occlusion, and the time between stroke and start of alteplase infusion are given in Table 1. The sex and age of the patients and the etiology of the vessels' occlusions did not influence the frequency of recanalization.

Immediately after treatment, partial and complete recanalization (per digital subtraction angiography) did not occur in combined internal carotid and middle cerebral artery trunk occlusions, occurred in 38% of isolated middle cerebral artery trunk occlusions, and occurred in 100% of middle cerebral artery branch occlusions. At 12–24 h after the stroke, the frequencies of recanalization as assessed by transcranial Doppler monitoring and/or a third angiogram were 15%, 57%, and 100%, respectively. Parenchymal hemorrhage occurred in 3 patients (8%) and hemorrhagic infarction without clinical deterioration in

Table 1. Potential determinants of partial and complete recanalization

	Total	Recanalization at			
		8 h		24 h	
		(n)	(%)	(n)	(%)
All patients	40	14	(35)	20	(50)
Dosage					
70 mg	7	3	(43)	3	(43)
100 mg	33	11	(33) NS	17	(52) NS
Occlusion					
ICA	1	1		1	
ICA/M1	13	0	(0)	2	(15)
M1	21	8	(38)*	12	(57)*
M2	5	5	(100)*	5	(100)*
Interval					
⩽3 h	11	5	(45) NS	7	(64) NS
>3⩽4 h	13	5	(39) NS	7	(54) NS
>4 h	16	4	(25) NS	6	(38) NS

ICA, internal carotid artery; M1, middle artery (MCA) trunk; M2, MCA branch; Recanalization, reperfusion grade 2 or 3 at 8 or 24 h after stroke; NS, statistically not significant; *, $p<0.05$ in comparison with ICA/M1 occlusion by Fisher's exact probability test.

Table 2. Effects of partial and complete reperfusion

	Total	Recanalization at	
		8 h (*n*)	24 h (*n*)
All Patients	40	14	20
Outcome			
Good	17	11**	16**
Poor, fatal	23	3	4
Hemorrhage			
PH	3	1 NS	2 NS
HI	9	4 NS	7 NS
Infarct Extent			
Small	21	11**	16**
Large, total	19	3	4
Increase of hypodense CT area			
No	22	11**	14 NS
Yes	18	3	6

PH, parenchymal hemorrhage; HI, hemorrhagic infarction
NS, statistically not significant; **, $p = 0.01$ by Fisher's exact probability test

9 patients (23%). Good clinical outcome and small infarction volume correlated with partial and complete recanalization at 8 h and 24 h after stroke ($p < 0.01$). Recanalization can prevent further increase in the infarct volume.

The potential effects of recanalization at 8 and 24 h after stroke on clinical outcome, cerebral hemorrhagic transformation, and development of infarct extension as documented by CT are given in Table 2. Hemorrhage was not observed in patients receiving 70 mg alteplase.

Discussion

Spontaneous recanalization of major cerebral arteries after thromboembolic occlusion has been observed by angiography in 27%–59% of patients during the first days after the stroke [1, 2, 5, 11, 17]. Angiographically proven data of the frequency of spontaneous recanalization during the first hours after symptom onset are still unavailable, though. Serial transcranial Doppler ultrasound recordings after MCA occlusion have shown spontaneous reperfusion 1 day later in 4 of 23 patients (17%) [12]. The frequency of partial and complete recanalization in our series was remarkably higher with 50% at 8 h and 65% at 24 h after the stroke in the patients with MCA trunk or branch occlusion. This suggests that recanalization was at least partly caused by the treatment. Studies with two-chain rt-PA (duteplase) [7, 15, 21] and intra-arterial urokinase [13, 14] have shown similar recanalization rates. Consistent with other studies [7, 14], recanalization was more frequent in the smaller vessels. This may result from more efficient thrombolysis of smaller distal thrombi. On the other hand, we did not observe immediate recanalization of the distal ICA in the combined ICA/MCA occlusion. This could be related to stagnant blood flow within the ICA preventing rt-PA from reaching the thrombus. In future studies, local application of plasminogen activator in this condition has to be tested.

The frequency of recanalization was unaffected by the time interval between symptom onset and start of treatment within 6 h. Only 7 patients received 70 mg rt-PA. This number is too small to determine whether 100 mg of rt-PA is more effective than 70 mg.

Ischemic infarcts were observed in all patients except one in whom rt-PA led to complete MCA trunk recanalization 5 h after the stroke. Despite early reperfusion, infarcts occurred in 13 patients which mostly involved the terminal blood supply area of the striatum. This observation and similar findings by Saito and coworkers [17] and Bozzao and colleagues [3] underline the significance of collateral blood flow. Increasing tissue pressure due to the ischemia-associated edema may disturb the collateral blood supply which then may cause an increase of infarct volume during the first days after the onset of symptoms. In our series, early reperfusion prevented the infarcts from getting larger. In consequence, complete and partial recanalization, even when achieved later than 6 h (but within 24 h) after symptom onset, was associated with small infarcts and good clinical outcome.

The observation that hemorrhages did not occur with 70 mg rt-PA but with 100 mg may be interpreted as a dose-dependent effect. The number of 7 patients, however, is too small to draw any definite conclusions. In comparison to other serial CT observations in non-anticoagulated stroke patients [10], intracerebral hemorrhages were less frequent in our patients.

We conclude from our observations that rt-PA can be given together with heparin by intravenous infusion with acceptable safety within the first 6 h after stroke. Whether recanalization can be achieved or not depends on the site and presumably on the composition of the thrombus. Thromboembolic occlusion of the distal ICA may probably be better treated by local rt-PA application. Recanalization within the first 24 h after the stroke can prevent extended infarction in the ICA territory with its resulting major neurological deficits.

References

1. Allock JM (1967) Occlusion of the middle cerebral artery: Serial angiography as a guide to conservative therapy. J Neurosurg 27:353–363
2. Bladin PF (1964) A radiologic and pathologic study of embolism of the internal carotid-middle cerebral arterial axis. Radiology 82:615–625
3. Bozzao L, Fantozzi LM, Bastianello S, Bozzao A, Fieschi C (1989) Early collateral blood supply and late parenchymal brain damage in patients with middle cerebral artery occlusion. Stroke 20:735–740

4. Chehrazi BB, Seibert JA, Kissel P, Hein L, Brock JM (1989) Evaluation of recombinant tissue plasminogen activator in embolic stroke. Neurosurgery 24:355–360
5. Dalal PM, Shah PM, Sheth SC, Deshpande CK (1965) Cerebral embolism: Angiographic observations on spontaneous clot lysis. Lancet 1:61–64
6. del Zoppo GJ, Ferbert A, Otis S, et al (1988) Local intra-arterial fibrinolytic therapy in acute carotid territory stroke. Stroke 19:307–313
7. del Zoppo GJ, Poeck K, Pessin MS, et al (1992) Recombinant tissue plasminogen activator in acute thrombotic and embolic stroke. Ann Neurol 32:76–87
8. Forsting M, Krieger D, von Kummer R, Hacke W, Sartor K (1992) The prognostic value of collateral blood in acute middle cerebral artery occlusion. In: 2nd International Symposium on Thrombolytic Therapy in Acute Cerebral Ischemia (this Proceeding)
9. Hennerici M, Hacke W, von Kummer R, Hornig C, Zangemeister W (1991) Intravenous tissue plasminogen activator for the treatment of acute thromboembolic ischemia. J Cerebrovasc Dis 1 (Suppl):124–128
10. Hornig CR, Dorndorf W, Agnoli AL (1986) Hemorrhagic cerebral infarction: A prospective study. Stroke 17:179–185
11. Irino T, Taneda M, Takaku M (1977) Angiographic manifestations in postrecanalized cerebral infarction. Neurology 27:471–475
12. Kaps M, Teschendorf M (1991) Spontaneous recanalization in middle cerebral artery occlusion. In: Hacke W, del Zoppo GJ, Hirschberg M (eds) Thrombolytic therapy in acute ischemic stroke. Springer-Verlag, Berlin Heidelberg New York, p 231
13. Matsumoto K, Satoh K (1991) Topical intra-arterial urokinase infusion for acute stroke. In: Hacke W, del Zoppo GJ, Hirschberg M (eds) Thrombolytic therapy in acute ischemic stroke. Springer-Verlag, Berlin Heidelberg New York, p 207
14. Mori E, Tabuchi M, Yoshida T, Yamadori A (1988) Intracarotid urokinase with thromboembolic occlusion of the middle cerebral artery. Stroke 19:802- -812
15. Mori E, Yoneda Y, Tabuchi M, et al (1992) Intravenous recombinant tissue plasminogen activator in acute carotid artery territory stroke. Neurology 42:976–982
16. Pessin MS, del Zoppo GJ, Estol C (1990) Thrombolytic agents in the treatment of stroke. Clin Neuropharmacol 13:271–289
17. Saito I, Segawa H, Shiokawa Y, Taniguchi M, Tsutsumi K (1987) Middle cerebral artery occlusion. Correlation of computed tomography with clinical outcome. Stroke 18:863–868
18. Theron J, Courtheoux P, Casco A, et al (1989) Local intra-arterial fibrinolysis in the carotid territory. AJNR 10:753–765
19. von Kummer R, Forsting M, Sartor K, Hacke W (1991) Intravenous recombinant tissue plasminogen activator in acute stroke. In: Hacke W, del Zoppo GJ, Hirschberg M (eds) Thrombolytic therapy in acute ischemic stroke. Springer-Verlag, Berlin Heidelberg New York, p 161
20. von Kummer R, Hacke W (1992) Safety and efficacy of intravenous tissue plasminogen activator and heparin in acute middle cerebral artery. Stroke 23:646–652
21. Yamaguchi T, Hayakawa T, Kikuchi H, Abe T (1991) Thrombolytic therapy in embolic and thrombotic cerebral infarction: A cooperative study. In: Hacke W, del Zoppo GJ, Hirschberg M (eds) Thrombolytic therapy in acute stroke. Springer-Verlag, Berlin Heidelberg New York, p 168

Intravenous Tissue Plasminogen Activator in Acute Thromboembolic Stroke: A Placebo-Controlled, Double-Blind Trial

T. Yamaguchi[1], T. Hayakawa[2], and H. Kikuchi[3]
for the Japanese Thrombolysis Study Group

Dramatic improvement of clinical symptoms and signs is not infrequent in patients with acute ischemic stroke. Such a syndrome has been called the "spectacular shrinking deficit," and its mechanism is presumed to be the rapid migration of an embolus to the distal branches of a cerebral artery after initially lodging in the main trunk [6, 7]. Supporting evidence for the mechanism and the frequency of this phenomenon has recently been reported by Minematsu and coworkers [5]. The existence of such patients encouraged us to carry out a clinical trial of thrombolytic therapy in acute ischemic stroke prior to the appearance of ischemic findings on computed tomography (CT).

Accordingly, a placebo-controlled, double-blind, multicenter clinical trial of the intravenous infusion of recombinant tissue plasminogen activator (rt-PA, duteplase, Sumitomo Pharmaceutical Co., Japan) was performed in patients with acute brain embolism.

Subjects and Methods

The present study was conducted during the 12-month period from May, 1990 to April, 1991 at multiple neurological and neurosurgical services around Japan where emergency angiography and CT were available on a 24-h basis. Patients with a clinical diagnosis of embolic stroke who satisfied all of the following inclusion criteria were enrolled in the study: 1) no ischemic findings on CT, 2) interval from onset to treatment < 6 h, 3) angiographic evidence of carotid axis occlusion, and 4) < 80 years of age. A diagnosis of thromboembolic stroke was made if the patient met at least two of the following criteria [12]: 1) abrupt onset of symptoms with an initial maximal neurological deficit, 2) history or evidence of embolization to other sites of the body, 3) presence of a potential source of emboli, and 4) angiographic features such as occlusion of the distal internal carotid artery (ICA), the middle cerebral artery (MCA) trunk, or its

[1] Cerebrovascular Division, National Cardiovascular Center, Suita, Osaka, Japan
[2] Department of Neurosurgery, Osaka University Medical School, Osaka, Japan
[3] Department of Neurosurgery, Faculty of Medicine, Kyoto, Japan

G.J. del Zoppo, E. Mori, W. Hacke (Eds.)
Thrombolytic Therapy in Acute Ischemic Stroke II

branches. Informed consent was obtained from the patients (or their relatives) before treatment.

The test drug contained either 20 million international units (MIU) of rt-PA or an identical inactive placebo. Both drugs were prepared by Sumitomo Pharmaceutical Company and were randomized by an independent controller (S. Naito, M.D., Tokyo Teishin Hospital). Patients were randomly assigned to one of the test drugs in sequential order of entry into the trial.

Immediately after the initial diagnosis of thromboembolic stroke was made and no changes were noted on CT, cerebral angiography was performed via the femoral approach using the Seldinger technique. When arterial occlusion was found in the carotid axis, the test drug, dissolved in 200 ml of physiological saline, was infused over 60 min with the angiography catheter being left in the abdominal aorta. Repeat angiography was carried out immediately after the completion of intravenous infusion.

CT scan was repeated 24 h later and again on days 3, 7, and 28 to evaluate infarct size and hemorrhagic transformation. Angiograms were reviewed by a qualified neuroradiologist who was independent from the Study Group (T. Okudera, M.D., Akita Brain and Vessel Research Center) and blind to the treatment given. The posttreatment and pretreatment angiograms were compared and classified into the following five categories [11]: grade 0, unchanged; grade 1, only slight migration of embolus without improvement of perfusion; grade 2, partial reopening of the occluded artery and $<50\%$ reperfusion of the arterial territory; grade 3, partial reopening and $>50\%$ reperfusion of the arterial territory; and grade 4, complete reopening and reperfusion.

In addition to the angiographic findings, therapeutic efficacy was evaluated by the improvement of neurologic deficits. Neurologic symptoms and signs were recorded before and after angiography, at 24 h posttreatment, and on days 3, 7, 14, and 28. The Hemispheric Stroke Scale (HSS) by Adams and colleagues [1] was applied for neurological evaluation. The subdomains of this scale include: 1) level of consciousness (inverted score of the Glasgow Coma Scale; 0–12 points), 2) higher brain functions including speech (0–40 points), and 3) sensorimotor function (0–48 points). The total score is 0 points in a normal individual and 100 points in a patient with the severest neurological deficits.

To assess improvement due to treatment, comparison of the scores and the percent reduction of the HSS were made between the rt-PA and placebo groups at the final evaluation. In addition, we minimized the bias caused by direct application of the score itself or its percent reduction by arbitrarily assigning a weighting to the original percent change on the basis of the initial HSS score. If the initial score was $\geqslant 91$, a weighting of 1.0 was given, and if it was between 81 and 90 the weighting was 0.95. Then, the weighting was reduced by 0.05 for every subsequent 10 points. For example, when a patient with an initial HSS score of 66 points had a final score of 33 points, the weighted percent reduction was 43% instead of 50%. The improvement rating was determined from this weighted percent reduction of the HSS score. Patients showing 70% or more reduction were rated as markedly improved, those with 40%–69% reduction were moderately improved, and those with 10% – 39% reduction were slightly improved. In addition, those with 0±9% change were rated as unchanged, and those with a 10% or more increase in the HSS score were defined as showing deterioration.

Continuous data were expressed as the mean ± standard deviation (SD) and Student's *t*-test was used for statistical analysis. Groups were compared by Wilcoxon's 2-sample test or the chi-square test where appropriate. A value of $p < 0.05$ was considered to be statistically significant.

Results

One hundred twelve patients were entered into the study. Fourteen patients were excluded before breaking the key code because of protocol violations (5 had delayed commencement of therapy, 5 had occlusion of the vertebrobasilar axis or no arterial occlusion, 1 had a history of cerebral hemorrhage, and 3 had additional treatments after test drug infusion). Therefore, a total of 98 patients were subjected to analysis, of whom 51 were treated with rt-PA and 47 with placebo. Baseline clinical characteristics such as sex, age, body weight, interval from onset to treatment, concomitant disorders, past history, site of occlusion, number of occluded vessels, and posttreatment management (decompression surgery, anti-edema agents, anticoagulants, etc.) were not significantly different between the two groups. The number of patients with multi-vessel occlusion was somewhat greater in the rt-PA group ($p < 0.1$, chi-square test). There were no significant differences between the two groups in the inverted Glasgow Coma Scale score (3.7±2.8 in the rt-PA group and 3.9±2.9 in the placebo group) and the HSS score (66.2±19.4 in the rt-PA group and 68.9±20.1 in the placebo group).

Reperfusion of various grades was found on posttreatment angiography (60 min after the beginning of infusion) in both groups (Table 1). When 50% or more reperfusion (grades 3 and 4) was defined as successful, 21.3% (10) and

Table 1. Grade of reperfusion immediately after completion of treatment (60-min infusion)

		Grade of reperfusion*				
	n	4	3	2	1	0
Placebo	46	0	2 (4.4)	7 (19.6)	4	33
rt-PA	47	2	8 (21.3)**	7 (36.2)	10	20

( ), cumulative % reperfusion
* $p < 0.005$, rt-PA > placebo (Mann-Whitney U-test);
** $p < 0.05$, vs. placebo (χ^2 test)

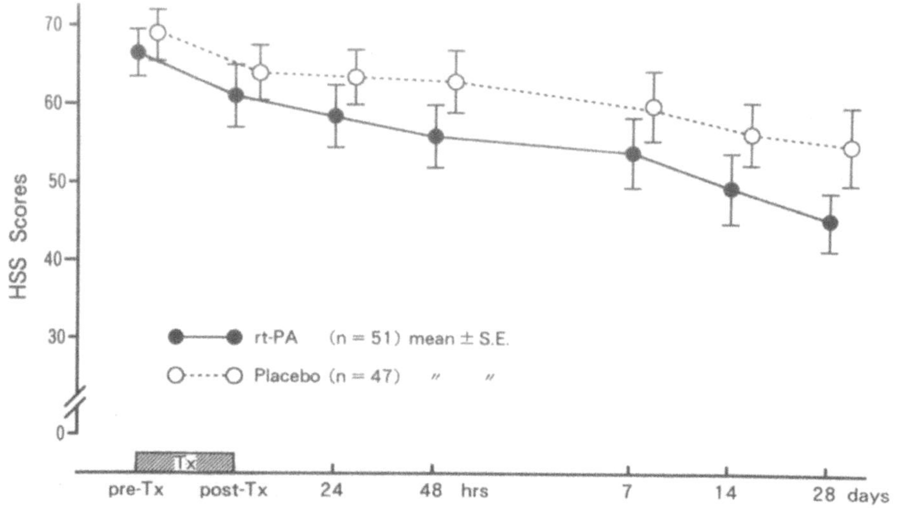

Fig. 1. Changes in the mean scores of the Hemispheric Stroke Scale in the rt-PA and placebo groups. No significant difference in the scores was obtained between the two groups, although those of the rt-PA group were lower than those of the placebo group

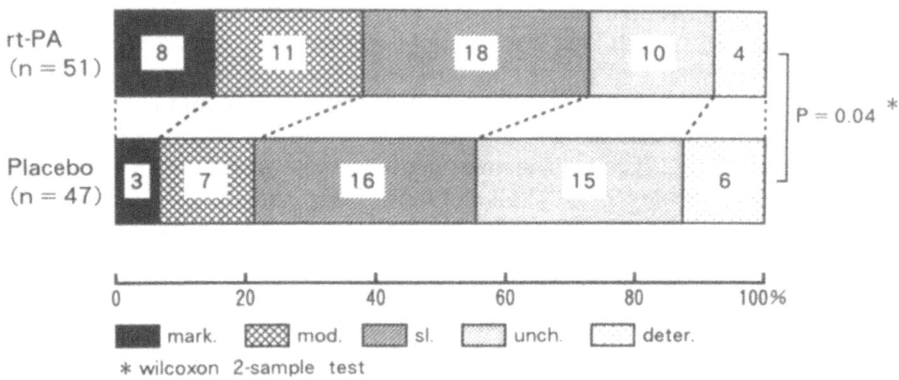

Fig. 2. Improvement ratings from the weighted percent reduction of the Hemispheric Stroke Scale. The rt-PA group had a better outcome than the placebo group. Criteria for the improvement rating were described in the text: ***mark***, markedly improved; ***mod***, moderately improved; ***sl***, slightly improved; ***unch***, unchanged; ***deter***, deteriorated

4.4% (2) of the patients showed successful reperfusion in the rt-PA and placebo-treated groups, respectively ($p<0.05$, chi-square test). Similar results were obtained when reperfusion was stratified by the site of occlusion into ICA and MCA occlusion ($p<0.05$, Wilcoxon's 2-sample test).

Changes in the HSS scores at each time of evaluation are shown in Fig. 1. Although the mean score of the rt-PA group was lower than that of the placebo group after treatment, no significant difference was noted at any time of evaluation because of the large standard error of the data. However, the improve-

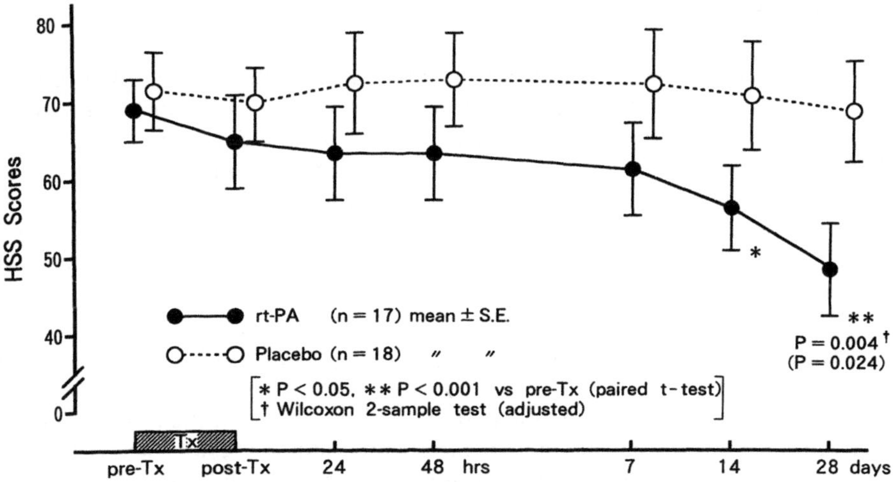

Fig. 3. Changes in the mean scores of the Hemispheric Stroke Scale in patients with internal carotid artery occlusion. The mean score in the rt-PA group was significantly lower than in the placebo group at 4 weeks after onset

ment ratings determined from the weighted percent reduction of the HSS score demonstrated that the rt-PA group had a more favorable outcome than the placebo group ($p = 0.04$, Wilcoxon's 2-sample test, Fig. 2). In a subset analysis of 35 patients with ICA occlusion, the mean score of the 18 placebo-treated patients did not decrease throughout the study period, while that of the 17 rt-PA-treated patients demonstrated a significant reduction at 4 weeks after treatment ($p = 0.004$ and $p = 0.024$ for non-adjusted and adjusted by the number of observations, respectively; Wilcoxon's 2-sample test; Fig. 3).

Among 47 patients treated within 4 h of onset, the rt-PA-treated patients demonstrated a significantly more favorable outcome than the placebo- treated patients ($p = 0.008$), but there was no difference in outcome between the patients treated either way after 4 h.

Hemorrhagic transformation was seen in 24 of the 51 rt-PA-treated patients (47.1%) and 22 of the 47 placebo-treated patients (46.8%). The frequency of massive hemorrhage was also almost the same in both groups (4 and 5 patients, respectively).

Five patients (8.8%) in the rt-PA group and 7 (12.7%) in the placebo group died during the study period, and no significant difference was noted between the groups. In the rt-PA group 2 patients died from brain herniation, and 1 patient each died of heart disease, pneumonia, and ruptured aortic aneurysm. The causes of death in the placebo group were brain herniation (4 cases), cardiac failure (1 case), pneumonia (1 case), and diabetic ketoacidosis (1 case).

Discussion

The intra-arterial application of a fibrinolytic agent into the occluded cerebral artery has been demonstrated to be effective in achieving thrombolysis [4, 8]. As this method is rather invasive, we performed a clinical trial to assess the efficacy of intravenous administration of a thrombolytic agent.

Although there have been a considerable number of reports emphasizing the efficacy and safety of rt-PA in ischemic stroke patients, most of them are still limited to uncontrolled, dose-finding pilot studies [2, 10, 11]. The only previous placebo-controlled, double-blind study performed in patients with acute carotid territory ischemic stroke demonstrated the efficacy and safety of 20 or 30 MIU of rt-PA delivered intravenously, although the number of subjects was relatively small [9].

The present placebo-controlled, double-blind trial enrolled the relatively large number of 98 patients and demonstrated similar results with regard to the efficacy and safety of rt-PA. Although the previous trial utilized two different doses of rt-PA (20 and 30 MIU), we used only a dose of 20 MIU in order to minimize hemorrhagic complications and to increase the number of subjects in each group. In addition, our preliminary open trial showed that the reperfusion rates were not much different between patients treated with 20 and 30 MIU (complete and >50% reperfusion; 24% vs. 31%, and <50% reperfusion; 57% vs. 42%, respectively). The effective reperfusion rate (>50% reperfusion) at 60 min after rt-PA infusion was slightly lower than that reported by Mori and colleagues [9], but it was still significantly higher than in the placebo group.

The subjects of the present study were restricted to thromboembolic stroke patients who met our diagnostic criteria [12]. The reasons for this restriction were as follows: in embolic stroke patients, 1) there is clinical evidence that early reperfusion can cause dramatic improvement [5], 2) the time of onset is easily recognized [12], 3) the frequency of a full hemispheric syndrome is high, making changes in symptoms and signs easily detectable [3, 12], 4) clinical severity does not vary as much as in thrombotic stroke, and 5) atherosclerosis of the cerebral arteries is generally less severe than in thrombotic stroke, so reocclusion in situ may rarely occur.

The lower reperfusion rate in patients with ICA occlusion than in those with MCA occlusion was consistent with the results of previous studies with and without fibrinolytic therapy [9]. Immediate reopening of an arterial occlusion during intravenous infusion over 60 min may be difficult in ICA occlusion, because emboli lodging at the distal end of the artery are larger than those lodging in MCA. However, the significantly better outcome of rt-PA-treated patients with ICA occlusion suggests that sufficient reperfusion may have occurred within a short time after posttreatment angiography was performed.

The incidence of hemorrhagic transformation (both petechial and massive) detected by frequent CT examination was not different between the two groups. Thus, use of rt-PA less than 6 h after embolic stroke does not increase the risk of hemorrhagic transformation, which often affects the outcome for these patients.

Concerning the therapeutic window for thrombolytic therapy, previous studies in a limited number of acute occlusive stroke patients have shown that initiation of rt-PA within 6 h of onset resulted in significant reperfusion without an increase in the frequency of massive hemorrhagic infarctions [2, 9–11]. The neurological outcome was better than in placebo-treated in these studies. Our study of embolic stroke treated within 6 h also showed a better outcome for rt-PA therapy than for placebo, although subset analysis of patients treated within 4 h revealed a higher level of efficacy.

In conclusion, the present study suggested the efficacy of 20 MIU of intravenous rt-PA in producing rapid thrombolysis and reperfusion with a better clinical outcome in patients with carotid axis embolic stroke, provided that it is given within 6 h of onset.

References

1. Adams RJ, Meador KJ, Sethi KD, Grotta JC, Thompson DS (1987) Graded neurological scale for use in acute hemispheric stroke treatment protocols. Stroke 18:665–669
2. Brott TG, Haley EC, Levy DE, et al (1992) Urgent therapy for stroke. Part I. Pilot study of tissue plaminogen activator administered within 90 minutes. Stroke 23:632–640
3. Cerebral Embolism Task Force (1989) Cardiogenic brain embolism. Arch Neurol 46:727–743
4. Hacke W, Zeumer H, Ferbert A, Bruckmann H, del Zoppo GJ (1988) Intra-arterial thrombolytic therapy improves outcome in patients with acute vertebrobasilar occlusive disease. Stroke 19:1216–1222
5. Minematsu K, Yamaguchi T, Omae T (1992) Spectacular shrinking deficit: Rapid recovery from a major hemispheric syndrome by migration of an embolus. Neurology 42:157–162
6. Mohr JP, Barnett HJM (1986) Classification of ischemic strokes. In: Barnett HJM, Stein BM, Mohr JP, Yatsu FM (eds) Stroke: Pathophysiology, diagnosis and management, Volume 1. Churchill Livingstone, New York, p 281
7. Mohr JP, Gautier JC, Hier DB, Stein BM (1986) Middle cerebral artery. In: Barnett HJM, Stein BM, Mohr JP, Yatsu FM (eds) Stroke: Pathophysiology, diagnosis and management, Volume 1. Churchill Livingstone, New York, p 377
8. Mori E, Tabuchi M, Yoshida T, Yamadori A (1988) Intracarotid urokinase with thromboembolic occlusion of the middle cerebral artery. Stroke 19:802–812
9. Mori E, Yoneda Y, Tabuchi M, et al (1992) Intravenous recombinant tissue plasminogen activator in acute carotid artery territory stroke. Neurology 42:976–982
10. von Kummer R, Hacke W (1992) Safety and efficacy of intravenous tissue plasminogen activator and heparin in acute middle cerebral artery. Stroke 23:646–652
11. Yamaguchi T, Hayakawa T, Kikuchi H, Abe T (1991) Thrombolytic therapy in embolic and thrombotic cerebral infarction: A cooperative study. In: Hacke W, del Zoppo GJ, Hirschberg M (eds) Thrombolytic therapy in acute ischemic stroke. Springer-Verlag, Berlin Heidelberg New York, p 168
12. Yamaguchi T, Minematsu K, Choki J, Ikeda M (1984) Clinical and neuroradiological analysis of thrombotic and embolic cerebral infarction. Jpn Circ J 48:50–58

The European Cooperative Acute Stroke Study (ECASS)

M. Kaste[1], C. Fieschi[2], W. Hacke[3], E. Lesaffre[4], M. Verstraete[5], and J. Fröhlich[6]

Stroke represents the third most common cause of death and is a major reason for hospitalization in the developed countries. It afflicts approximately 700000 Europeans annually. Stroke is a tragic occurrence to its victims and it also causes enormous financial costs. To date, no therapy is available to improve the outcome of patients with ischemic stroke. Stroke therapies have been aimed at the prevention of future cerebrovascular attacks. The significant mortality and morbidity associated with stroke necessitate development of acute therapeutic interventions to limit stroke mortality and morbidity.

Clinical data indicate that thrombosis is a primary cause of brain infarction. Thrombi may originate in atherosclerotic lesions in neck and brain arteries or they may enter the intracranial circulation from extracranial sources such as atherosclerotic lesions of carotid bifurcation or the cardiac system. Restoring cerebral blood flow into the ischemic brain tissue by recanalization of the occluded artery might help to decrease the extent of infarction as has been the case in the thrombolytic treatment of acute myocardial infarction. Encouraging reports of a successful recanalization with improved outcome following intra-arterial infusion of thrombolytic agents have recently been reported [1, 2, 4]. Intra- arterial therapy cannot, however, be an acute therapy for such a large patient group as patients with brain infarction. Thrombus-selective agents such as tissue plasminogen activator, a serine protease included in the endogenous thrombolytic system, are effective in intravenous thrombolytic therapy in acute myocardial infarction [7]. Intravenous thrombolytic therapy, if proven effective in acute brain infarction, would be more suitable for the large group of ischemic stroke patients than intra-arterial therapy.

[1] Department of Neurology, University of Helsinki, Helsinki, Finland
[2] Department of Neurology, University of Roma "La Sapienza", Roma, Italy
[3] Department of Neurology, University of Heidelberg, Heidelberg, Federal Republic of Germany
[4] Department of Epidemiology, School of Public Health, Catholic University of Leuven, Leuven, Belgium
[5] Center for Thrombosis and Vascular Research, Department of Medical Research, University of Leuven, Leuven, Belgium
[6] Dr. Karl Thomae GmbH, Boehringer Ingelheim Deutschland GmbH, Biberach an der Riss, Federal Republic of Germany

G. J. del Zoppo, E. Mori, W. Hacke (Eds.)
Thrombolytic Therapy in Acute Ischemic Stroke II

The object of this study is to evaluate the clinical efficacy and safety of the recombinant t-PA alteplase in patients with ischemic stroke. Treatment with the study drug will be initiated within 6 h from the onset of symptoms.

The study is a double-blind, randomized, placebo-controlled, multicenter trial to evaluate the clinical efficacy and safety of intravenous recombinant tissue plasminogen activator (rt-PA, alteplase) in patients with acute ischemic hemispheric stroke where the thrombolytic therapy can be initiated within 6 h from the onset of symptoms. Each patient will undergo cerebral CT scan before the therapy, but no angiographic evaluation is included in the trial. The primary outcome event will be improved functional outcome of patients.

Patients meeting study entry criteria and completing informed consent requirements will be randomized equally to the treatment with either alteplase or placebo. Each participating center will be supplied with a balanced randomization schedule of its own. The patients will receive a 60- min intravenous infusion of the study drug or placebo, with 10% of the total dose given as a bolus over 1–2 min. The total dose will be 1.1 mg/kg body weight not to exceed 100 mg. Enrollment will be 300 patients per treatment group.

A total of 40–50 European centers, either neurological acute care centers or stroke units, will take part in the study. The study aims to finish patient recruitment within 18–24 months after the first patient has been entered. The recruitment of patients is expected to start in Autumn, 1992.

Subjects and Methods

The hypothesis to be tested by this study is that treatment of patients with the study drug will result in improved clinical outcome when compared to a comparable placebo-treated group.

The *primary hypotheses* state that: 1) There is a difference between the alteplase and placebo groups in activities of daily living defined as a difference of 15 points in the Barthel index [3] 90 ± 7 days after treatment. Death within 90 days will be counted as the lowest possible score (= 0) in the Barthel index. 2) There is a difference between the two groups in clinical impression of outcome defined as a difference of one grade in the modified Rankin Scale [8] 90 ± 7 days after treatment. Deaths within 90 days will be scored as grade 6 in the modified Rankin Scale.

The *secondary hypotheses* state that: 1) There is a difference between the two groups in the clinical course assessed by the long-term score of Scandinavian Stroke Scale [6] (SSS) from baseline to 90 ± 7 days. 2) There is a difference between the two groups in fatality rate within the first 30 days. 3) There is a difference between the two groups in quality of life defined as combination of the Barthel index and modified Rankin Scale 90 ± 7 days after treatment. Deaths will be excluded.

Other measures of efficacy will be evaluated: 1) Differences between the two groups in the clinical course will be assessed by the long-term score of the SSS from baseline to 2, 8±1, and 24±2 h, and 7±1 and 30±2, and 90±7 days. 2) In addition to the SSS, the NIH Stroke Scale will be assessed at baseline, 24±2 h, and 90±7 days, and at each time point a correlation between the NIH and the SSS will be assessed. 3) Differences between the two groups in the duration of hospital stay of surviving patients will be examined.

Safety parameters are important in this study. The incidence of cerebral hemorrhage, space occupying infarction, adverse events and differences in laboratory parameters will be compared between the two groups.

The patient population will be selected on the basis of both clinical and CT inclusion and exclusion criteria.

Clinical *inclusion criteria* require that patients be 18–80 years of age, have a clinical diagnosis of moderate to severe ischemic hemispheric stroke, have a body weight maximally 100 kg, have onset of symptoms within 6 h of initiation of the therapy with the study drug, have symptoms for at least 1 hour and still present at the time of randomization, and complete informed consent.

The noncontrast cerebral CT requirements before a patient can be included in the study are a normal CT, circumscribed slight hypodensity in less than 1/3 of the middle cerebral artery (MCA) territory, or effacement of cortical sulci or the Sylvian fissure in less than one-third of the MCA territory.

Clinical *exclusion criteria* include the following: unknown exact time of stroke onset; coma; severe stupor; hemiplegia plus fixed eye deviation suggesting that a major brain infarction has already matured; complete global aphasia, or the patient only has minor stroke symptoms (>50 points out of maximal 58 of the SSS); or a rapid improvement of the symptoms at the time of randomization meaning that he/she most likely will make an excellent recovery irrespective of therapy. Presumed vertebrobasilar stroke including isolated hemianopia or ataxia will be excluded, as will patients with clinical presentation suggestive of subarachnoid hemorrhage, even if the initial CT scan is normal. Patients with known active seizure disorder or a first seizure within 6 h, or hypertension (systolic blood pressure >200 mm Hg, or diastolic blood pressure >115 mm Hg) will be excluded. A previously known intracranial hemorrhage is an exclusion criterion, as also are a previous stroke within 3 months, or other disabling stroke; presumed septic embolus and pericarditis; known infective endocarditis; presence of ventricular thrombus or aneurysm related to a recent acute myocardial infarction. Any condition associated with an increased risk of hemorrhage after thrombolytic agents is an exclusion criterion. Pregnancy, lactation or parturition within the previous 30 days are also exclusion criteria. Serious, advanced or terminal illnesses and any other conditions which the investigator feels could interfere with the performance of valid neurological assessment or follow-up will exclude the patient from this study.

Baseline laboratory values will be drawn, but the results of the analyses will only be waited for if there are clinical reasons to suspect that glucose is <2.75 mmol/l (50 mg/l) or >22.0 mmol/l (400 mg/l), platelets <10000/mm^3, or Hct <25.

If the pretreatment CT reveals a high density lesion consistent with intracranial hemorrhage of any degree, diffuse swelling of the affected hemisphere with space occupying effects on the lateral ventricle or narrowing of the perimesencephalic cisternae, or acute hypodense parenchymal lesion(s) in more than 1/3 of the MCA territory, the patient will be excluded.

Administration of the Study Agents

The intravenous (IV) infusion of the study drug (alteplase, Boehringer Ingelheim, FRG) will take place immediately following the CT demonstration that no intracranial hemorrhage is present provided that no other reason for exclusion is apparent and all inclusion criteria have been fulfilled. The rt-PA dose will be 1.1 mg/kg, not to exceed 100 mg. Ten percent of the total drug will be given as an IV bolus over 1–2 min followed by a 60-min IV infusion of the remainder of the dose. The placebo treatment will be administered in an identical manner.

Subcutaneous heparin to prevent deep venous thrombosis may be given immediately, but intravenous heparin is prohibited before and during the study drug administration and the initial 24 h thereafter. Administration of oral anticoagulants, antiplatelet agents, hemorrheologic agents, and brain protective drugs is prohibited during the initial 24 h after completion of the study drug administration. Thereafter, administration of antiplatelet agents is recommended but administration of hemorrheologic agents is discouraged. Other drugs may be used according to the needs of the patient.

Study Design

Other measures such as angiographic evaluation, nuclear magnetic resonance imaging, single photon emission tomography, etc., may be allowed according to clinical and scientific indications. They must not, however, delay the randomization of a patient or the initiation of the study drug administration in any circumstance.

Statistical Considerations and Patient Accruals

The sample size has been determined by a simulation study utilizing typical histograms of the Barthel index and the modified Rankin Scale as an anticipated data model for the placebo patients to be recruited in this trial. The necessary sample size to achieve 80% power with a two-sided two-sample Wilcoxon rank-sum test with significance level at 0.025 is at least 240 evaluable patients per treatment group for both primary endpoints, respectively. After 120 evaluable patients per group will have completed the 90±7-day observation period, an interim analysis will be performed at a two-sided significance level of 0.001. The final significance remains at 0.025 [5].

Enrollment will be 300 patients per treatment group to ensure that the alteplase and placebo groups have 240 evaluable patients. An exclusion log for patients actively screened but not entered in the trial will be kept to provide information about the patient population where the included patients come from.

Study Center Eligibility and Study Administration

There will be 40–50 trial centers, either neurological acute care centers or stroke units, from Scandinavia, Germany, Switzerland, Austria, the Benelux countries, Italy, France, England, Spain and Portugal. To be eligible for the study, a center must be able to treat a pilot patient with alteplase according to the official study procedure within the first two months. Thereafter, the monthly recruitment rate minimum will be one randomized patient for any center to continue its participation in the trial.

The organization of the study includes Steering Committee, Ethical and Safety Monitoring Committee, CT Scan Reading Panel, Publication Committee, Regional and National Coordinators and Clinical Monitors of the manufacturer. An independent center will perform data consistency checks, safety updates, and statistical analysis of all trial data.

Summary

This trial represents a double-blind, randomized, placebo-controlled, multicenter Phase III study of safety and efficacy of intravenous rt-PA (alteplase) in acute ischemic hemispheric stroke where thrombolysis is initiated within 6 h from the onset of symptoms. No angiographic evaluation is included in the trial. Primary endpoints will be activities of daily living (Barthel Index) and clinical impression of outcome (modified Rankin Scale) at 90 days and secondary endpoints neurological outcome assessed by Scandinavian Stroke Scale from baseline to 90 days, fatality rate within the first 30 days, and quality of life defined as combination of the Barthel Index and modified Rankin Scale at 90 days. Safety will be evaluated by the incidence of CT scan documented cerebral hemorrhage and space occupying infarction, adverse events and differences in laboratory parameters. Each patient will undergo diagnostic cerebral CT scan to rule out a hemorrhagic lesion. Subjects will be women and men, and age 18 through 80 completed years. Patients meeting study entry criteria and completing informed consent requirements will receive a 60-min IV infusion of the study drug, with 10% of the total dose given as a bolus over 1–2 min. The total dose will be 1.1 mg/kg, not to exceed 100 mg. Subcutaneous heparin may be given but intravenous heparin, antiplatelet agents, hemorrheologic agents, brain protective drugs and oral anticoagulants are prohibited during the initial 24 h after the termination of the study drug infusion. Thereafter, administration of antiplatelet agents is recommended. Enrollment will be 300 patients per treatment group, and 40–50 European neurological acute care centers or stroke units will take part in the trial.

The study will start as soon as the Ethical Review Boards of the participating centers and the medical authorities of the participating countries have accepted the study protocol. This will probably take place in the second half of 1992. The study is expected to last 1 to 1/2 to 2 years. After the present trial and other randomized double-blind trials in progress, we shall hopefully know the relative benefits and risks of the thrombolytic treatment with intravenous recombinant tissue plasminogen activator in acute ischemic brain infarction.

References

1. del Zoppo GJ, Ferbert A, Otis S, et al (1988) Local intra-arterial fibrinolytic therapy in acute carotid territory stroke. Stroke 19:307–313
2. Hacke W, Zeumer H, Ferbert A, Bruckmann H, del Zoppo GJ (1988) Intra-arterial thrombolytic therapy improves outcome in patients with acute vertebrobasilar occlusive disease. Stroke 19:1216–1222
3. Mahoney FI, Barthel DW (1965) Functional evaluation: The Barthel Index. Maryland State Med 14:61–65
4. Mori E, Tabuchi M, Yoshida T, Yamador A (1988) Intracarotid urokinase with thromboembolic occlusion of the middle cerebral artery. Stroke 19:802–812
5. Peto R, Pike MC, Armitage P, et al (1976) Design and analysis of randomized clinical trials requiring prolonged observation of each patient. I. Introduction and design. Br J Cancer 34:585–612
6. Scandinavian Stroke Study Group (1985) Multicenter trial of hemodilution in ischemic stroke – background and study protocol. Stroke 16:885–890
7. The TIMI Study Group (1989) Comparison of invasive and conservative strategies after treatment with intravenous tissue plasminogen activator in acute myocardial infarction. Results of the thrombolysis in myocardial infarction (TIMI) phase II trial. N Engl J Med 320:618–627
8. van Swieten JC, Koudstaal PJ, Visser MC, Schouten HJA, van Gijn J (1988) Interobserver agreement for the assessment of handicap in stroke patients. Stroke 19:604–607

On the Estimation of the Sample Size for the ECASS Study

E. Lesaffre[1], I. Scheys[1], J. Fröhlich[2], and E. Bluhmki[2]

Recently a stroke trial – called the ECASS study – was set up. It is a double-blind, randomized, parallel study designed to compare the effect of alteplase and placebo on patients with acute ischemic stroke. The primary outcome of the study is the patient's status at month 3 assessed by the Barthel index [5]. This index is a measure of quality-of-life, assessing the ability of the patient to perform his daily activities. A Barthel index score of 0 corresponds to complete dependence of the patient on others. We additionally introduced a score of 0 in case of death of the patient. A score of 100 implies that the patient can perform all his daily activities without any assistance. The latter can, but does not necessarily, imply complete neurologic recovery of the patient. Several versions of the Barthel index exist [2, 3]. The original scale increases or decreases with steps of 5, 10 or 15. Our version is a modified Barthel index, but for convenience we still call it the Barthel index.

Sample size calculations, now common practice in the planning of (controlled) clinical trials, are usually made by the use of standard tables or, more recently, also by computer software. These tables are constructed by making standard assumptions about the distribution of the primary endpoint. For a comparison of means, with the two-sample *t*-test in mind, these assumptions are usually: location shift and normality. However, here the nonparametric two-sample Wilcoxon rank sum test is needed to compare the distributions of the Barthel index between the two treatment groups. Unfortunately, for this test no useful sample size tables are available and no adequate software has been written. Therefore, often the above classical assumptions are made even when they cannot be fulfilled. In the section "Sample Size Calculations for the ECASS Study" we show what effect these assumptions have on the estimation of the sample size for the ECASS study. In the section "Calculating the Power of the Wilcoxon Test Using Bootstrap Methods" we illustrate our approach which involves bootstrap methods. But first we review some classical concepts

[1] Biostatistical Centre, Department of Epidemiology, Catholic University of Leuven, Leuven, Belgium
[2] Boehringer Ingelheim Deutschland GmbH, Biberach an der Riss, Federal Republic of Germany

G. J. del Zoppo, E. Mori, W. Hacke (Eds.)
Thrombolytic Therapy in Acute Ischemic Stroke II

such as the location shift assumption, the power of a study and the Wilcoxon test.

The Classical Assumptions for the Sample Size Calculation – Location Shift and Normality

Let us suppose that, except for location, the distribution of the endpoint in the ECASS study is the same for the placebo as for the alteplase group. That is, assume that the density of the Barthel index for the placebo group is given by $f_0(x)$, then the density of the alteplase group is given by $f_0(x\text{-}\Delta)$. This implies that the density $f_0(x)$ is shifted on the x-axis by a distance Δ to obtain the density of the Barthel index for the alteplase group. This is called the *location shift assumption.* If $f_0(x)$ is the normal density, then we obtain the classical two-group model upon which most sample size calculations for continuous responses are based. In Fig. 1 this assumption is graphically illustrated. The distance Δ measures the displacement of the normal density $f_0(x)$ due to the administration of alteplase. Thus, it measures the effect of the active treatment compared to the placebo treatment.

For every significance test there are two types of error. Take for instance the two-sample t-test. A type I error then occurs when one concludes from the test that on the average the active treatment results in a different Barthel index than the placebo treatment, while in fact both treatments give the same result. This error is controlled by the significance level usually taken as 0.05 or 0.01. A type II error occurs if the test claims that there is no therapeutic effect of the active treatment while alteplase is in reality better than placebo. 1 minus the probabil-

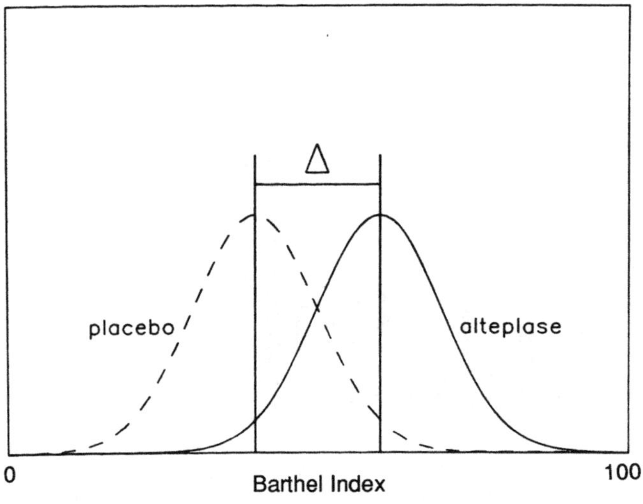

Fig. 1. Pictorial representation of the location-shift assumption with normal densities

ity of a type II error is called the *power* of the significance test. For the two-sample *t*-test and for a given standard deviation of the normal distributions (assumed to be equal), the power increases with increasing $|\Delta|$. Further, for a given Δ the power of the *t*-test decreases with increasing standard deviation. Finally, the power of the test also increases with the size of the study.

Thus, the determinants of the power are the sample size, the difference Δ and the standard deviation. The latter two are related to the choice of the endpoint and the inclusion and exclusion criteria, respectively. Once these are chosen only the sample size can change the power. Every well-designed study minimizes the probability of making a type II error and so has a high power for the specified clinical difference, usually 80% – 90%. The task is then to determine the sample size which corresponds to such a (prespecified) power. This is done by methods explained in the sections on sample size calculations and calculations using the bootstrap methods.

The Two-Sample Wilcoxon Rank Sum Test

The Barthel index does not have a normal distribution (for the patient population under consideration). This became evident during the preparation of the trial. Figure 2 shows the histogram of the Barthel index of treated and non-treated patients in a previous stroke trial. It was believed that this figure represents well the histogram of the placebo patients since the active medication didn't influence the Barthel index in a significant way. Thus, the two-sample

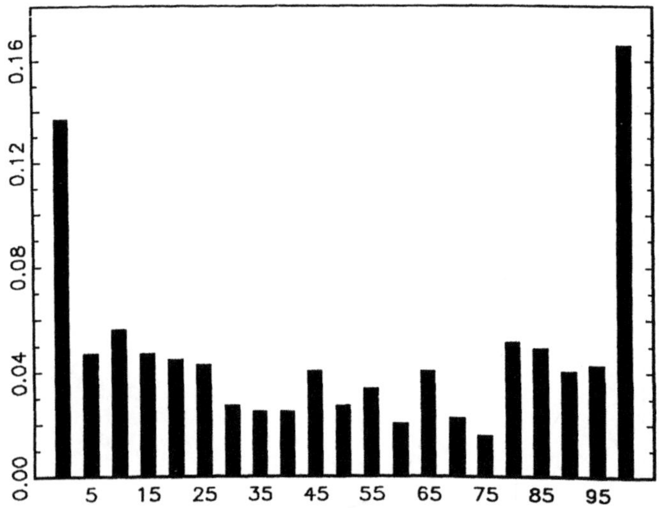

Fig. 2. Histogram of the Barthel index at about 3 months after onset of treatment based on results from another placebo-controlled trial. This histogram was used as data model for the calculation of the sample size of the ECASS study

t-test was replaced by the two-sample Wilcoxon rank sum test.

For the two-sample Wilcoxon rank sum test the data are replaced by their ranks. Here the Barthel index of every patient, irrespective of treatment, is ranked in increasing order. The ranks of patients of one treatment group (say of the active treatment) are then summed up to give the Wilcoxon test statistic W. A large (small) value of W indicates that the distribution of Barthel index of patients from, say, the active treatment is more located to the right (left). However, to be useful one needs to know whether W is significantly too large (or too small) to be explained as a result of chance. For this, tables of significance are available, or if the sample is large then asymptotic results are employed to calculate the significance.

Sample Size Calculations for the ECASS Study – The Classical Approach

At the start of the study planning, not much information was available about the distribution of the Barthel index. Figure 2 was released later. Therefore, initially, the classical method was employed to determine the necessary sample size of the study. We will describe this approach below and indicate the problems involved with it.

It was anticipated that the investigational treatment of the ECASS study should at least improve the patient's condition with $\Delta = 15$ points on the Barthel index scale compared to placebo. As test statistic W was chosen. To establish the sample size we looked in the literature and found that 40 might be a good choice for the standard deviation of the Barthel index under placebo treatment. Since sample size tables are lacking for the Wilcoxon test, we proceeded via the two-sample t-test with a standardized difference of $\Delta_s = 15/40 = 0.38$. Based on a two-sided significance level of 0.05 with a power of 80%, 115 patients are required in each arm of the study. Further, taking into account the relative efficiency of 95% of the two-sample Wilcoxon test to the two-sample t-test [6], about 240 evaluable patients are needed in the study. This method, though commonly used, has several major drawbacks.

First, the Barthel index is a constructed score and has an ordinal character. Thus, it is not at all clear what the meaning is of an average and a standard deviation [1]. Further, in the above calculations one implicitly assumes that the underlying distribution is normal. In other words, more assumptions are made for the calculation of the sample size than for the analysis afterwards.

Second, it is not immediately clear how to interpret the clinically relevant difference of 15 points improvement on the Barthel scale. Indeed, the Barthel index is bounded between 0 (= complete disability or death) and 100 (= complete independence). So, if a patient scores 100 under placebo, e.g., for a spontaneous recovery, then under investigational treatment no extra improvement can be seen, at least not by the Barthel index. Moreover, pilot studies and clinical experience indicated that the investigational treatment has possibly no effect on mortality. Consequently, depending on the inclusion and exclusion criteria, a large number of patients might not show any benefit from the investigational treatment when assessed by the Barthel index. Hence, if one roughly expects an individual improvement of 15 points of the Barthel index, then this corresponds to a lower difference on an average basis. When the initial sample size calculations were finished, evidence for this phenomenon became available from at least three other just completed, placebo-controlled trials. In one of the three, 43% of the patients had a Barthel index of 100 at 4 months after the onset of treatment and 21.5% of the patients did not survive. Then a $\Delta = 15$ implies an average improvement ascribable to treatment of only 4.1 on the Barthel scale. For such a difference and with the same significance level and power, 3,148 patients are needed. The discrepancy was not that dramatically high for the two other anticipated situations. In fact, the final calculations were done on the histogram given in Fig. 2, which does not contain that many deaths and patients with a Barthel index of 100. However, it illustrates the amount of error one can make by taking the classical assumptions for granted.

Third, the location-shift model implies that, on a certain scale, the difference in effect of the investigational medication and placebo is constant, or at least that the investigational medication shifts the distribution of Barthel scores under placebo to the right (or to the left if the investigational medication would be harmful), thereby keeping the shape of the distribution. However, the boundedness of the Barthel index renders the location-shift assumption questionable, certainly if the proportion of cases on each edge of the score interval is high as in our situation. For example, a location-shift assumption would imply here that under investigational treatment all patients will survive, which cannot be and was not expected.

Calculating the Power of the Wilcoxon Test Using Bootstrap Methods

If the classical assumptions, i.e., location-shift and normality, cannot be assumed, the mathematics involved to theoretically calculate the sample size or power become extremely complex and therefore no sample size tables are available anymore. Instead, one could use the computer to approximate the necessary sample for a particular power.

Let us first look how it could be done under the location-shift model. Suppose the Barthel index is known for a sample of patients treated with placebo and that a clinically relevant difference between the active treatment and placebo is expressed by Δ. A second sample, called the pseudo sample, can then be derived by adding to the Barthel index of the placebo patient the value Δ [assume that all values remain in the interval (0, 100)]. For these two samples the Wilcoxon rank sum statistic is calculated which yields an estimate of the necessary sample size (for more details see [4]). A recently proposed variant of this is the *bootstrap estimator.* In practice it comes down to regard the drawn control sample and the constructed pseudo sample as the populations of interest. Thus, one assumes for the sake of the calculations that these are not samples but represent all the present and future observations. Based on this assumption one then repeatedly draws samples with replacement from these two *hypothetical* populations. For every pair of samples, the Wilcoxon statistic is tested for its significance. If one performs this, say, 1000 times, an estimate of the power is provided by the proportion of significant Wilcoxon statistics at a chosen level, e.g., 0.05. This can be repeated for different anticipated study sizes so that by interpolation techniques the necessary sample size N_B is obtained. The procedure is somewhat more involved than the previous but a simple computer program is sufficient to obtain N_B. More importantly, it can be shown that the procedure provides a good estimate of the correct sample size.

For other than location-shift assumptions, the same procedure can be applied, with the only restriction being that the pseudo sample must have values in the interval (0, 100).

For the sample size calculation of the ECASS study we have taken as significance level 0.025 since two primary endpoints were involved, the Barthel index and the modified Rankin scale [7]. The former is assumed to differentiate well the badly recovered patients; the second appears to do well for the well recovered patients. The study size was then calculated with a particular data model for the placebo patients in mind. For the Barthel index three data models were at our disposal. All three show a U- shaped histogram, but they have different proportions of patients at the values 0 (p_0) and 100 (p_{100}). It was not anticipated that active medication would alter the rate of survival. Further, in all three data models the histogram of the Barthel index was fairly uniform over the interval (5, 95). So, besides the true effect of treatment, the most important determinants of the power and the sample size are the proportions p_0 and p_{100}. Indeed, for these patients either it is not expected to see improvement (the majority of the patients with a Barthel index of 0 are deaths) or it cannot happen (for patients with a Barthel index of 100 under placebo). To determine the sample size also the relevant clinical effect of the active treatment must be known. If treatment is able to improve the patient's condition with 15 points on the Barthel scale compared to placebo, then that effect is worth considering, according to the neurologists. It is not realistic to assume that every patient will improve under active treatment (as seen above also). A more realistic expression of this postulated effect is, therefore: if the patient would survive under placebo with a Barthel index between 0 and 85, then under active treatment he would also survive and on the average he would improve with 15 points. Those with 90 or more under placebo are expected to have about 100 (not more) under active treatment. For a power of 80%, about 250 patients in each arm are needed. This was based on the model shown in Fig. 2 and the stated clinically relevant effect. However, as seen above, for another data model more than 3000 patients are needed.

The second primary endpoint is the modified Rankin index. This index ranges from 0 to 6; 0 corresponds to no clinical symptom and 6 corresponds to death. The relevant effect which one doesn't want to miss is an increase of 1 for the surviving patients, again in comparison to the effect of what placebo would have given. For this clinically relevant effect, 2×250 patients is sufficient to achieve a power of 80% with a significance level of 0.05.

Final Remarks

Since the study is about a life-threatening disease, one could argue to split up the primary endpoint into two primary end-points, namely survival/death after treatment and the Barthel index among survivors. However, this was difficult to do since we were not able to detect with a reasonable probability clinically important differences in the mortality rate between placebo and alteplase. For instance, at a significance level of 0.025 and with a power of 80%, 2×375 patients are needed if the percentage of deaths under placebo is 20% and under active treatment 30%, or vice versa. For 20% and 25% deaths, 2×1,365 patients are needed. In both cases the sample size requirements fall beyond the budget of the trial. Further, splitting up the primary endpoint in two assessments can complicate the global assessment of alteplase if by chance the effect of alteplase on the mortality rate is in one direction (even if not in a significant way) and its effect on the survivors in terms of the Barthel index is in the opposite direction.

We have shown that the Barthel index posed nonclassical problems for the calculation of the sample size. One could have chosen another endpoint which differentiates better the patients such that a U-shaped distribution is avoided. But also based on the Barthel index one can think of other endpoints. For instance one can consider as outcome the percentage of patients above a certain Barthel index value, say 50. For the data model shown in Fig. 2, about 50% of the patients fall above 50. Under the assumed effect for the alteplase group (15-point increase) 60% of the patients will fall above 50. A binomial test can then be applied. This approach is much simpler than what we have applied in the above sections and, therefore, also much more attractive from this point of view. However, there are two difficulties with this approach. First, for all cutpoints the binomial test will need (many) more patients for the same assumed effect of the active treatment and for the same power and significance level. Next, and even more important, there is no logical choice for the cutpoint. So, it is not unlikely that during the planning phase of the study, one cutpoint is chosen and afterwards, when faced with the results of the trial, one realizes that possibly another cutpoint should have been chosen.

References

1. Anderson B (1990) Methodological errors in medical research. Blackwell Scientific Publications, Oxford
2. Collin C, Wade DT, Davies S, Horne V (1988) The Barthel ADL index: A reliability study. Int Disabil Stud 10:61–63
3. Granger CV, Albrecht GL, Hamilton BB (1979) Outcome of comprehensive medical rehabilitation: Measurement of PULSES Profile and Barthel Index. Arch Phys Med Rehabil 60:145–154
4. Lesaffre E, Scheys I, Fröhlich J, et al (1993) Calculation of power and sample size with bounded outcome scores. Stat Med (In Press)
5. Mahoney FI, Barthel DW (1965) Functional evaluation: The Barthel Index. Maryland State Med 14:61–65
6. Siegel S (1956) Statistics for the behavioral sciences. International Student Edition, McGraw-Hill Series in Psychology, Tokyo,
7. van Swieten JC, Koudstaal PJ, Visser MC, Schouten HJA, van Gijn J (1988) Interobserver agreement for the assessment of handicap in stroke patients. Stroke 19:604–607

Australian Streptokinase Trial (ASK)

G.A. Donnan[1], S.M. Davis[2], B.R. Chambers[3], P.C. Gates[4], G.J. Hankey[5], E.G. Stewart-Wynne[5], D. Rosen[6], R.R. Tuck[6], and J.J. McNeil[7]

A multicenter randomized controlled trial will be conducted to test the hypothesis that the intravenous administration of the thrombolytic agent streptokinase within 4 h of the onset of acute ischemic stroke will result in a significant reduction in subsequent morbidity and mortality. Six hundred eligible patients from 20 to 30 centers will be randomized to receive either 1.5×10^6 units of streptokinase or placebo infused over 60 min. Patients will be accrued over a 3-year period and the results analyzed on an intention-to-treat basis. Primary end-points will be death and 3-month disability on Barthel index or, if no significant difference in death rates between treatment and placebo groups exists, the primary end-point will be improvement in Modified Canadian Neurological Score (MCNS) among the living.

The *primary aim* of this study is to test, by randomized, double-blind, placebo-controlled trial, the hypothesis that intravenous streptokinase administered within 4 h of acute ischemic stroke will significantly reduce subsequent morbidity and mortality.

Secondary aims are: 1) to establish the natural history of hemorrhagic transformation in acute ischemic stroke as documented by CT scan 7–10 days postinfarction, and 2) to establish a model for future multicenter randomized clinical trials of therapy in acute ischemic stroke in an Australian setting.

Subjects and Methods

The efficacy of intravenous streptokinase in reducing morbidity and mortality after acute ischemic stroke will be assessed in 600 patients by using a double-blind, randomized, placebo-controlled trial technique. Patients will be randomized to receive either streptokinase or placebo.

Department of Neurology, [1]Austin, [2]Royal Melbourne and [3]Repatriation General Hospitals, Melbourne, Victoria; [4]Geelong Hospital, Geelong, Victoria; [5]Royal Perth Hospital, Perth, Western Australia; [6]Royal Prince Alfred Hospital, Sydney, New South Wales; and the [7]Department of Social and Preventive Medicine, Monash University, Victoria, Australia

G.J. del Zoppo, E. Mori, W. Hacke (Eds.)
Thrombolytic Therapy in Acute Ischemic Stroke II

Patients who fulfill the entry criteria will be entered from 20 to 30 centers. The study inclusion criteria dictate that: 1) the patient be between 18 and 85 years of age inclusively; 2) neurological deficit be present for less than 4 h (if at all unclear – i.e., if the patient awoke with the deficit – and was last awake greater than 4 h prior, the patient is INELIGIBLE); 3) no intracranial hemorrhage or tumor is present on CT scan; and 4) the informed consent has been obtained from the patient or patient's relative.

Exclusion criteria which lead to patient ineligibility are: 1) warfarin, heparin or other anticoagulant given within 48 h (aspirin is not a contraindication); 2) streptokinase administration within the previous 12 months; 3) acute stroke within the previous 3 months; 4) previous stroke in the same hemisphere which will interfere with the neurological assessment; 5) active peptic ulcer disease; 6) recent major trauma within the previous 3 months or surgery within the previous 10 days; 7) pregnancy or within 4 weeks postpartum; 8) uncontrolled hypertension SBP > 200 mm Hg DBP > 120 mm Hg; 9) severe systemic disease with poor prognosis; 10) proliferative diabetic retinopathy; 11) mild neurological deficit with Modified Canadian Neurological Score (MCNS) greater than 9.0; and 12) recovery of neurological deficit prior to registration to a Modified Canadian Neurological Score greater than 9.0.

Administration of the Study Agents

For those patients eligible to receive treatment, streptokinase will be administered intravenously at a dosage of 1.5 million units in 100 ml normal saline infused over a period of 60 min, or matched placebo will be given in like manner. Placebo, prepared to have a similar appearance to streptokinase, will be provided by Behringwerke, Germany, in association with Hoechst, Australia.

Should blood pressure fall below 100 mm Hg systolic during the infusion, therapy will be stopped and intravenous Haemaccel® administered until pressure is above 100 mm Hg systolic at which time infusion may recommence. If hypotension occurs the infusion should be slowed. If the hypotension persists despite Haemaccel®, the infusion will be terminated.

Therapy must be completed within 3 h or the infusion abandoned. Cardiprin® 100 mg (aspirin, Reckitt and Colman) will be given orally within 4 h of streptokinase administration and continued at 100 mg/day for the duration of the study.

All patients will receive standard medical treatment at the discretion of the participating center physician with the exception that no heparin or warfarin or similar anticoagulants may be administered within 48 h of study therapy.

Randomization Procedures

Patients eligible for participation in this study will be randomized to streptokinase or placebo. Randomization will be coordinated by the main randomization center (Department of Neurology, Royal Melbourne Hospital). The center will be contactable by telephone on a 24-h basis to provide registration numbers for patient allocation and/or advice about entry criteria. Patients will be stratified based on severity of deficit at time of registration to *Group 1*: Moderate (Modified Canadian Neurological Score of 4.0 or greater and less than or equal to 9.0); or *Group 2*: Severe (Modified Canadian Neurological Score less than 4). Each group will then be randomized separately. Patients with MCNS > 9.0 will not be eligible.

Study Design

The study is being conducted in two phases: 1) The pilot phase was conducted to establish with even more certainty the safety of streptokinase administration, particularly with regard to hemorrhagic transformation. It was an open study which involved 7 centers with a total of 52 patients, each patient receiving streptokinase 1.5 million units intravenously within 4 h of the ictus. 2) The subsequent main randomized, double-blind, placebo-controlled, multicentered trial will involve up to 30 hospitals throughout Australia.

Assessments

Baseline assessment will be performed at the time of study entry (4 h or less after the ictus). Patient history and clinical examination will establish whether any other exclusion criteria, apart from time delay from ictus, are present. Blood for baseline hematological tests will be taken as would be done for standard management of stroke patients (see below). A non-contrast CT scan will then be performed to exclude the presence of unsuspected cerebral hemorrhage as is already standard management practice. Neurological score (Modified Canadian Neurological Score) will be recorded prior to and following therapy administration. The subtype of stroke [hemispheric (cortical signs present), lacunar (motor and/or sensory signs only) or brainstem] will be categorized for post hoc analysis. Infusion of either streptokinase or placebo (will follow registration through the randomization center). Chest X-ray, electrocardiograph, and full blood examination including clotting profile, renal function tests, red blood grouping, blood glucose as well as a ward glucose test will be performed.

Following treatment, all patients will be examined daily for the next 3 days, then again at time of second CT scan. Should clinical deterioration occur, a repeat CT scan will be performed within 24 h as would occur in usual practice.

If hemorrhagic transformation or hematoma formation has occurred, the Coordinating Center will be notified within 24 h. A routine CT scan performed at 7–10 days, together with the clinical examination, will be used to confirm stroke subcategorization for those patients whose clinical deficit has not completely resolved (this second scan is also current standard management in Australia Stroke units). It will also be used to detect the development of hemorrhagic infarction or frank cerebral hemorrhage otherwise undiagnosed.

All patients will be reviewed at 3 months. The primary end-points of death, functional score (Barthel index) and neurological score (Modified Canadian Neurological Score) will also be documented. Further neurological or cardiac events will also be recorded.

Statistical Considerations and Patient Accrual

Six hundred patients will be randomized, half to active treatment and half to placebo. Assuming a 50% incidence of unfavorable outcomes in the control group (defined as death or a disability Barthel index less than 3), then this study will have a power of 85% to identify a reduction in this percentage to approximately 38% ($p < 0.02$, two-sided).

Based on our pilot data, this number of patients will be accrued in a period of 36 months but perhaps earlier, given that recruitment is likely to improve as publicity generated by the study leads to earlier hospital presentation of acute stroke patients. Including the 3-month follow-up assessment, checking and analysis of data, the total duration of the study will be 4 years.

Statistical analysis will be undertaken in the Department of Social and Preventive Medicine, Monash University, under the guidance of Prof. J. J. McNeil and in collaboration with Dr. J. Simes of the NH&MRC Clinical Trials Unit. The study will be conducted with cases included on an intention-to- treat basis. A comparison between patients with an unfavorable outcome (death, or disability < 100 on Barthel index) will be made using statistical tests for categorical data. If no statistically significant difference exists between treatment groups with death as the primary end-point alone, analysis with the improvement in neurological score in the living as the primary end-point will be undertaken. The Safety Monitoring Committee will inform the Steering Committee if any significant detrimental or markedly beneficial effect of therapy is found prior to its completion, and the Steering Committee will then decide if the trial should be suspended. Analyses of the effect of stroke category, age, and delay time in therapy administration upon the outcome will be performed using multiple logistic regression.

Ethical Aspects and Safety Assessments

The study will be conducted according to the ethical guidelines of the National Health and Medical and Research Council (NH&MRC) and the Helsinki Declaration. All patients will be fully informed concerning the nature of the study and written consent will be obtained before entry into the study. Any patient may withdraw from the study without prejudicing their routine management. Approval for the study will be sought from Ethics Committees of each participating center.

The dose regimen of streptokinase is identical to that used safely in myocardial infarction studies and coexistent use of anticoagulants will not occur. The Safety Monitoring Committee will independently review all data of the open pilot study and the main randomized study. CT scans showing hemorrhagic infarction and frank cerebral hemorrhage from the pilot study will be reviewed by the Radiology Committee. During the main study, the Safety Monitoring Committee will advise the Steering Committee at any time if full data analysis for safety aspects is required (see statistical considerations). They will receive reports following recruitment of each 50 patients and at 12 monthly intervals.

Should the study be terminated early because of a significantly adverse or beneficial effect of treatment, all participating centers will be immediately notified and information concerning the reasons for early study termination will be made available to all active participants.

Study Center Eligibility and Study Administration

Study centers must have sufficient access to CT facilities to perform the first scan within 4 h of the ictus. A neurologist/stroke physician nominated by the Steering Committee must be in a position to supervise patient management. Ethics Committee approval must be obtained from all participating institutions and Clinical Trial Notification completed. The study will be administered by the Steering Committee. The Coordinating Center (Department of Neurology, Austin Hospital) will be responsible for central data accrual and data analysis in conjunction with the Department of Social and Preventive Medicine, Monash University. The Randomization Center (Department of Neurology, Royal Melbourne Hospital) will coordinate randomization procedures in other centers.

Addendum

Steering Committee Members:

Dr. G.A. Donnan (Chairman), Dr. S.M. Davis, Dr. B.R. Chambers, Dr. P.C. Gates, Dr. G.J. Hankey, Dr. E.G. Stewart-Wynne, Dr. D. Rosen, Dr. R.R. Tuck, Prof. J.J. McNeil

Safety Monitoring Committee:
Dr. R. Collins (Chairman), Coordinator ISIS Trials, Oxford OX2 6HE, United Kingdom
Dr. R. Stark, Alfred Hospital, Department of Neurology, Prahran Victoria 3181, Australia
Assoc. Prof. R. Moulds, Department of Clinical Pharmacology, Royal Melbourne Hospital, Parkville Victoria 3050, Australia

Data Analysis Committee:
Prof. J. J. McNeil, Alfred Hospital, Prahran Victoria 3181, Australia
Dr. A. Forbes (statistician), Alfred Hospital, Prahran Victoria 3183, Australia

Radiology Committee:
Prof. O. Hennessy (Chairman), Radiology Department, Austin Hospital, Heidelberg Victoria 3084, Australia
Prof. B. Tress, Radiology Department, Royal Melbourne Hospital, Parkville Victoria 3050, Australia
Dr. R. O'Sullivan, Department of Radiology, Austin Hospital, Heidelberg Victoria 3084, Australia

Coordinating Center:
Dr. A. Gilligan (Clinical Coordinator, 1992), Ms. D. Jones (Data Manager), Department of Neurology, Austin Hospital, Heidelberg Victoria 3084, Australia

Randomization:
Dr. S. M. Davis (Chairman), Mr. S. Rossiter, Department of Neurology, Royal Melbourne Hospital, Parkville Victoria 3050, Australia
Ms. Kay Hynes, Clinical Trial Pharmacist, Austin Hospital, Heidelberg Victoria 3084, Australia

Consultants:
Clinical Trials Consultants:
Dr. John Marler, NIH Project Coordinator, NINDS Bethesda, MD USA
Dr. John Simes, NH&MRC Clinical Trials Unit, University of Sydney, NSW, Australia

Hematology Consultant: Dr. Alex Gallus, Flinders Medical Centre, Adelaide, SA, Australia

Thrombolytic and Antithrombotic Therapy in Acute Ischemic Stroke. Multicenter Acute Stroke Trial – Italy (MAST-I)

The MAST-I Collaborative Group

Stroke is a major cause of death and disability, and it consumes a large proportion of health resources. Numerous treatments have been suggested for acute ischemic stroke but so far none has been shown to be effective in large randomized controlled trials. Thrombolytic treatment, which is so effective in acute myocardial infarction, has been evaluated in numerous individual stroke patients and some small pilot studies. Its efficacy now needs to be tested in a large multicenter trial.

Most acute ischemic strokes can be attributed to a thromboembolic event of cardiac or supracardiac origin. Therefore, it could be hypothesized that in these patients early recanalization will limit or prevent extension of the cerebral injury. Although it is recognized that the pathogenesis is not similar in all respects, an analogy can be made with acute myocardial infarction. In this latter condition it is well established that thrombolytic treatment significantly decreases early and late mortality [11]. A potential benefit could likewise be expected in ischemic stroke. Several reports published since the introduction of CT scans for patients with stroke have suggested that thrombolysis may be of some use performed both by intravenous or intra-arterial treatments [5, 10]. This has been confirmed by recent pilot studies [3, 6, 13]. Streptokinase and tissue plasminogen activator (t-PA) [1, 12] appear equally effective and safe in acute myocardial infarction; moreover, fewer strokes, especially early cerebral hemorrhages, were seen in streptokinase-treated than in t-PA- treated patients [8]. Thus streptokinase seems one of the most successful thrombolytic treatments which could be tested in acute stroke trials.

Antiplatelet and anticoagulant treatments were combined with a thrombolytic agent to further reduce mortality in patients with acute myocardial infarction and to prevent reinfarction and stroke [7]. There is, however, little direct evidence on the usefulness of antithrombotics (heparin or antiplatelet drugs) in acute cerebral infarction. Aspirin is the most widely tested antiplatelet agent for the prevention of cerebral ischemia and is equally efficacious in TIA and stroke [2]. Therefore, it is expected that this treatment alone

Presented by L. Candelise, Istituto di Clinica Neurologica, Università degli Studi di Milano, Milano, Italy

G. J. del Zoppo, E. Mori, W. Hacke (Eds.)
Thrombolytic Therapy in Acute Ischemic Stroke II

or in combination with a thrombolytic would be able to improve the short-term prognosis of stroke patients.

The aim of the Multicenter Acute Stroke Trial – Italy (MAST-I) is to determine whether there is a favorable risk-to-benefit ratio for thrombolytic and antiplatelet treatment in patients with acute ischemic stroke and, more specifically, to demonstrate a significant reduction of 6- month mortality and disability by both streptokinase and aspirin.

Subjects and Methods

All patients hospitalized for sudden development of a focal neurologic deficit attributable to stroke in carotid or vertebrobasilar vascular territories are eligible. Patients are excluded if: 1) they present severe coma without any purposeful motor response to noxious stimuli, 2) randomization and treatment is impossible within 6 h of onset of symptoms, 3) the CT scan indicates cerebral hemorrhage (intraparenchymal hemorrhage or hemorrhagic infarctions), or 4) the symptoms of neurologic deficit resolve completely by the time of randomization. Patients who have a clear indication for or a clear contraindication to the use of thrombolytic or antiplatelet therapy, and patients who are already receiving treatment with oral anticoagulants are not randomized. A register is being kept of eligible but non-randomized patients.

MAST-I is a multicenter, unblinded, but controlled randomized trial. Its general aspects are shown in Fig. 1. A factorial design will be used to allow evaluation of the two treatments in a single study. Therefore, patients will be assigned in equal proportion to the following 4 groups: streptokinase, aspirin, streptokinase plus aspirin, and control. Allocation to one of the 4 treatment groups will be random according to a centralized randomization list, stratified by center, with access by telephone operating 24 h a day, 7 days a week. The study was launched in 1991 by the Istituto di Clinica Neurologica and the Istituto di Ricerche Farmacologiche "Mario Negri," both located in Milan, Italy, and is being conducted in about 60 Italian centers. A Steering and Executive Committee supervises the daily conduct of the trial and adherence to the protocol; a Clinical Reviewing Committee reviews the intrahospital events in blind fashion. Follow-up is performed centrally, independent of the Steering Committee, and blinded with respect to treatment allocation. The 6-month follow-up data will be obtained by telephone. The latter method was successfully used in the Italian Hemodilution Trial [9] in which the inter-rater agreement and the agreement between the telephone and direct examination assessments was very good [4].

The protocol must receive the approval of the Ethical Committee of each collaborating center. The decision whether to request informed consent is left to the local investigator in order to follow the best practice for the individual patient, considering local requirements and advice from local Ethical Committees. An independent Monitoring Committee reviews the results periodically,

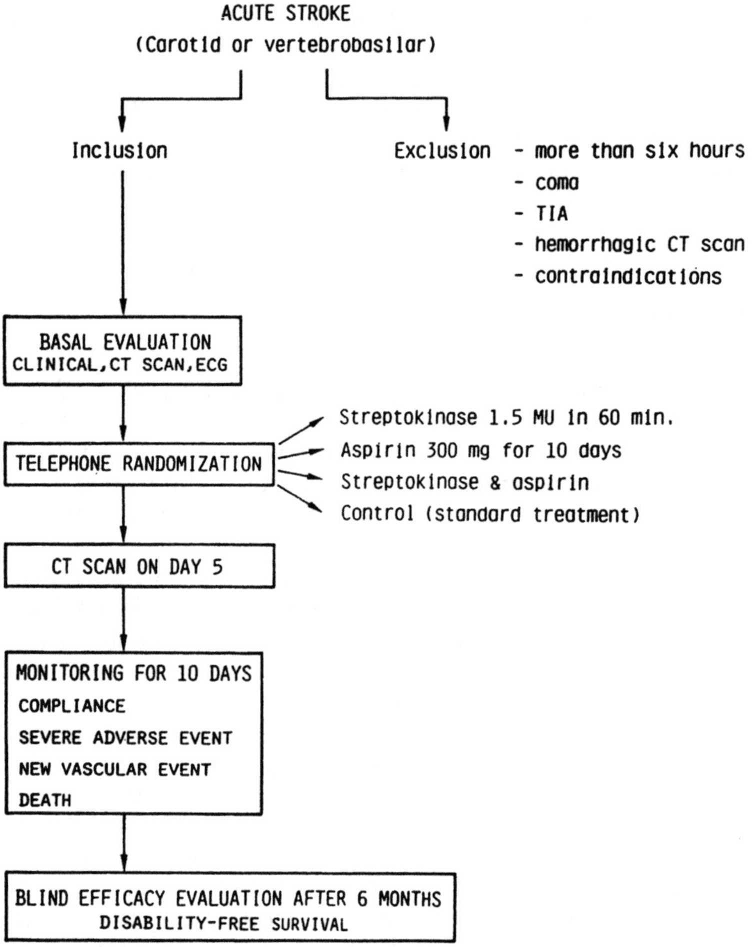

Fig. 1. MAST-I: Trial organization and treatments

conducts the interim analyses and gives recommendation to the Steering and Executive Committee if the results indicate the trial should be stopped. At least one arm of this study will be suspended if a difference is shown of over 3 standard deviations in favor or disfavor of the thrombolytic or antiplatelet therapy.

Administration of the Study Agents

Streptokinase (Kabikinase, Pierrel, Italy), 1.5 M U in 100 ml physiological saline, is delivered intravenously and started immediately after randomization and terminated after 60 min. Aspirin tablets (300 mg, Ascriptin, Rorer, Italy) are taken once daily, the first immediately after randomization and then every day until day 10 post-streptokinase. Whenever the patient is unable to swallow, parenteral aspirin (100 mg, Flectadol, Maggioni Winthrop, Italy) in 100 ml physiological saline is infused intravenously over 60 min, and substitutes for the aspirin tablet (even for only one administration). No placebo is used. All patients (in the treated and control groups) are given the standard treatment according to the local policy. Thrombolytics, oral anticoagulants, intravenous heparin and antiplatelet treatment must be avoided for the first 10 days; when used they must be considered protocol deviations. Subcutaneous calcium heparin is allowed for patients at risk of deep venous thrombosis, but no more than 5000 units (0.2 ml) three times a day. After 10 days, long-term antithrombotic treatments (aspirin, ticlopidine, anticoagulants) are left to local practice, but large-scale use is encouraged for secondary prevention.

Assessment

A standard baseline form (Fig. 2) is used to record a short pertinent history, detailed neurologic and general examinations, and CT scan diagnosis before telephone randomization. The patient is evaluated each day during the first 10 days after randomization to check compliance to aspirin therapy, the occurrence of severe adverse events like anaphylactic reaction, severe bleeding and cerebral hemorrhage, and the occurrence of new ischemic cerebrovascular episodes, acute myocardial infarction and death (Fig. 2). The CT scan is repeated in each patient on day 5, and in case of sudden and unexpected neurologic worsening. All new events, the causes of deaths, and the CT scans are re-evaluated blindly at a central facility.

The clinical status of each patient is assessed centrally with a modified Rankin scale at 6 months to evaluate the degree of disability. The follow-up data are obtained by telephone interview conducted by a single, appropriately trained investigator who is blind to the allocation of treatment. Preferably the patient is interviewed; otherwise, it is the person responsible for his care.

Statistical Considerations and Patient Accrual

Sample size requirements were derived from estimates that about 50% of untreated patients would be dead or seriously disabled at 6 months, with the intent to detect a 20% reduction of death or dependence at 6 months, and an alpha and beta type error of 5%, in a two-sided comparison. A trial including 1500 patients has a very good chance of detecting such an effect. The protocol will include two separate primary analyses. These will evaluate the effects of both streptokinase and aspirin on 6-month mortality and severe disability (Rankin score greater than 2). No separate analysis for survival will be conducted. All randomized patients will be kept in the analysis according to the

Center code | _ | _ | _ |

Centre ____________________

DEMOGRAPHIC DATA

Patient code | _ | _ | _ | _ |

Surname and name ____________________ Married name ____________________

Date of birth | _ | _ || _ | _ || _ | _ | Sex M | _ | F | _ |

Address ____________________

Postal code ________ City ____________________ Phone ____/____________

Relative ____________________ (surname and name) Phone ____/____________

General Practitioner ____________________ (surname and name) Phone ____/____________

RANDOMIZATION DATA

Onset of symptoms hour | _ | _ | minute | _ | _ | date | _ | _ || _ | _ || _ | _ | (when unknown, indicate mid-point between last known norr and discovery of symptoms)

Neurologic deficit

Stupor	1
Drowsiness	2
Severe motor plus non motor	3
Severe motor alone	4
Slight motor plus non motor	5
Slight motor alone	6
Only non motor	7

TRIAL TREATMENT

PLEASE STICK THE LABEL

Non motor deficit (only if neurologic deficit is 3, 5, 7)

- Dysphasia | _ |
- Visuospatial | _ |
- Sensory | _ |
- Visual field | _ |
- Brain stem/cerebellar | _ |

Side of motor deficit yes, right | _ | yes, left | _ | no | _ |

Blood pressure systolic | _ | _ | _ | mmHg diastolic | _ | _ | _ | mmHg

ECG Heart rate/min | _ | _ | _ | **Atrial fibrillation** yes | _ | no | _ |

CT scan hour | _ | _ | minute | _ | _ | date | _ | _ || _ | _ || _ | _ | normal/uncertain | N | infarct | I |

TIME OF RANDOMIZATION hour | _ | _ | minute | _ | _ | date | _ | _ || _ | _ || _ | _ |

Name of person completing this form ____________________ date | _ | _ || _ | _ || _ | _ |

Fig. 2. MAST-I: Randomization form

Treatment

Streptokinase administered according to protocol yes [ ] no [ ] if no, dose infused [|] ml

Cause of interruption:

haemorrhage	[ ]	persistent hypotension (systolic BP<90 mmHg for > 1h)	[ ]
allergic reaction	[ ]	other	[ ]

Aspirin administered according to protocol yes [ ] no [ ]

Aspirin i.v. (at least one administration) [ ]

If discontinued: date (day month) [| ‖ |]

Cause of interruption:				
	haemorrhage	[ ]	gastro-intestinal toxicity	[ ]
	allergic reaction	[ ]	other	[ ]

Concomitant treatment (1st administration)

			Start (day month)	End (day month)
Glycerol	[ ]	date	[| ‖ |]	[| ‖ |]
Mannitol	[ ]	date	[| ‖ |]	[| ‖ |]
Calcium heparin (low doses)	[ ]	date	[| ‖ |]	[| ‖ |]

Deviation to the protocol for a possible use of:

			day month	day month
Thrombolytics	[ ]	date	[| ‖ |]	[| ‖ |]
Anticoagulants	[ ]	date	[| ‖ |]	[| ‖ |]
Antiplatelets	[ ]	date	[| ‖ |]	[| ‖ |]

CT scan (between 4th and 6th day) date [| ‖ |]

normal	[1]	haemorrhagic infarct	[3]	other intracranial bleeding	[5]
infarct	[2]	haemorrhage	[4]	other	[6]

Neurologic deficit (in 10th day)

Coma	[0]
Stupor	[1]
Drowsiness	[2]
Severe motor plus non motor	[3]
Severe motor alone	[4]
Slight motor plus non motor	[5]
Slight motor alone	[6]
Only non motor	[7]
Normal	[8]

Diagnosis TIA [1] Lacunar stroke [2] Non lacunar stroke [3]

Intra-hospital assessment (within 10th day)

			day month
Anaphylactic shock *	[ ]	date	[| ‖ |]
Systemic haemorrhage*	[ ]	date	[| ‖ |]
New stroke with haemorrhage*	[ ]	date	[| ‖ |]
New stroke with infarct	[ ]	date	[| ‖ |]
Myocardial infarction	[ ]	date	[| ‖ |]
Death	[ ]	date	[| ‖ |]

* contact trial office immediately

Cause of death

cerebral	[1]	sudden death	[3]	infection	[5]
cardiac	[2]	polmonary embolism	[4]	other	[6]

Name of person completing this form ______________________ date [| ‖ | ‖ |]

Fig. 3. MAST-I: Intrahospital form

intention-to-treat principle. A secondary efficacy analysis will be done. Secondary analyses will also be performed on new vascular events and causes of death. Subgroup analysis will be conducted according to the main baseline prognostic variables identified.

Characteristics of MAST-I

Because many patients are recruited in multicenter clinical trials, a scrupulous approach is mandatory to avoid loss of contact with the single patients and to reduce protocol deviations. The clinicians involved in a multicenter trial are more interested in treating their patients than in collecting data for research. The MAST-I design and administration is, therefore, very simple and practicable within the framework of busy routine clinical practice. However, this pragmatic approach makes close supervision of the conduct of the study necessary and also scrupulous analysis of the data from each patient. Quality control measures in MAST-I include the following: 1) All baseline forms are screened centrally by neurologists who are also directly involved in the study in the participating center. 2) Any questionable entries or problematic evaluations are discussed directly with clinicians involved in recruitment of the patients. 3) The main intrahospital events are attributed centrally on the basis of the copy of clinical records, and all CT scans are reviewed centrally under blinded conditions. 4) The follow-up is always assessed centrally in order to avoid intracenter variability and reduce the bias due to unblinded conditions. 5) All centers will receive at least one site visit during the study, and they will all send participants to 6-monthly meetings organized to assess progress of the study.

References

1. Gruppo Italiano per lo Studio della Sopravvivenza nell'Infarto Miocardico: GISSI-2 (1990) A factorial randomized trial of alteplase versus streptokinase and heparin versus no heparin among 12, 490 patients with acute myocardial infaction. Lancet 336:65–70
2. Antiplatelet Trialist's Collaboration (1988) Secondary prevention of vascular disease by prolonged antiplatelet treatment. Br Med J 296:320–331
3. Brott T, Haley C, Levy D, et al (1990) Safety and potentional efficacy of tissue plasminogen activator (tPA) for stroke (Abstract). Stroke 2:181
4. Candelise L, Pinardi G, Aritzu E (1990) Stroke disability assessed by telephone interview: Reliability and reproducibility (Abstract). J Neurol 237:143
5. del Zoppo GJ (1988) Thrombolytic therapy in cerebrovascular disease. Stroke 19:1174–1179
6. del Zoppo GJ, Poeck K, Pessin MS, and 16 coauthors of the rt-PA Acute Stroke Study Group (1992) Recombinant tissue plasminogen activator in acute thrombotic and embolic stroke. Ann Neurol 32:78–86
7. ISIS-2 (Second International Study of Infarct Survival Collaborative Group) (1988) Randomized trial of intravenous streptokinase, oral aspirin, both, or neither among 17, 187 cases of suspected acute myocardial infarction. Lancet 13:349–360

8. ISIS-3 (Third International Study of Infarct Survival Collaborative Group) (1992) A randomized comparison of streptokinase vs. tissue plasminogen activator vs. anistreplase and of aspirin plus heparin vs. aspirin among 41, 299 cases of suspected acute myocardial infarction. Lancet 339:753–770
9. Italian Acute Stroke Study Group (L.Candelise principal investigator) (1988) Haemodilution in acute stroke: Results of the Italian haemodilution trial. Lancet 1:318–321
10. Sloan MA (1987) Thrombolysis and stroke: Past and future. Arch Neurol 44:748–768
11. Sundt T, Sharbrough F, Anderson R, Michenfelder J (1974) Cerebral blood flow measurements and electroencephalograms during carotid endarterectomy. J Neurosurg 41:310–320
12. The International Study Group (1990) In-hospital mortality and clinical course of 20, 891 patients with suspected acute myocardial infarction randomized between alteplase and streptokinase with or without heparin. Lancet 336:71–75
13. von Kummer R, Hutschenreuter M, Wildemann B, Hacke W (1989) Thrombolytic therapy with intravenous recombinant tissue plasminogen activator in acute occlusions of intracranial arteries. J Cereb Blood Flow Metab 9(Suppl):5721

Appendix

The following investigators and centers are collaborating (provisional list):

Steering and Organizing Committee: E. Aritzu[1], L. Candelise[1], A. Ciccone[2] G. Landi[1], S. Ricci[3], M.C. Roncaglioni[2], G. Tognoni[2] ([1] Istituto di Clinica Neurologica, Universita' degli Studi, Milano; [2] Istituto di Ricerche Farmacologiche "Mario Negri", Milano; [3] Clinica Neurologica, Perugia).

Data Management Office: E. Negri, F. Colombo (Istituto di Ricerche Farmacologiche "Mario Negri", Milano).

Neuroradiologic Reviewing Committee: E. Boccardi, C. De Grandi, G. Scialfa (Divisione di Neuroradiologia, Ospedale "Niguarda Ca' Granda", Milano).

Clinical Reviewing Committee: C. Argentino (Dipartimento di Scienze Neurologiche, Universita' "La Sapienza", Roma); V. Bertele' (Clinica Medica Generale, Ospedale Luigi Sacco, Milano); A.P. Maggioni (Divisione di Cardiologia, Ospedale Fornaroli, Magenta, Milano); P. Perrone (Ospedale di Legnano, Divisione Neurologica, Legnano, Milano).

Data Monitoring Committee: H.J.M. Barnett (The John Robarts Research Institute, London, Ontario, Canada); J. Bogousslavsky (Centre Hospitalier Universitaire Vaudois, Lausanne, C.H.); A.D el Favero (Clinica Medica, Policlinico, Perugia, Italy); U. Loi (Corte d'Appello, Palazzo di Giustizia, Milano, Italy); R. Peto (Clinical Trial Service Unit, Oxford, U.K.); C. Warlow (Western General Hospital, Edinburgh, U.K.)

Centers: Ancona, Ospedale Torrette, Clinica Neurologica; Ancona, Ospedale Sestilli, Divisione Neurologica, Divisione Radiologica, Divisione Geriatrica; Antella (FI), Ospedale S. Maria Annunziata, Medicina Interna 1a, 2a, 3a; Aosta, Ospedale Regionale, Divisione Neurologica; Arezzo, Divisione Medicina Interna, Divisione Radiologica; Bari, Universita' degli Studi- Policlinico, Ia Clinica Neurologica; Bassano del Grappa, Divisione Neurologica; Bergamo, Ospedali Riuniti, Divisione Neurologica 1a; Bergamo, Ospedali Riuniti, Divisione Neurologica 2a; Bologna, Ospedale Bellaria, Divisione Neurochirurgia 1a; Busto Arsizio (VA), Divisione Neurologica; Caltanissetta, Divisione Neurologica; Carpi (MO), Divisione Neurologica; Catania, Ospedale "Garibaldi", Divisione Neurologica; Cesena (FO), Ospedale Bufalini, Divisione Medicina, Divisione Neurofisiopatologica; Como, Ospedale S. Anna, Divisione Medicina A; Como, Ospedale S. Anna, Divisione Medicina B; Como, Ospedale S. Anna, Divisione Neurologica; Como, Ospedale Valduce, Divisione Neurologica, Divisione Radiologica; Crema (CR), Divisione Neurologica; Empoli, Divisione di Medicina; Grosseto, Divisione Neurologica; Grottaglie (TA), Divisione Medicina; Imola (BO), Ospedale Nuovo, Divisione Medicina Generale; Lecco (CO), Divisione Neurologica; Melegnano (MI), Ospedale Vizzolo Predabissi, Divisione Neurologica; Merate (CO), Divisione Neurologica, Servizio Radiodiagnostica; Messina, Policlinico Universitario, 1a Clinica

Neurologia; Milano, Ospedale Fatebenefratelli, Divisione Neurochirurgica; Milano, Ospedale Niguarda, Divisione Neurologica, Divisione Medicina Generale 2, Divisione Medicina Generale 5; Milano, Medicina "Vergani"; Milano, Ospedale Policlinico, Clinica Neurologica; Milano, Ospedale Policlinico, Medicina d'Urgenza; Milano, Ospedale Sacco, Divisione Neurologica; Milano, Ospedale S. Carlo, Divisione Medicina 6° piano, Divisione Neurologia; Milano, Ospedale S. Raffaele, Divisione Neurologica; Modena, Ospedale Civile; Modena, Ospedale Policlinico, Clinica Neurologica, Servizio Neuroradiologia; Palermo, Ospedale Civico, Divisione Neurologica; Palermo, Villa Sofia, Divisione Neurologica; Parma, Istituto di Neurologia, Cattedra di Neuroradiologia, Medicina d'Urgenza; Pavia, Istituto Neurologico "C. Mondino", Divisione 3a; Policlinico S.Matteo Presidio Belgioioso; Ospedale C. Mira; Perugia, Clinica Neurologica, Divisione Neuroradiologia; Pesaro, Divisione Neurologica; Pistoia, Ospedale Del Ceppo, Divisione Neurologica; Pozzilli (IS), Istituto Scientifico Sanatrix, Divisione Neurologica, Reparto di Anestesiologia e Terapia Intensiva; Prato, Divisione Neurologica; Ravenna, Divisione Neurologica; Reggio Emilia, Arcispedale, Divisione Neurologica, Divisione di Radiologia; S. Benedetto del Tronto (AP), Divisione Neurologica, Divisione Geriatrica; Saronno (VA), Divisione Neurologica; Seriate (BG), Ospedale Bolognini, Divisione Neurologica; Sesto S. Giovanni (MI), Ospedale, Divisione Medica "Campari"; Spoleto (PG), Ospedale Civile "S. Matteo degli Infermi" Divisione Neurofisiopatologia – Medicina Generale Geriatria; Taranto, Divisione Neurologica; Terni, Divisione Neurologica, Divisione Neuroradiologica; Trento, Ospedale S. Chiara, Divisione Neurologica; Treviglio (BG), Divisione Medicina 2a; Trieste, Ospedale Maggiore, Divisione Neurologica; Varese, Divisione Medicina Generale; Vicenza, Ospedale, Divisione Neurologica; Zingonia (BG), Policlinico S. Marco, Divisione Neurologica, Divisione Cardiologica.

Discussion Summary: Clinical Trials in Progress

Chaired by G. Boysen

In opening the discussion, Dr. Brott was asked by Dr. del Zoppo to clarify the clinical significance of a 4-point change on the NIH scale as it would appear for the individual patients. Dr. Brott explained that in the pilot study the mean score at entry was 14 points on the NIH scale, which ranges from 0 (no neurological signs) to 50 points. Here a 4-point improvement would correspond to the ability to hold up the arm and the leg against gravity for 10 s in a patient who was not able to do so before. The median improvement in the pilot study was 8 points, so that 4 points would mean a comparably small improvement. Dr. Ferbert inquired if one would include a patient with hemiplegia due to lacunar infarction in the randomized study. To this Dr. Brott replied that this was indeed a question discussed in planning the study. These patients, however, were also to be included, since in the emergency room a distinction could not be made about the clinical criteria and, moreover, there is no evidence that there is a subtype of focal ischemia which would not respond to thrombolytic therapy.

Following his presentation of the rt-PA Acute Stroke Study Group data, Dr. Alberts was asked if the documented recanalization rate was comparable to spontaneous lysis. A comparison with the data presented by Dr. Fieschi in the first session was not possible because in that study follow-up angiograms were done after 24 h or after one week. The 65% late recanalization frequency was comparable to that reported from studies in myocardial infarction. A physician inquired about the rate of embolic infarction and about the correlation between recanalization and clinical improvement in the rt-PA Acute Stroke Study Group trial. The rate of embolic infarctions was approximately 60%, but no correlation was found between recanalization and clinical improvement. In that study the fatality rate of 12.5% in patients with MCA occlusions was surprisingly low, although patients with hemiplegia and eye deviation were excluded at the outset. Such patients are known to have a higher mortality rate.

In the discussion of Dr. von Kummer's presentation of data from the Heidelberg Study, Dr. Verstraete pointed out that the low reocclusion frequency after lysis of MCA occlusions as compared to the higher reocclusion frequency of

Department of Neurology, Rigshospitalet, Copenhagen, Denmark

G.J. del Zoppo, E. Mori, W. Hacke (Eds.)
Thrombolytic Therapy in Acute Ischemic Stroke II

the coronary vessels (approximately 50%) may be due to the fact that in cardiogenic cerebral embolism the vessels as such are healthy in contrast to in situ thrombotic occlusions in coronary artery disease. Dr. von Kummer agreed. In his study the frequency of cardiogenic embolism was about 80%. He reported experiencing a high frequency of immediate reocclusion specifically in atherothrombotic occlusions of the basilar artery. When asked by Dr. Busse about the necessity and additional risk of another arteriogram 24 h after infusing the thrombolytic agent, Dr. von Kummer noted that just 9 patients underwent angiograms at 24 h. Transcranial Doppler examination appeared sufficient for follow-up checks. However, no complications could be attributed to the arteriograms.

In response to his presentation, the results of a double-blind, placebo- controlled multicenter trial of intravenous rt-PA, Dr. Yamaguchi was asked by Dr. Poeck about the treatment of the placebo group and the ethical aspects of substituting physiologic saline for the thrombolytic agent in that group. Dr. Yamaguchi replied that since no established therapy existed in cardioembolic stroke, he saw no ethical problems in employing a placebo group. From the audience the question was raised whether patients with hemorrhagic infarctions did deteriorate clinically. It was noted that only patients with massive hemorrhage became worse and that this was observed equally in the placebo and the rt-PA groups. Additionally, heparin was not used in either group. Finally, Dr. Yamaguchi stressed the point that most events were caused by cardiogenic embolism. Differentiation between atherothrombotic and cardioembolic occlusions was performed primarily on clinical grounds.

In the follow-up presentation of the current status of the ASK trial, Dr. Wolpert noted that none of the data presented was angiographically controlled. What was the likelihood under those circumstances that patients who did not have acute embolic stroke would be treated?

Dr. Donnan replied that the deliberate policy of the ASK group was to give streptokinase (SK) within 4 h, which would obviate the use of an angiogram. There is no evidence currently that there is any difference in therapeutic effect in large vessel versus small vessel disease. Patients one would clinically classify as having lacunes would therefore be included.

The presentation of the ECASS protocol raised similar issues. Dr. Ferbert noted that in its design the Barthel Score was to be used but that it cannot be applied acutely. Dr. Kaste clarified that it would be used only after three months. In the ECASS Study, the Scandinavian Stroke Scale and the NIH Scale will be used for acute evaluation. Further, Dr. Kaste commented on the angiographic evaluation. For acute myocardial infarction, intra-arterial treatment with thrombolytic agents and angiographic evaluation were used in concert at the outset to define the vascular anatomy and vascular outcome; in later clinical studies angiography was not necessary. The question could be reversed as to how one can diagnose acute myocardial infarction without angiography as it is quite the same thing with a stroke, as it is a clinical diagnosis. Dr. Kaste noted that if treatment will ever be effective, it must be clear that if an angiographic evaluation is needed, a thrombolytic approach will never be a treatment for large population groups. It would only be for selective centers highly prepared for emergency angiography.

Dr. Furlan, from the audience, commented further on the angiography controversy. He noted that at this stage with so many unknowns, it is not certain what one is treating without angiography, because, as most studies have shown, there is a 20% – 30% incidence of negative angiograms (those not demonstrating a symptomatic vascular occlusion). To treat such patients and not know whether a vessel is in fact occluded would make interpretation of the results quite difficult.

Dr. Alberts suggested that in the MAST-I Trial the mortality was about 24% which was quite high and about double that observed in the rt-PA Acute Stroke Study Group study. Dr. Candelise explained that in the multicenter controlled clinical study with hemodilution the acute mortality was also approximately 20%, similar to the early findings of MAST-I, which most probably has reflected that many patients with severe strokes were treated.

In trials employing streptokinase, hypotension may be observed, the development of which in acute stroke patients may be a worry. Dr. Alberts was concerned whether any neurological deterioration accompanied hypotension in the experience of the ASK trial reported by Dr. Donnan. Dr. Donnan indicated that hypotension is a serious problem, which was seen in 17% of treated patients. In two patients hypotension was associated with clinical deterioration, but, fortunately, recovery occurred within a period of hours. Because of this experience, the ASK trial has adopted a different policy for the administration of streptokinase. If the blood pressure drops 20 mm Hg a plasma expander is administered. With this change, the study will then examine the effect of streptokinase plus whatever is necessary to support the blood pressure versus placebo in acute stroke.

Dr. Poeck commented on the episodes of severe ecchymoses seen in Dr. Donnan's study, which may reflect the development of a systemic thrombolytic state. In reply to why urokinase was not used in the ASK trial, Dr. Donnan noted that the reasons were practical ones. He stated, "I was impressed, as was Livia Candelise, with the data from the cardiac studies, and I saw all of you other people struggling away with t-PA and realized that we needed to look at a cheaper drug that potentially might be even more effective than t-PA!"

Dr. Yamaguchi, when asked whether any symptomatic patients with patent arteries received rt-PA (duteplase), replied that this was an unusual situation. Dr. Caplan, in pursuit of the issue of vascular diagnosis, noted that "thrombolytic drugs, as far as we know, are working by opening up closed vessels. Now, if we give them to people who do not have closed vessels, there is no reason to think that they are going to work. There is no hypothesis. One of the virtues of studies like this is that we do not want to do harm. So it would be nice to know that if we gave it to a person who had open vessels, it would not hurt him. But I do not see how we are going to learn much unless we know what the cases are. I can understand the problems in some parts of the world in getting evaluation, but I think right now, since we have echocardiography and transcranial Doppler sonography, there is a way to classify these patients by noninvasive techniques. Later we can compare the Australian, Japanese, French-Canadian, and European [study] groups to say what they are; otherwise, we are not going to be able to evaluate the studies."

Dr. Overgaard, from the audience, asked generally about dose regimens among the various studies. In Dr. Yamaguchi's trial there was no apparent difference in hemorrhage between rt-PA-treated and saline-treated control groups and Dr. von Kummer's trial indicated that 100 mg rt-PA (alteplase) was more effective for reperfusion than 70 mg rt-PA. The MAST-I trial and the Australian trial employed relatively high doses of streptokinase and also added aspirin which were quite near to the established acute myocardial infarction dose regimens. One rt-PA (alteplase) (TTATTS) trial will examine 0.9 mg/kg and the ECASS will employ 1.1 mg/kg. Both regimens are about 20%–30% lower than the dose of alteplase employed in acute myocardial infarction trials. It is possible that t-PA trials with low-dose rt-PA would be compared with high-dose SK trials. In Dr. Overgaard's opinion an rt-PA dose of 1.3 mg/kg should be examined.

Dr. del Zoppo noted that dose–rate comparability is an important issue, but for practical reasons, based upon thrombus lysis assays, ad hoc comparisons would not be meaningful. In the rt-PA Acute Stroke Study Group study, the highest dose used when the study was terminated did not exceed the limits for hemorrhagic transformation. If the study had been extended, the value of high dose-rate rt-PA (duteplase) might be apparent now.

T. Brott noted that when the current NIH randomized trial was planned two doses were favored. A second higher dose was seriously discussed with the FDA, but was not employed. Most recently, he noted that the concern about the doses being insufficient was shared and efforts to explore the evaluation of a second dose are underway.

Regarding the use of angiograms, angiograms were employed in the pilot study of 74 patients, in 75% of whom evidence of thrombus or embolus was observed (after rt-PA infusion). Dr. Brott indicated that "the cardiac literature has shown us that angiography is a rocky road with respect to what we are really doing." In the TIMI I trial recanalization was twice as frequent with t-PA compared to streptokinase, which led to enthusiasm for the former, although subsequent mortality outcome studies have shown that this difference does not translate into dichotomous outcome. Angiograms were performed immediately following therapy. Dr. von Kummer indicated a change in the rate of recanalization in the Heidelberg Study as a function of time with rt-PA. "With streptokinase, which has more of a systemic anticoagulant effect, particularly when combined with heparin, one would have to ask, when [does one] do the second angiogram? [Does one] need three or four angiograms and how [does one] make inferences about recanalization with only one second angiogram done 1 h after the end of therapy? I think it will throw us back on our clinical end-points because those clinical end-points are the rock solid end-points for the cardiac studies today."

Dr. Mohr responded: "Could I offer the suggestion that subgroup analysis be preplanned? We went through Dante's Inferno over claims that we were doing post hoc analysis in the Nimodipine Study and I think that everything other than the angiographic studies are throwing the dice for very high stakes. If the clinical measures, which are convenient to use quickly, do not prove very sensitive, and if the disease being treated is not responding, it is possible that no real effect will be seen and a whole line of inquiry and therapy will disappear again. So I would just like to plea for having a biologically relevant marker of effect, because I strongly suspect that the trials are going to have a hard time to show a benefit."

Other Applications of Fibrinolytic Agents in the Central Nervous System

Acute Central Retinal Artery Occlusion and the Role of Thrombolysis

H.-J. Freitag[1], H. Zeumer[1], and V. Knospe[2]

Central retinal artery occlusion (CRAO) is one of the major causes for monocular blindness in the elderly. The diagnosis is easily achievable by means of clinical signs and symptoms and ophthalmoscopy. Spontaneous improvement is a rare event and treatments using vasoactive drugs are poorly effective. Up to now fibrinolysis seems to be the only rational treatment for CRAO. In 1992 Schmidt and colleagues [1] reported on successful treatments of CRAO employing superselective microcatheter techniques with local application of urokinase into the ophthalmic artery. The most surprising result was the observation that vision may recover even more than 6 h after retinal stroke.

Subjects and Methods

Since January, 1991 we treated each consecutive patient exhibiting with the signs of CRAO or occlusion of a major branch of the retinal artery [2].

Patients exhibiting impaired coagulation and those with severe carotid stenosis were excluded. After a neurological examination and after cranial CT had ruled out recent infarction or hemorrhage, all patients received a bolus injection of 5000 IU heparin followed by 1000 IU/h. In 20 patients the tip of the (Tracker 18) catheter was navigated into the orifice of the ophthalmic artery. This was followed by an infusion of 10 mg of recombinant tissue plasminogen activator (rt-PA, alteplase) per hour, usually continued for 2 h. In only 4 cases was 30 mg over 3 h administered. In all patients the catheterization of the ophthalmic artery was fast and easily done. Controls were performed clinically and ophthalmoscopically. The treatment was finished if vision improved and re-established flow was seen in the retinal arteries. Low-dose heparinization was continued for 3 days.

No bleeding or angiography-related complications occurred. However, one hypertensive patient presented with a progressing hemiparesis 12 h later which

[1] Department of Neuroradiology, [2]Department of Ophthalmology, University Hospital Hamburg Eppendorf, Hamburg, Federal Republic of Germany

G. J. del Zoppo, E. Mori, W. Hacke (Eds.)
Thrombolytic Therapy in Acute Ischemic Stroke II

was due to a lacunar infarction at the internal capsula as demonstrated by CT. Symptoms cleared within 1 week.

Results

As demonstrated in Fig. 1 the time interval between onset of clinical symptoms and fibrinolysis ranged between 5 and 50 h. Vision of hand movement or less was the initial finding in 12 patients. Four patients were able to count fingers and 4 others had a vision of 0.1 or more. In 16 cases the central retinal artery and in 4 cases a major branch of the retinal artery were occluded. The bar diagram (Fig. 1), in which the X-axis represents the delay of treatment, demonstrates the pre- and posttreatment vision. Nine patients reported significant vision improvement or an expansion of the visual field during the local fibrinolysis. In 1 patient, after initial improvement in vision testing 24 h later showed some degree of deterioration. In 9 patients, the improved vision remained unchanged. In 5 patients, vision improved less than 3 vision grades, 6 showed an improvement of 3 or more vision grades. In 2 patients, the last eye was involved. Despite late onset of treatment and only minimal improvement of vision, the patients regained their peripheral visual field including the capability to orientate in space, which was an enormous advantage in comparison to complete blindness. In total, almost 50% of our patients had a benefit from the treatment.

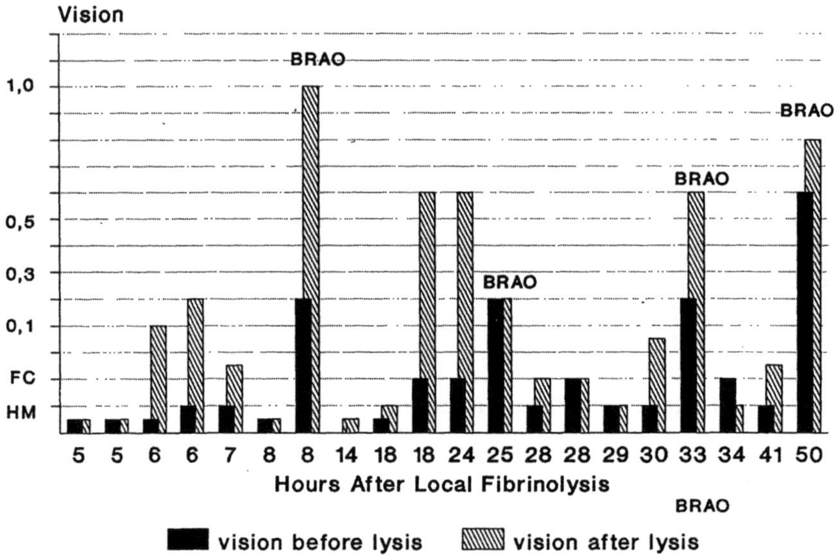

Fig. 1. Clinical results after treatment of CRAO with local fibrinolysis. *BRAO,* branch occlusion

Discussion

Recent results have shown that the bad prognosis of CRAO can be significantly improved by using fibrinolytic therapy. Since the ophthalmic artery is an end- artery, central retinal artery "occlusions," in our opinion, are not really complete obstructions of the lumen. Probably some minimal remaining flow protects the neuronal structure and allows it to regain function after flow has been re-established.

Microcatheter techniques are safely and easily performed in the carotid artery. Since only 10 mg of rt-PA per hour are applied, the treatment does not lead to measurable changes in hemostasis. After treatment, catheters can be removed and the patient can be taken care of on the ward as if only a diagnostic angiography had taken place. By now, safety is the major reason for using rt-PA, but there is no evidence of superiority in comparison to urokinase [3]. Obviously, the patients are not jeopardized by any risk of hemorrhage. On the other hand, the possibility of secondary embolization in the middle cerebral artery territory is possible. Schumacher and colleagues observed such a complication, which could be successfully treated using local fibrinolytic therapy through the same catheter [1].

From our recent experience, we can draw the following conclusions:

1) The prognosis of branch occlusions is much better than that of central retinal artery occlusion. Even 50 h after occlusion, major improvement is possible.

2) If at the beginning of treatment some remaining vision still exists, the prognosis concerning improving vision is much better. If even light is not perceived, an improvement of vision is rarely achievable.

3) The delay of treatment after loss of vision obviously plays a minor role.

These conclusions are also true for the cohort from Freiburg.

References

1. Schmidt D, Schumacher M, Wakhloo AK (1992) Catheter fibrinolytic therapy with urokinase in central retinal artery occlusion. Am J Ophthalmol (In Press)
2. Zeumer H, Freitag HJ, Knospe V (1992) Intravascular thrombolysis in CNS cerebrovascular disease. Neuroimaging (In Press)
3. Zeumer H, Freitag HJ, Zanella F, et al (1992) Local intra-arterial fibrinolytic therapy in stroke patients: Urokinase versus rtPA. Neuroradiology (UnPub)

Current Status of Fibrinolysis for the Rapid Dissolution of Subarachnoid and Intraventricular Clot

B. Weir

The half century coming to a close will hopefully have witnessed the discovery, description, elucidation, treatment and prophylaxis of a previously unknown disease entity – cerebral vasospasm from aneurysmal rupture and subarachnoid bleeding. Lysed red blood cells were shown to have vasoconstrictive activity in 1944. In 1949, autogenous erythrocytes incubated at body temperature for 4 days produced maximal pleocytosis in the spinal fluid of dogs as well as considerable protein elevation. During the same year it was shown in humans dying of ruptured aneurysms that almost one-third of cases showed cerebral infarcts consistent with temporary spasm of supplying vessels showing evidence of previously having been surrounded by blood clot. Two years later, cerebral vasospasm was demonstrated angiographically and it was shown to be a reversible process. The same year it was suggested that it would be logical to raise systemic blood pressure in patients having compromised cerebral hemodynamics following a variety of strokes. By the 1960's it was generally accepted by neurosurgeons that the development of angiographic vasospasm was a prognostic factor for poor outcome. In that decade experimental studies showed that the application of autologous blood could cause primate arteries to go into spasm both acutely and chronically. The following 10 years witnessed the working out of the time course of vasospasm. It was demonstrated that spasm was not a continuous process that was present from the moment of aneurysmal rupture. Instead, it was seen to develop progressively over several days, reaching a maximum about 1 week following the aneurysmal rupture. Experimental evidence accumulated that vasospasm was related to exposure of cerebral arteries to erythrocyte breakdown products.

With the advent of computed tomographic (CT) scanning, a powerful new tool was available to visualize the blood clot and its devastating consequences following the rupture of an aneurysm. First in Japan, and then independently in the United States, it was shown that the principal determinant of the development of symptomatic vasospasm was the volume of subarachnoid blood clot seen immediately after the rupture. Various surgeons conjectured that early removal of clot might abort the development of symptomatic vasospasm. During the 1980's there was suggestive evidence that rigorous early clot re-

Department of Surgery, University of Alberta, Edmonton, Alberta, Canada

G. J. del Zoppo, E. Mori, W. Hacke (Eds.)
Thrombolytic Therapy in Acute Ischemic Stroke II

moval with early aneurysm clipping might reduce the incidence of vasospasm, but there were no prospective randomized trials of this hypothesis. Most aneurysm surgeons began to use deliberate intravascular volume expansion and hypertension as needed when delayed ischemic neurologic deficits developed. In the late 1980's, calcium antagonists were shown to be associated with an improved outcome. With the advent of good animal models of delayed ischemia associated with severe diffuse spasm, it was possible to work out the pathophysiology in greater detail [14].

The evidence that mechanical removal of blood might be associated with improved outcome following aneurysm surgery has been recently reviewed. The evidence that mechanical suction removal or washout by cistern drainage were effective in the prophylaxis of vasospasm was at best suggestive [15]. Beginning with Kennady's study in 1969, there was preliminary evidence that fibrinolytic agents might accelerate the removal of blood from the subarachnoid space. When a primate model of subarachnoid hemorrhage which reliably produced chronic vasospasm became available, it was possible to evaluate mechanical clot removal. Nosko and then Handa demonstrated the efficacy of clot removal in preventing chronic vasospasm 7 days after the original clot application [15].

Findlay has recently reviewed the natural clearance of subarachnoid clot [1]. If the volume of blood clot released at the time of aneurysm rupture is sufficiently great it will readily clot. The amount of fibrinolytic activity in cerebrospinal fluid is normally very limited. Plasminogen activators are probably released from the irritated meninges and slowly allow fibrinolysis to proceed. Hemolysis also occurs in the subarachnoid space and is usually complete about 10 days after the subarachnoid hemorrhage. It is this breakdown of erythrocytes that liberates the spasmogenic oxyhemoglobin in the highest concentrations directly around the conducting arteries in the subarachnoid space. Some red blood cells are not broken down but are engulfed by macrophages. An unknown number may return to the systemic circulation by direct passage across arachnoid villi. The rationale for subarachnoid fibrinolytic treatment for the prevention of cerebral vasospasm has recently been reviewed [2, 3].

Experimental Studies

In a series of experiments conducted using a primate model of chronic cerebral vasospasm, Findlay and colleagues at the University of Alberta investigated whether or not the intrathecal instillation of a fibrinolytic agent could prevent the development of vasospasm. The safety and efficacy of the thrombolytic agent tissue-type plasminogen activator (t-PA) in the elimination of subarachnoid clot and prevention of chronic vasospasm were evaluated in a blinded, randomized, placebo-controlled trial. Monkeys were randomly assigned to one of two groups of 12 subjects. Each group underwent baseline angiography and coagulation analysis followed by right-sided craniectomy and application of blood clot around the arteries. A reservoir was inserted with its catheter placed into the subarachnoid space. Twenty-four hours later one group (the t-PA group) received 0.5 mg of t-PA in 0.5 ml of buffer via the reservoir every 8 h three times, while the placebo group received the same volume of physiological saline. On day 7, angiography was again done and the animals sacrificed.

One animal from the placebo group developed a delayed ischemic neurological deficit on day 5 after clot application. Moderate to severe vasospasm was present on day 7 in the arteries surrounded by clot of the animals in the placebo group, while in the t-PA group only mild narrowing of the anterior cerebral artery was seen. No deterioration in coagulation status occurred in either group. All animals in the placebo group had a large amount of subarachnoid clot remaining at the time of sacrifice, but 11 of the 12 animals in the t-PA group were completely free of clot. The results of electron microscopic studies of the cerebral arteries correlated with angiography, and there was no histological evidence of brain inflammation associated with the intrathecal use of t-PA [8].

To further test the safety of a large intrathecal dose of t-PA, 6 cynomolgous monkeys were given 10 mg of t-PA through a reservoir after craniectomy and dissection of the basal cisterns. Bleeding occurred briefly at the incision in 2 animals; otherwise the clinical condition of all 6 remained normal throughout the postoperative period. Systemic fibrinolysis did not occur and gross and microscopic examination of the brain revealed no abnormality. Subsequently, the efficacy of unilateral administration of t-PA suspension (0.5 mg) with slow-release gel t-PA (1.25 mg) in lysing a bilateral subarachnoid clot and preventing vasospasm in a randomized, placebo-controlled trial was studied. Sixteen monkeys were divided randomly into 2 equal groups, each of which underwent baseline angiography, followed by craniectomy and induction of clot application on both sides. Before closure on the right side either t-PA or an equal volume of placebo was injected. On day 7 angiography was repeated, and the animals were sacrificed. One of the animals in the placebo group developed a cerebral infarction on day 5. In the placebo group significant vasospasm occurred in all major right- and left-sided anterior cerebral vessels, but no vasospasm occurred in the t-PA-treated animals. Whereas clot averaging 1.13 g was found in all animals in the placebo group, only a small fragment of clot was found in a single t-PA-treated animal. The gel had no adverse microscopic effects on the brain. Intrathecal thrombolysis with t-PA was considered to be safe and effective in preventing vasospasm in primates [4].

In another study, 16 monkeys were divided into 4 groups of 4 each, each of which received a different dose of sustained-release gel t-PA. Cerebral angiography 7 days later showed that, whereas no vasospasm occurred in the groups receiving 0.5 or 0.75 mg of t-PA, mild to moderate vasospasm occurred in the groups receiving 0.125 or 0.25 mg of t-PA. Gross subarachnoid clot remained in all of the animals in the 0.125 and 0.25 mg dose groups, in 2 of the animals in the 0.5 mg dose group, and none of the animals in the 0.75 mg dose group. It was therefore concluded that 0.75 mg of gel t-PA is sufficient to comletely lyse a 4.25 ml subarachnoid hemorrhage and prevent vasospasm in this primate model [6].

The effect of intrathecal t-PA administered at times from 0 to 72 h after subarachnoid hemorrhage on the development of cerebral vasospasm in primates was then examined. Thirty monkeys were randomly assigned into one of five groups: a control group that underwent subarachnoid hemorrhage alone, and 0-, 24-, 48-, and 72-h treatment groups that received 0.75 mg of t-PA at those times after baseline cerebral angiography and subarachnoid hemorrhage on the right side. Seven days later angiography was repeated and the animals were euthanized. One animal in the 72-h group developed a delayed ischemic deficit on day 7 after subarachnoid hemorrhage. In the control and 72-h groups, significant vasospasm occurred in the arteries originally surrounded by clot, but no significant vasospasm developed in the 0-, 24-, and 48-h groups. Although a large subarachnoid clot remained in the control animals, most clot had been dissolved in all treatment groups. Lysing of subarachnoid hematoma with intrathecal t-PA within 72 h of subarachnoid hemorrhage was effective in preventing vasospasm [5].

This work at the University of Alberta was confirmed in a canine model by Seifert and colleagues in Hannover. The efficacy of t-PA in preventing delayed cerebral vasospasm after experimental subarachnoid hemorrhage using a single intracisternal bolus injection of this agent in a canine model was investigated. With a single injection of 25 μg of t-PA into the cisterna magna 48 h after the first and 6 h after the second injection of blood in the two- hemorrhage model, angiographic spasm of the basilar artery was completely prevented in all animals so treated. In the control group, severe vasospasm occurred. Autopsy studies demonstrated that the subarachnoid blood clots were removed by intracisternal t-PA application. Also, the signs of vasculopathy present in all animals of the control group were not seen in the t-PA group. This demonstrated that a single, intracisternal bolus injection of t-PA was highly efficacious in preventing angiographic as well as histological vasospasm [12].

Clinical Experience

On the basis of these animal experiments showing the efficacy of t-PA in the prevention of vasospasm, various neurosurgical centers around the world began human trials. Mizoi and coinvestigators in Sendai, Japan, evaluated the efficacy of postoperative intrathecal injections of t-PA in preventing cerebral vasospasm in cases with a diffuse severe subarachnoid hemorrhage. All of their first 10 cases were graded Group 3 according to the classification of Fisher and associates, and the CT number (Hounsfield number) of the subarachnoid clot was over 75. After clipping the aneurysm and mechanically removing as much clot as possible, three cisternal drainage catheters were inserted into both sylvian cisterns and the prepontine cistern, and continuous ventricular drainage was performed. Postoperatively, t-PA (0.5 mg/2.5 ml) was infused as a bolus both basal cisterns and the lateral ventricle twice daily for about 6 days. Angiography and cerebral blood flow studies using single photon emission computed tomography were performed on day 4 or 5 and between days 7 and 10 after aneurysmal rupture. None of their first 10 cases showed severe angiographic vasospasm or delayed ischemic neurological deficits. They considered that the intrathecal bolus injection of t-PA produced a marked reduction in vasospasm [10].

From the University of Alberta, Findlay and collaborators reported on 15 patients who underwent surgery within 48 h of aneurysm rupture and who were administered t-PA directly into the basal subarachnoid cisterns after minimal surgical clot removal and aneurysm clipping. Preoperatively, 13 patients had diffuse or localized thick subarachnoid blood clots on computerized tomography, and two had diffuse thin clots. The t-PA was given as a single intraoperative injection of 7.5 mg to 1 patient, 10 mg to 9 patients, or 15 mg to 5 patients. Postoperative cisternal drainage was employed in three patients. All patients except one demonstrated partial to complete cisternal clot clearance on CT scans within 24 h after surgery. The patient who showed no clot reduction was the only patient in this series to develop symptomatic vasospasm and died 8 days after rupture. No vasospasm was seen on follow-up cerebral angiography in 6 of the 14 responding patients, although mild-to-moderate arterial narrowing was seen in at least one major cerebral artery in the remaining 8 patients. Severe angiographic vasospasm was not seen, although the patient who died did not undergo repeat angiography. One patient developed a large extradural hematoma within several hours of craniotomy, probably due to the t-PA. Intrathecal fibrinolytic treatment appeared effective in clearing subarachnoid clot and reducing vasospasm, and was considered to be associated with acceptable risks if given to patients with large-volume subarachnoid hemorrhages at high risk for severe vasospasm [7].

Thirty patients were reported by Ohman and colleagues from Helsinki, Finland, who had single, angiographically verified aneurysmal subarachnoid hemorrhage and who were studied for the effect of intrathecal thrombolytic therapy with t-PA on outcome, angiographic vasospasm, and computerized tomography findings after surgery. The patients were operated within 3 days after the hemorrhage. CT showed blood only in the basal cisterns and patients had the aneurysm(s) treated in one operation. The patients were divided into groups of 10, with patients receiving 3, 10, or 13 mg of t-PA in a single intracisternal injection after the clipping. There were no differences between the treatment groups in overall outcome. One patient from the 3-mg t-PA group developed a postoperative intracerebral hemorrhage, while one patient from the 10-mg t-PA group had a postoperative epidural hematoma. The only death in the 13-mg t-PA group was caused by inclusion of a segment of pericallosal artery in the clip. In all groups a reduction was observed in the amount of blood seen on the postoperative CT scans compared to the preoperative CT scans. The greater reduction in SAH grade on CT scan between the 10-mg and 13-mg t-PA groups was statistically significant. The difference in the severity of angiographic vasospasm between the 3-mg and 13-mg t-PA (less spasm) groups was also significant [11].

The results of another preliminary trial of intracisternal t-PA in 10 patients were reported by Zabramski and colleagues from Phoenix, Arizona (USA). All patients were clinically Grade III or IV and had thick clots or layers of blood in the basal cisterns and major cerebral fissures. Ventriculostomy and surgery for clipping of the aneurysms were performed within 48 h. In only 1 patient, 10 mg t-PA was instilled into the subarachnoid cisterns prior to closing the dura. In the other 9 patients, a small catheter was left in the subarachnoid space and t-PA [5 mg in 4 cases or 1.5 mg (0.5 mg every 8 h for 3 infusions) in 5 cases] was instilled 12–24 h after surgery. Minor local bleeding complications were noted in all patients receiving 5 or 10 mg t-PA. Oozing was noted at the operative incision site in 4 of 5 patients and at the ventriculostomy site in 2 patients. One patient developed a small epidural hematoma that was treated by delayed drainage. No bleeding complications were noted in the patients receiving the lower regimen of t-PA (3 infusions of 0.5 mg each). Analysis of cisternal cerebrospinal fluid samples demonstrated high t-PA levels for 24–48 h. Angiography 7–8 days after rupture disclosed mild to moderate spasm in 9 patients, while 1 patient with hemorrhage from a posterior inferior cerebellar artery aneurysm had severe focal spasm of the vertebral arteries that was asymptomatic. The results of serial t-PA levels suggested to them that the lower dosage regimen with divided dosages at 8-h intervals is well tolerated and that even lower dosages may be effective [17].

At a recent meeting of the American Association of Neurological Surgeons, Usui and colleagues reported a comparative study of the efficacy of intrathecal thrombolytic therapies with urokinase and t-PA on vasospasm. During 5 years (1986–1990), 100 ruptured intracranial aneurysms were treated surgically within 48 h after bleeding, 43 patients received continuous cisternal irrigation with 60 000 U urokinase/day for 7 days, 15 were treated with intermittent cisternal administration of 25 000 to 600 000 IU t-PA every 8 h for 5 days, and 42 received no thrombolytic therapy. In these 3 groups, they analyzed angiographic vasospasm, infarction on CT scan, and outcome. The vasospasm was assessed by comparing the diameters of the main cerebral arteries measured on angiograms obtained on days 0–1 and on days 6–13. The latter angiograms showed vessel diameters reduced to 80.0%, 80.0%, and 65.6% in the urokinase, t-PA, and control groups, respectively. The degree of vasospasm in the urokinase and t-PA groups was significantly less than that of the control group. Infarctions due to vasospasm were found in 19% of 42 patients in the urokinase group, 10% of 10 in the t-PA group, and 29% of 34 in the control group. There were no significant differences in outcome of the 3 groups when patients were in preoperative neurological Grades 1 or 2, although among patients in Grades 3 to 5, 50% of 18 patients, 30% of 10, and 21% of 23 had a good outcome in the respective urokinase, t-PA, and control groups. The incidence of infarction was less and the outcome better in the urokinase group than in the control group, but not significantly. The results of their study suggested that thrombolytic therapies significantly reduced the degree of vasospasm and that they could prevent infarction and improve outcome [13]. At the same meeting, Yoshimoto gave an update on the Sendai experience and presented data on 30 cases, which confirmed their earlier report on 10 patients. In addition, he compared the 30 patients with thick clot who were at high risk from vasospasm with a less sick group of patients with smaller clots. Despite this imbalance in prognostic factors, the patients receiving t-PA did as well as the patients who were considered to be at lesser risk. There were no fatal infarctions in the thick clot patients treated by t-PA. Severe diffuse vasospasm appeared to have been effectively prevented by repeated intrathecal instillations [16].

Another important contribution to the management of ruptured aneurysm patients may be in the rapid dissolution of intraventricular clot by catheter instillation of boluses of t-PA. Findlay and colleagues reported a dramatic case of early lysis of an intraventricular blood cast [9]. At the University of Alberta an additional half dozen patients with intraventricular clot have been effectively treated by this maneuver.

Summary

Intrathecal instillation of fibrinolytic agents obviously is a two-edged sword. The plasminogen activator cannot tell good clot from bad clot. There is clearly a risk of causing postoperative hemorrhage at the craniotomy site if excellent intraoperative hemostasis is not obtained. It remains to be demonstrated whether or not the risk-benefit ratio of using t-PA for the prophylaxis of vasospasm by the early dissolution of subarachnoid clot, and the treatment of intracranial hypertension and perhaps hydrocephalus by the early dissolution of intraventricular clots, can be bought at an acceptable price without aggravating the tendency towards postoperative intracranial hemorrhage, which is a natural complication following any type of craniotomy and has a certain irreducible rate of occurrence in the best of hands. It goes without saying that the offending aneurysm must be completely clipped and that the operating surgeon must be certain that he has clipped the lesion responsible for the hemorrhage in cases of multiple aneurysms or aneurysms and associated arteriovenous malformations. We would recommend a cautious approach at the present and only use t-PA in the presence of a significant subarachnoid clot where aneurysm clipping is considered to have been definitive and hemostasis is perfect. Prospective randomized trials are underway and, hopefully, there will be confirmation of the very encouraging results already shown in the preliminary open trials.

References

1. Findlay JM (1990) Intrathecal thrombolytic therapy in the prevention of vasospasm following subarachnoid hemorrhage. In: Sawaya R (ed) Fibrinolysis and the central nervous system. Hanley and Belfus, Philadelphia, p 203

2. Findlay JM (1991) Subarachnoid fibrinolytic treatment for the prevention of cerebral vasospasm. Semin Neurol 11:400–410
3. Findlay JM, Macdonald RL, Weir BKA (1991) Current concepts of pathophysiology and management of cerebral vasospasm following aneurysmal subarachnoid hemorrhage. Cerebrovasc Brain Metab Rev 3:336–361
4. Findlay JM, Weir BKA, Gordon P, Grace M, Baughman R (1989) Safety and efficacy of intrathecal thrombolytic therapy in a primate model of cerebral vasospasm. Neurosurgery 24:491–498
5. Findlay JM, Weir BKA, Kanamaru K, Grace M, Baughman R (1990) The effect of timing of intrathecal fibrinolytic therapy on cerebral vasospasm in a primate model of subarachnoid hemorrhage. Neurosurgery 26:201–206
6. Findlay JM, Weir BKA, Kanamaru K, et al (1989) Intrathecal fibrinolytic therapy after subarachnoid hemorrhage: Dosage study in a primate model and review of the literature. Can J Neurol Sci 16:28–40
7. Findlay JM, Weir BKA, Kassell NF, Disney LB, Grace MGA (1991) Intracisternal recombinant tissue plasminogen activator after aneurysmal subarachnoid hemorrhage. J Neurosurg 75:181–188
8. Findlay JM, Weir BKA, Steinke D, Tanabe T, Gordon P, Grace M (1988) Effect of intrathecal thrombolytic therapy on subarachnoid clot and chronic vasospasm in a primate model of SAH. J Neurosurg 69:723–735
9. Findlay JM, Weir BKA, Stollery DE (1991) Lysis of intraventricular hematoma with tissue plasminogen activator. Case report. J Neurosurg 74:803–807
10. Mizoi K, Yoshimoto T, Fujiwara S, Sugawara T, Takahashi A, Koshu K (1991) Prevention of vasospasm by clot removal and intrathecal bolus injection of tissue-type plasminogen activator: Preliminary report. Neurosurgery 28:807–813
11. Ohman J, Servo A, Heiskanen O (1991) Effect of intrathecal fibrinolytic therapy on clot lysis and vasospasm in patients with aneurysmal subarachnoid hemorrhage. J Neurosurg 75:197–201
12. Seifert V, Eisert WG, Stolke D, Goetz C (1989) Efficacy of single intracisternal bolus injection of recombinant tissue plasminogen activator to prevent delayed cerebral vasospasm after experimental subarachnoid hemorrhage. Neurosurgery 25:590–598
13. Usui M, Hoya K, Kuroki T (1992) The efficacy of intrathecal thrombolytic therapies with urokinase and tissue plasminogen activator on vasospasm and outcome following SAH. Presented at the 1992 Annual Meeting of the American Association of Neurological Surgeons, San Francisco, California, April 11–16
14. Weir B (1990) The history of cerebral vasospasm. Neurosurg Clin North Am 1:265–276
15. Weir B (1990) The effect of clot removal on cerebral vasospasm. Neurosurg Clin North Am 1:377–385
16. Yoshimoto T (1992) Vasospasm. Presented at the 1992 Annual Meeting of the American Association of Neurological Surgeons, San Francisco, California, April 11–16
17. Zabramski JM, Spetzler RF, Lee RS, et al (1991) Phase I trial of tissue plasminogen activator for the prevention of vasospasm in patients with aneurysmal subarachnoid hemorrhage. J Neurosurg 75:189–196

Discussion Summary: Other Applications of Fibrinolytic Agents in the Central Nervous System

Chaired by B. Copeland

In the discussion of Dr. Zeumer's paper on central retinal artery occlusion and the therapeutic effects of thrombolysis, three major points were raised. The first was the time course of revascularization. Dr. Zeumer was asked how long it took to demonstrate clinical and angiographic revascularization. It was Dr. Zeumer's experience that normally one would see clinical or angiographic improvement within 1 h. In the 70% of patients who revascularized, there was some evidence of clinical improvement within the first hour. It has been his experience that if no change in the patient's condition is noted within the first hour, there is little likelihood of successful treatment.

The second point raised was the efficacy of intravenous t-PA. Dr. Zeumer pointed out that previous studies had indicated efficacy equivalent to that of intra-arterial infusions; however, greater doses are required. The point is, one trades off the risk of embolization with intra-arterial catheterization with the risk of hemorrhage from the greater doses required by intravenous administration.

The third point raised was about the intrinsic nature of the vascular pathology that predisposes to central retinal artery occlusion. It was asked whether branch occlusions were more commonly embolic, as opposed to central retinal artery occlusions which may be more commonly thrombotic. Dr. Zeumer said that the diameter of the central retinal artery is consistent with a thrombotic mechanism and that the vast majority of their patients had significant atherosclerotic vascular disease. He pointed out, however, that the cause of central retinal artery occlusion in many patients remains obscure, particularly in the young. It is quite possible that vasculitis plays a role in this group of patients.

In the discussion of Dr. Weir's paper on the use of thrombolytic agents in subarachnoid hemorrhage, the question of time course was again raised. He was asked why vasospasm appeared to be a delayed phenomenon when the blood could easily be seen on the initial CT scan studies. Dr. Weir explained that it seems likely that the breakdown products of erythrocytes, particularly oxyhemoglobin, is the cause of the vascular smooth muscle response. He

Division of Neurosurgery, Scripps Clinic & Research Foundation, La Jolla, CA, USA

G. J. del Zoppo, E. Mori, W. Hacke (Eds.)
Thrombolytic Therapy in Acute Ischemic Stroke II

pointed out that CSF concentrations of oxyhemoglobin correlate well with the degree of vasospasm and pointed out that the release of oxyhemoglobin requires time for the erythrocytes to break down.

Dr. Weir was asked whether the use of thrombolytic agents induced new bleeding. He indicated that in an untreated group of patients one could expect 3 to 5% incidence of new bleeding, and that although there did not appear to be any increase in the patients in their study, the numbers remain insignificant to reach conclusions at this time.

Lastly, a technical point was raised about the administration of the thrombolytic agents into the subarachnoid space. It was asked how extensive the lavage must be and how best to administer the t-PA. Dr. Weir reiterated his concerns with the use of subarachnoid catheters and explained that the 15-min time course of the lavage was arbitrarily chosen. He stated that in vitro work has demonstrated a necessity that the rt-PA bind chemically with blood products. Fifteen minutes seems like a reasonable time course and the initial results would seem to justify this approach.

Insights into the Pathogenesis of Cerebral Ischemia Relevant to Fibrinolysis

Deterioration of Acute Stroke*

K. Asplund

Terminology and Definitions

There is no agreement on the terminology or definitions to characterize a stroke patient who deteriorates soon after the onset of symptoms. The terms progressing (or progressive) stroke, stroke-in-progression, evolving stroke, stroke-in-evolution, and deteriorating stroke have all been used. Deteriorating stroke is often used to encompass not only cerebral but also systemic causes of deterioration [13]. It is attractive to use this term because it describes the phenomenon without giving commitments as to the cause, and it challenges us to seek for underlying mechanisms, including systemic ones, without predetermined minds. "Deteriorating stroke" is therefore used in the present article.

Deteriorating (or progressing) stroke is poorly delineated in both qualitative and quantitative terms. The upper time limit for worsening of symptoms to occur is often operationally set at 48 or 72 h after onset. These time limits originate from the work by Jones and Millikan in 1976 and 1980, who observed that the great majority of stroke patients who deteriorated reached the maximal degree of deficit within 48 h if the carotid artery territory was affected [19] and within 72 h if the vertebrobasilar territory was involved [20]. However, as stated in a review by Price, "... the time when a patient is declared unlikely to progress is somewhat arbitrary..." [29].

Worsening of motor function or speech are consistently encompassed by the definitions given in the literature, but there is less agreement if other neurological domains such as level of consciousness, sensory function, ocular movements and cognitive functions should be included. If a broad, noncommitting term like "deteriorating stroke" is used, it is reasonable to include any clinically significant neurological worsening. A tentative definition, in line with most of the previous proposals [3, 7, 12, 13, 26, 29] is:

---

* This study was supported by grants from the Swedish Medical Research, Council (27X-07192), the National Association Against Heart and Chest Diseases, King Gustaf V's 80th Anniversary Fund, King Gustaf V's and Queen Victoria's Foundation, the Year 1987 Stroke Fund, and the Samverkansnämnden

Department of Medicine, University Hospital, Umeå, Sweden

G. J. del Zoppo, E. Mori, W. Hacke (Eds.)
Thrombolytic Therapy in Acute Ischemic Stroke II

Deteriorating stroke is a stepwise or smooth worsening of neurological symptoms or signs – motor or sensory functions, speech (except dysarthria), ocular movements and level of consciousness – that occurs after the first hour and not later than 72 h after onset of stroke.

This definition means that symptoms or signs evolving very early after onset are not included. The mechanisms are, in all likelihood, fundamentally different when deterioration occurs within the first few hours or at a later time after an initial stable course. As discussed later, our knowledge about the underlying mechanisms are scanty. A pragmatic approach is to use definitions that encompass a broad spectrum of deteriorating stroke patients, then trying to identify specific clinical subgroups in post hoc analyses. Such analyses could be helpful when trying to formulate hypotheses for underlying pathophysiological mechanisms in subsets of patients with deteriorating stroke.

There is also little agreement on how much worsening counts as "deteriorating stroke." Clearly, the sooner after onset and the more detailed the examination is, and the more often it is repeated the more likely worsening is to be detected. In the study by Britton and Rödén [3], early deterioration occurred in 43% of the patients if one step on their 8-step motor/speech function scale was used as cut-off, whereas only 25% fulfilled the definition if a 2-step decline was required.

Occurrence and Clinical Characteristics

Table 1 shows patient series published in recent years, in which descriptions of the clinical course of stroke includes early deterioration. In addition to previously published studies, the present review includes data from the Umeå Stroke Unit collected during the years 1977–1986. The Unit admits patients directly from the emergency room in a manner that ensures a sample representative of all patients admitted acutely for stroke within the hospital catchment area [32]. Within this area, less than 5% of patients with manifest stroke are treated out of hospital [31]. The definition of deteriorating stroke described above has been applied. Details of diagnostic procedures and criteria, data collection and basic patient characteristics have been published previously [9, 32].

Despite varying definitions, study designs, and patient selections, some degree of deterioration has been reported to occur in similar proportions of patients (19%–43%) in the 7 studies included in Table 1.

As shown in Table 2, early progression of neurological signs is more frequent in hemorrhagic than in ischemic strokes. Based on the series of Jones and Millikan [19, 20], it is often stated that deterioration is more common when the posterior rather than the anterior circulation is involved. However, Hachinski and Norris, in a larger series of stroke patients, found no greater proportion of deterioration in brain stem compared with hemisphere infarction [13]. In patients with minor stroke, progression is frequent in lacunar as well as cortical brain infarctions. Deterioration is equally common in patients with and without a cardiac source of embolism (Table 2).

Table 1. Studies of deterioration early after stroke characteristics of patient series

Reference	Authors	Patient selection	Type of study	No. of patients	Mean age	Deterioration (%)
[19]	Jones and Millikan 1976	Brain infarction, carotid territory	Retrospective	179	NA	19
[20]	Jones et al. 1980	Brain infarction, vertebrobas territory	Retrospective	37	NA	43
[3]	Britton and Rödén 1985	Unselected stroke	Prospective	402	73	43
[13]	Hachinski and Norris 1985	Unselected stroke	Prospective	300	NA	37
[26]	Norrving and Cronqvist 1989	Minor stroke	Retrospective	122	58	30
[7]	Dávalos et al. 1990	Ischemic stroke	Prospective	98	NA	41
–	Own series 1992	Unselected stroke	Prospective	915	72	27

Table 2. Proportion of deteriorating stroke by type and site of brain lesion and concomitant disorders: Combined results of published patient series and own population-based series of 915 patients

Comparison	References	No of. patients	Deterioration (%)
Type of stroke:			
Hemorrhagic	[3, 13], own series	142	51
Ischemic	[3, 13], own series	1407	32
Site of lesion:			
Carotid	[19]	179	19
Vertebrobasilar	[20]	37	43
Hemispheric	[13]	262	38
Brain stem	[13]	38	32
Lacunar (minor stroke)	[26]	61	35
Cortical (minor stroke)	[26]	53	23
Concomitant disorders			
Cardiac source of embolism	[3], own series	250	39
No cardiac source of embolism	[3], own series	1057	31
Hypertension	[3], own series	630	31
No hypertension	[3], own series	673	33
Diabetes	[3], own series	207	34
No diabetes	[3], own series	1103	32

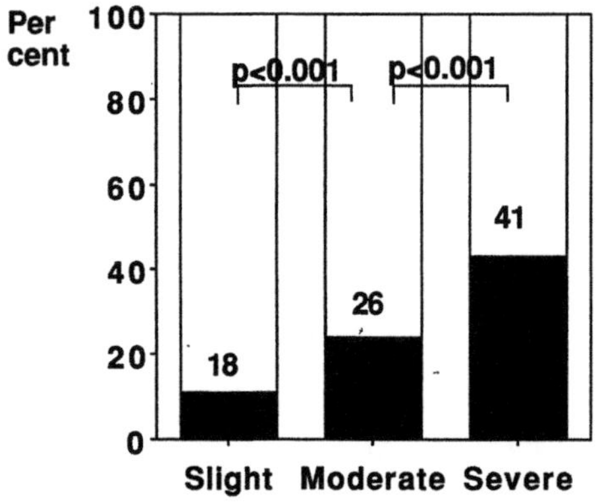

Fig. 1. Frequency of deteriorating stroke by severity of neurological symptoms and signs at admission to hospital

It is not finally settled whether or not large lesions or extensive neurological deficits at hospital admission predict progression. In the study by Britton and Rödén [3], only a very modest difference in neurological deficit was observed at admission to hospital between those patients who deteriorated within 4 days and those who did not. On the other hand, in a CT study, Dávalos and investigators found that patients with deterioration had larger infarcts within 8 h of onset than did patients who had stable deficits [7]. In our own patient series, the severity of symptoms and signs at arrival to hospital clearly predicted deterioration (Fig. 1).

Mechanisms

Many different mechanisms are likely to contribute to the progressive worsening of stroke. Some obvious explanations are:

1. Propagation of thrombus, as documented by angiography [13], at acute thromboendarterectomy [13] and at autopsy [21]. It should, however, be noted that serial assessments of indicators of platelet activation have failed to show major changes at the time of deterioration [17].
2. Hemorrhagic transformation of a brain infarct, amply demonstrated in CT scan studies [27].
3. Recurrent emboli, the rate of recurrence within the first few days probably being around 5% [5].
4. Re-bleedings in intracerebral hematomas as evidenced by repeated CT scans [6].

Common to all these potential mechanisms are, however, that a direct temporal relationship between the postulated underlying event and the deterioration has (with the exception of re-bleedings) rarely been documented.

The frequent occurrence of deterioration in many different types of stroke-ischemic and hemorrhagic, lacunar and cortical, embolic and nonembolic – suggests that mechanisms common to many diverse initiating factors are operating. The discussion here is restricted to three of these possibilities: first, delayed neuronal death; second, brain edema with mass effect; and third, microthrombus formation.

Pernicious arachidonic acid metabolites and oxygen metabolites have been implicated in the gradual propagation of neuronal damage [delayed neuronal death [28]] after an ischemic insult. These noxious metabolites can be produced by activated thrombocytes and leucocytes in the ischemic area but they may also be formed by dying neurons, glia cells, and endothelial cells. Excessive eicosanoid production in ischemic brain tissue, resulting in elevated levels of prostaglandins and leucotrienes and other lipoxygenase metabolites has been shown to persist for at least one week after the ischemic injury [10]. Whereas some eicosanoids are modulators of blood cell aggregation, others modify cerebral blood vessel tone and blood-brain barrier permeability and may promote the formation of brain edema [2]. It is also possible that some of the eicosanoids have direct neurotoxic effects [2]. There is now compelling evidence that excitatory amino acids may act as endogenous neurotoxins and lead to progressing neuronal death [24]. Dysregulation of the GABAergic and other neurotransmitter systems can modify the evolution of delayed neuronal death following ischemia [22].

In an illustrative experimental study of the significance of a mass effect, progressive worsening of neurological symptoms occurred over several hours when a balloon was inflated in the brain parenchyma [25]. Evidently, the mass itself (the balloon) initiates a sequence of events that leads to progressive neuronal dysfunction. The mass effect may be one of several reasons why patients with intracerebral hemorrhage progress more often than those with ischemic lesions

(Table 2). The role of brain edema in early deterioration remains, however, obscure. In a recent study by Dávalos and coworkers, the presence of a mass effect on initial CT scan (performed within 8 h) did not predict neurological deterioration [7].

An interesting recent extension of the concept of thrombus propagation as a cause of deteriorating stroke is the observation of thrombi in the microcirculation in and around ischemic brain areas. Such microthrombi are present in both experimental focal ischemia and in patients with cerebral infarction [16]. The longer the duration of ischemia and the larger the lesion, the more extensive is the formation of microthrombi [16]. This is in line with clinical observations that extensive neurological deficits at onset are associated with a high risk of deterioration (see above).

Treatment

The tradition to use heparin in patients who progress early and in whom intracerebral bleeding has been excluded is based on the assumption that thrombus propagation is an important contributing factor to deterioration. The only controlled trials of this therapeutic principle were published in the years 1958–1961; they all purported to show beneficial effects of heparin [1, 4, 11]. These trials have been heavily criticized: they were performed before the CT era, they were small (the largest included 128 patients), and they certainly did not meet present standards for clinical trial design.

The results of three studies published in recent years have challenged heparin as an effective treatment of deteriorating stroke: first, a randomized trial of heparin in patients with partial stable stroke showing no effect of heparin on late progression [8]; second, a report of a high rate of continued progression despite early heparin treatment in patients with deteriorating stroke [14]; and third, observations that clinical outcome in heparin-treated patients can not be predicted by the intensity of anticoagulation [30]. When comparing new and old studies, it should be emphasized that, even in the 1958–1961 studies, the proportion of patients who progressed during heparin treatment was high, only that it was much higher in nontreated patients [1, 4, 11].

As long as no new controlled trials have been performed, we have to rely on the information we have available, old-fashioned and incomplete as it may be. Taking the 232 patients included in the controlled trials from 1958– 1962 together [1, 4, 11], the odds ratio becomes 2.4 in favor of heparin over no treatment when the outcome variable is further progression or death (Fig. 2). The 95% confidence interval is 1.4–4.2, indicating a definite effect of heparin.

The ambivalence towards the use of heparin in patients with deteriorating stroke is highlighted by a survey of U.S. neurologists treating stroke patients [23]. Only 6% thought that heparin had been shown to be effective. Yet, 76% of the respondents thought that prevention of stroke progression was an important indication for heparin therapy. When asked if the results of a future

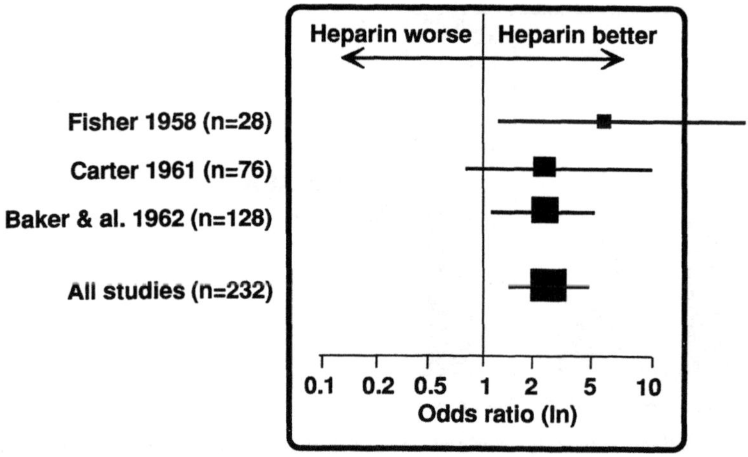

Fig. 2. Odds ratios with 95% confidence intervals for further progression or death during treatment with heparin vs no treatment in patients with progressing (deteriorating) stroke. If the 95% confidence interval does not include odds ratio 1.0, there is a statistical significance at the 5% level

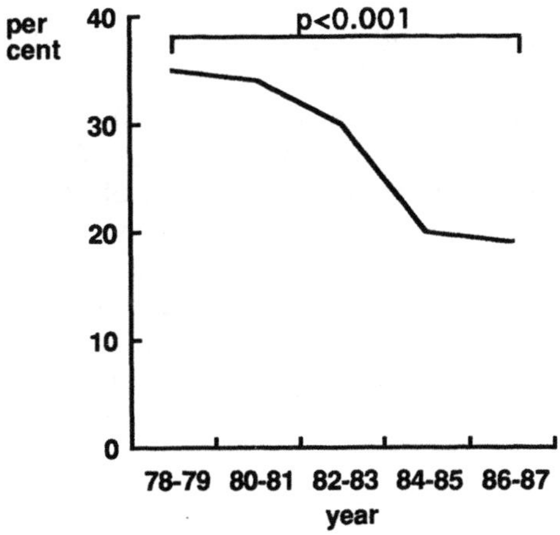

Fig. 3. Secular trends of the rate of early deterioration in a population-based sample of 915 stroke patients admitted to hospital during the years 1978–1987

heparin trial would be useful, all but one physician said yes. Large-scale randomized trials of heparin and heparinoids are now planned or in progress.

As alternatives to heparin, aspirin and other antiplatelet drugs are of particular interest because they may not only prevent macrothrombus propagation and recurrent embolism, but they can also reduce the number of microthrombi in ischemic brain tissue, as shown by studies in a middle cerebral artery occlusion stroke model in the rat [15]. In addition, these agents may inhibit propagation of cellular damage in ischemic brain tissue by interfering with arachidonic acid metabolism in platelets, leucocytes, endothelial cells and neurons. Modulators of neurotransmitter release, 21-aminosteroids, and other

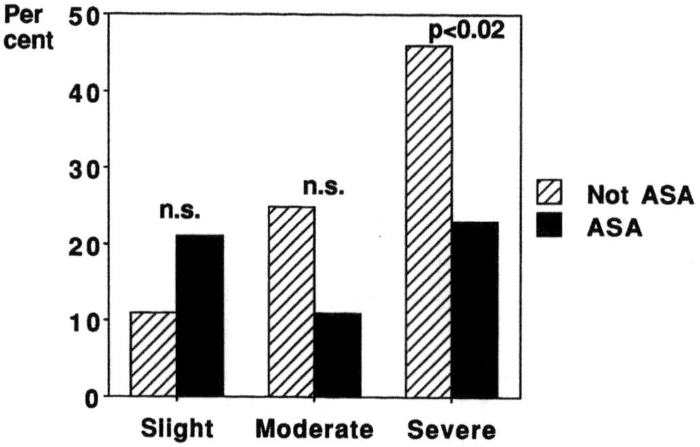

Fig. 4. Proportion of patients with early deterioration in relation to severity of neurological symptoms and signs on admission to hospital and treatment with acetyl salicylic acid (*ASA*, aspirin) at onset

scavengers of oxygen metabolites may serve the same purpose to reduce progressing neuronal damage.

In the acute phase of myocardial infarction, administration of aspirin has convincingly been shown to reduce infarct size and improve clinical outcome [18]. When we reviewed patients admitted to our stroke unit over a 10-year period (1978–1987), there was a marked decline in the proportion who showed early deterioration (Fig. 3). This was during a period when the use of aspirin and other antiplatelet drugs became increasingly common in people with various manifestations of atherothrombotic disorders. Indeed, stroke patients who were on aspirin on admission to hospital were at a lesser risk of deterioration than those who were not on aspirin. This was observed only in patients with severe symptoms and signs at onset and a high risk of deterioration if not on aspirin (Fig. 4). At least one study of immediate aspirin administration in patients with acute ischemic stroke is now in progress.

Summary

In seven different patient series, between 19% and 43% of stroke patients have been found to deteriorate early after admission to hospital. Deterioration is common in all types of stroke: intracerebral hemorrhage, large-vessel thrombotic stroke, cerebral embolism of cardiac origin, lacunar infarcts, and watershed infarct. It occurs most often in patients who already have severe symptoms on admission. Thrombus propagation, hemorrhagic transformation and recurrent embolism may all contribute to progression of neurological deficits in patients with ischemic stroke. Mechanisms common to many different initiating pathophysiological events may also be important, among them programmed (delayed) neuronal death, cerebral edema, and microthrombus formation. Aspirin (and similar drugs) may be beneficial in that they reduce formation of microthrombi, embolization and production of noxious arachidonic acid metabolites that probably contribute to programmed neuronal death and extension of ischemic brain damage. Clinical observations support the contention that aspirin reduces the risk for early deterioration.

References

1. Baker RN, Broward JA, Fang HC, et al (1962) Anticoagulant therapy in cerebral infarction. Report on a cooperative study. Neurology 12:828–835
2. Black KL (1984) Leucotriene C_4 induces vasogenic cerebral edema in rats. Prostaglandin Leukot Med 14:339–340
3. Britton M, Rödén (1985) Progression of stroke after arrival at hospital. Stroke 16:629–632
4. Carter AB (1961) Anticoagulant treatment in progressing stroke. Br Med J 2:70–73
5. Cerebral Embolism Task Force (1989) Cardiogenic embolism. The second report of the Cerebral Embolism Task Force. Arch Neurol 46:727–743
6. Chen ST, Chen SD, Hsu CY, Hogan EL (1989) Progression of hypertensive intracerebral hemorrhage. Neurology 39:1509–1514
7. Dávalos A, Cendra E, Teruel J, Martinez M, Genís D (1990) Deteriorating ischemic stroke. Risk factors and prognosis. Neurology 40:1865–1869
8. Duke RJ, Block RF, Turpie AG, Trebilcock R, Bayer N (1986) Intravenous heparin for the prevention of stroke progression in acute partial stable stroke: A randomized controlled trial. Arch Intern Med 105:825–828
9. Eriksson S, Asplund K, Hägg E, Lithner F, Strand T, Wester PO (1987) Clinical profiles of cerebrovascular disorders in a population-based patient sample. J Chron Dis 40:1025–1032
10. Feuerstein G (1989) Eicosanoids in deteriorating stroke. Ann NY Acad Sci 559:313–322
11. Fisher CM (1961) Anticoagulant therapy in cerebral thrombosis and cerebral embolism: A national cooperative study, interim report. Neurology 11:119–131
12. Gautier JC (1985) Stroke-in-progression. Stroke 16:729–733
13. Hachinski V, Norris J (1985) The deteriorating stroke. In: The acute stroke. FA Davis, Philadelphia, p 123
14. Haley EC, Jr., Kassell NF, Torner JC (1988) Failure of heparin to prevent progression in progressing ischemic infarction. Stroke 19:10–14
15. Heye N, Campos A, Kannuki S, Cervós-Navarro J (1991) Effects of triflusal and acetylsalicylic acid on microthrombi formation in experimental brain ischemia. Exp Pathol 41:31–36
16. Heye N, Paetzold C, Cervós-Navarro J (1991) The role of microthrombi and microcirculatory factors in localization and evolution of focal cerebral ischemia. Neurosurg Rev 14:7–16
17. Ho C-H, Hu H-H, Wong W-J (1989) The serial hemostasis-related changes in patients with cerebral infarction: Comparison between progressing and non-progressing stroke. Thromb Res 56:635–647
18. ISIS-2 (Second International Study of Infarct Survival) Collaborative Group (1988) Randomized trial of intravenous streptokinase, oral aspirin, both, or neither among 17, 187 cases of suspected acute myocardial infarction: ISIS-2. Lancet 13 August:349–360
19. Jones HR, Jr., Millikan CH (1976) Temporal profile (clinical course) of acute carotid system cerebral infarction. Stroke 7:64–71
20. Jones HR, Jr., Millikan CH, Sandok BA (1980) Temporal profile (clinical course) of acute vertebrobasilar system cerebral infarction. Stroke 11:173–177
21. Jörgensen L, Torvik A (1969) Ischaemic cerebrovascular diseases in an autopsy series. Part 2. Prevalence, location, pathogenesis, and clinical course of cerebral infarcts. J Neurol Sci 9:285–320

22. Lust WD, Assaf HM, Ricci AJ, Ratcheson RA, Sterau LL (1988) A role for gamma-aminobutyric acid (GABA) in the evolution of delayed neuronal death following ischemia. Metab Brain Dis 3:287–292
23. Marsh EE, Adams HP, Biller J, et al (1989) Use of antithrombotic drugs in the treatment of acute ischemic stroke: A survey of neurologists in practice in the United States. Neurology 39:1631–1634
24. Mohammed AA, Gotoh O, Graham DI, et al (1985) Effect of pretreatment with the calcium antagonist nimodipine on local cerebral blood flow and histopathology after middle cerebral artery occlusion. Ann Neurol 18:705–711
25. Nehls DG, Mendelow AD, Graham DI, Sinar EJ, Teasdale GM (1988) Experimental intracerebral hemorrhage: Progression of hemodynamic changes after production of a spontaneous mass lesion. Neurosurgery 23:439–444
26. Norrving B, Cronqvist S (1989) Clinical and radiologic features of lacunar versus nonlacunar minor stroke. Stroke 20:59–64
27. Okada Y, Yamagushi T, Minematsu K, et al (1989) Hemorrhagic transformation in cerebral embolism. Stroke 20:598–603
28. Petito CK, Pulsinelli WA (1984) Sequential development of reversible and irreversible neuronal damage following cerebral ischemia. J Neuropathol Exp Neurol 43:141–153
29. Price TR (1986) Progressing ischemic stroke. In: Barnett HJM, Mohr JP, Stein BM, Yatsu FM (eds) Stroke: Pathophysiology, diagnosis, and management. Churchill Livingstone, New York, p 1059
30. Slivka A, Levy D (1990) Natural history of progressive ischemic stroke in a population treated with heparin. Stroke 21:1657–1662
31. Stegmayr B, Asplund K (1993) Stroke in the population: Quality of routine data vs. a population-based registry. Neuroepidemiology (In Press)
32. Strand T, Asplund K, Eriksson S, Hägg E, Lithner F, Wester PO (1985) A non-intensive stroke unit reduces functional disability and the need for long-term hospitalization. Stroke 16:29–34

Early Spontaneous Recanalization of Thromboembolic Stroke

E. Mori and Y. Yoneda

It is well-known that spontaneous recanalization of the occluded arteries is often observed [4, 9, 12]. Several studies have documented a fairly high frequency of spontaneous recanalization for internal carotid artery (ICA) and middle cerebral artery (MCA) occlusion using serial angiography, spaced days or weeks apart [3, 8, 10, 11, 17, 23]. Spontaneous recanalization is at least partly responsible for patent cerebral arteries at the moment of initial angiographic examination [2, 6, 7, 13, 18–20]. Limited information about the incidence of early spontaneous recanalization indicates that spontaneous recanalization may occur within hours of ictus [4, 14, 21]. However, when or how early spontaneous recanalization occurs remains unclear. Before linking the use of thrombolytic agents with recanalization, a comprehensive understanding of the natural history of the occlusive lesion is necessary.

Our recently completed, placebo-controlled recombinant tissue plasminogen activator trial for thromboembolic stroke presents several clues about very early spontaneous recanalization [16]. This study yielded two data sets in terms of early spontaneous recanalization. One was the recanalization frequency in the placebo-treated patients demonstrated by serial angiograms, which represents the incidence of early spontaneous recanalization in a short period, and the other was vascular patency on a baseline angiogram, which may in part be attributed to spontaneous recanalization before the angiographic study. On the basis of the data derived from our trial, we address these issues of early spontaneous recanalization.

Subjects and Methods

The trial of two-chain recombinant tissue plasminogen activator (rt-PA, duteplase) for carotid artery territory thromboembolic stroke was undertaken between September, 1988 and October, 1990. Results of this trial have been reported in detail elsewhere [16]. The subjects for the patency study were 34 patients suspected to have acute carotid artery thromboembolism who had an

Neurology Service, Hyogo Brain and Heart Center at Himeji, Himeji, Japan

G. J. del Zoppo, E. Mori, W. Hacke (Eds.)
Thrombolytic Therapy in Acute Ischemic Stroke II

angiographic study in the course of this trial. The subjects for the spontaneous recanalization study were 12 patients who received a placebo infusion.

In this trial, patients who met the entry criteria were randomly assigned to one of the three regimens: 30 MIU rt-PA, 20 MIU rt-PA, and rt-PA placebo. Inclusion criteria were: acute embolic stroke in the carotid artery territory with appropriate clinical signs less than 6 h after onset; age under 80; absence of a baseline CT abnormality related to the ischemic events; and angiography-documented ICA or MCA occlusion.

Eligible patients received a baseline CT, underwent neurological assessment, gave blood for examination, and submitted to cerebral angiography. Angiography was performed by the femoral approach. Patients without angiographically proven occlusion were excluded from the trial at this time. A small dose of heparin was given during the angiographic procedure. The drug or placebo was dissolved in 200 ml of physiological saline and was given intravenously over 1 h. Angiography was repeated 30 and 60 min after the start of the infusion. Comparing the baseline and the post-infusion angiograms, recanalization was classified into 5 categories: Grade 0, unchanged; Grade 1, movement of thrombus without reperfusion; Grade 2, less than 50% partial recanalization; Grade 3, more than 50% partial recanalization; and Grade 4, complete recanalization. Grades 2, 3 and 4 were considered as the achievement of reperfusion. Anticoagulation or antiplatelet treatment was delayed until 24 h after the infusion. CT scans were repeated at predetermined intervals. Neurological status was assessed and followed up using a slightly modified version of the Hemispheric Stroke Scale (HSS) [1].

Results

The baseline angiography was performed from 1.5 to 6 (mean 4.0 ± 1.1) h after symptom onset. Three patients who had patent cerebral arteries did not enter the trial protocol. The final diagnosis of these patients was sensorimotor-type lacunar infarction ($n = 2$) or hypoglycemia with aphasia and right hemiparesis ($n = 1$). Therefore, vascular occlusion of the appropriate cerebral arteries was observed in 100% of patients who had a cerebral thromboembolism [cervical internal carotid artery ($n=1$); intracranial internal carotid artery ($n = 7$); middle cerebral artery, M1 ($n = 15$); middle cerebral artery, M2 ($n = 6$); anterior and middle cerebral artery, M2 ($n = 2$)], while the observed patency rate was 9% when all eligible patients were considered. Of the 31 included patients, 12 patients were assigned to the placebo group. In this group, time from onset to the baseline angiography was from 2.1 to 5.5 (mean 3.6 ± 1.1) h, and arterial lesions included distal internal carotid artery occlusions ($n = 4$), middle cerebral artery M1 segment occlusions ($n = 5$), and M2 segment occlusions ($n = 3$). Previous history included: transient ischemic attack in 1 patient, minor stroke in 2 patients, hypertension in 2 patients, diabetes mellitus in 3 patients, ischemic heart disease in 2 patients, mitral valvular disease in 4 patients, atrial fibrillation in 4 patients, dilated cardiomyopathy in 2 patients, and sick sinus syndrome with pacemaker in 2 patients.

No recanalization was noted on the second (30-min) angiograms. Partial recanalization of the occluded arteries was observed on the third (1-h) angiograms in 2 (17%) of 12 patients. In one patient, distal movement of the thrombus without reperfusion was noticed. In the rest of the patients, no angiographic changes of occlusions were apparent. Thus, results of the 1-h angiogram were summarized as distal internal carotid artery occlusions ($n = 3$), anterior cerebral/ middle cerebral artery M2 occlusions ($n = 1$), middle cerebral artery M1 occlusions ($n = 4$), M2 occlusions ($n = 3$), and M3 occlusions ($n = 1$).

Case 1. A right-handed 61-year-old man with known atrial fibrillation suddenly developed right-sided hemiplegia and loss of speech and comprehension 1.5 h prior to admission. On admission, he was drowsy and globally aphasic, and had a right homonymous hemianopia, leftward conjugate ocular deviation, right hemi-sensory deficits, dense right-sided hemiplegia, and an extensor plantar response. The modified HSS score was 87 points. A brain CT on admission was normal (Fig. 1). A left carotid angiogram performed 144 min after symptom onset demonstrated a complete occlusion at the siphon of the ICA (Fig. 2). The right carotid and right vertebral angiograms demonstrated an occlusion of the left anterior cerebral artery at the A1 segment, filling in the left anterior cerebral artery through the anterior communicating artery, and some collaterals from leptomeningeal anastomoses arising from the left posterior cerebral artery in the left middle cerebral artery territory. Infusion of the assigned regimen (inert placebo) was initiated 11 min after the left carotid angiography, and the second and third left carotid angiograms were performed 30 and 60 min after initiation of the infusion (185 and 215 min after symptom onset). Although no changes were noted in the second (30-min) angiogram, partial recanalization was apparent in the third (1-h) angiogram; thrombi which occluded the carotid siphon moved to the origin of the common branch of the superior division of the MCA, and the trunk of the MCA was recanalized, resulting in reperfusion of the inferior division of the MCA and lenticulostriate perforators. Occlusions in the A1 segment remain unchanged (Fig. 2). No neurological change was noticed after angiography and placebo infusion. The CT obtained 24 h after the treatment revealed a hematoma in the putaminal region with ventricular perforation and perifocal edema (Fig. 1). No neurological deterioration was noted. The patient improved to some degree, and was discharged 3 months later with right-sided hemiparesis and severe Broca's aphasia.

Case 2. A left-handed, 70-year-old woman with known mitral valvular disease and atrial fibrillation suddenly developed left-sided hemiparesis and difficulty with speech 1.5 h before admission. A neurological examination at the emergency room revealed nonfluent spontaneous speech, moderately disturbed comprehension, repetition, and confrontation naming, constructional disabili-

1
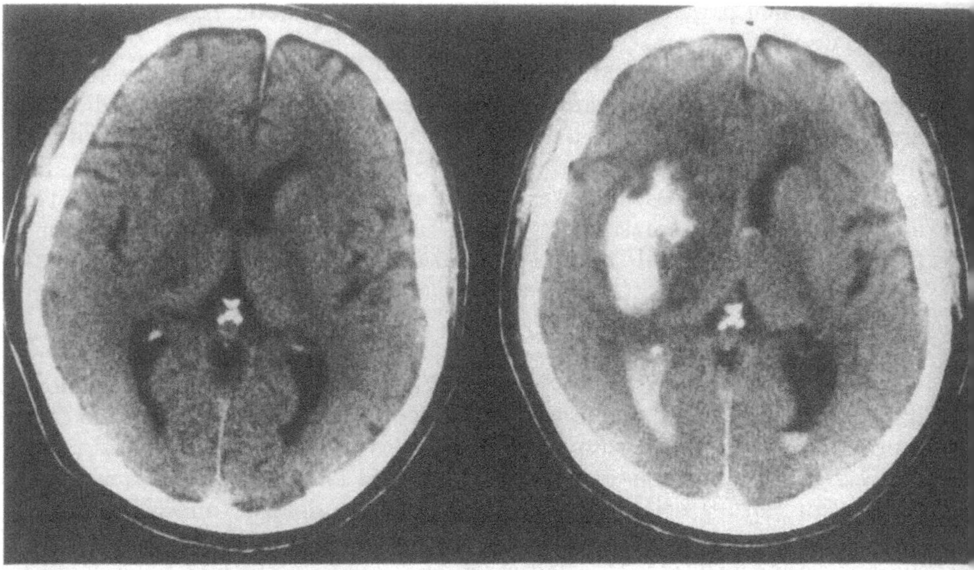

2
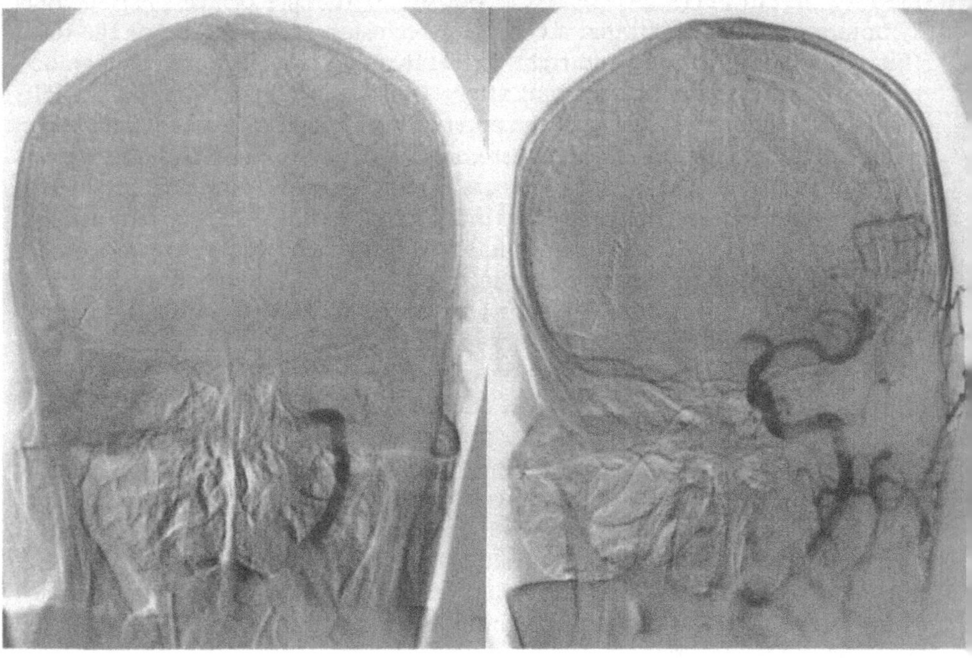

Fig. 1. CTs of Case 1. *Left*, baseline CT; *right*, 24 h later

Fig. 2. Angiograms of Case 1. *Left*, baseline left carotid angiogram; *right*, 1 h later

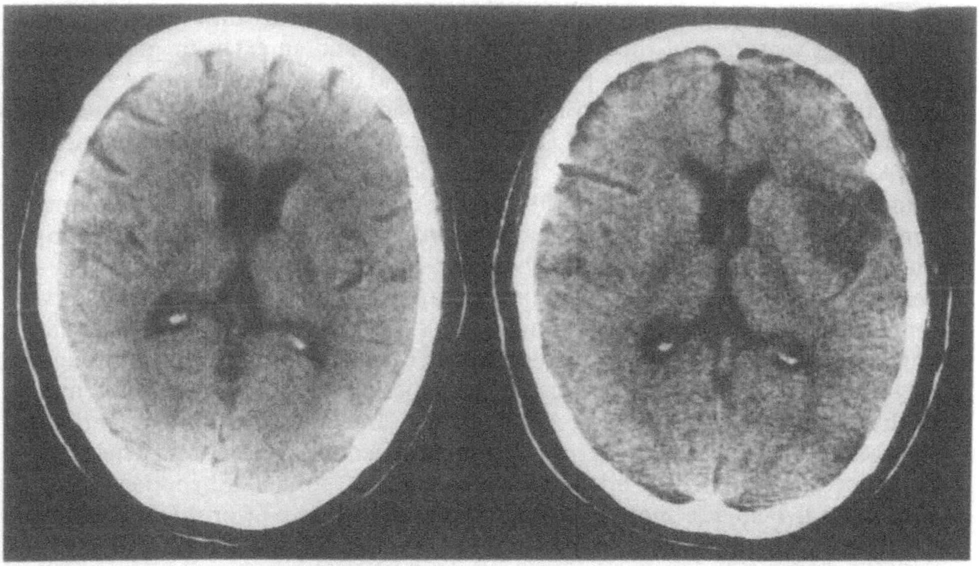

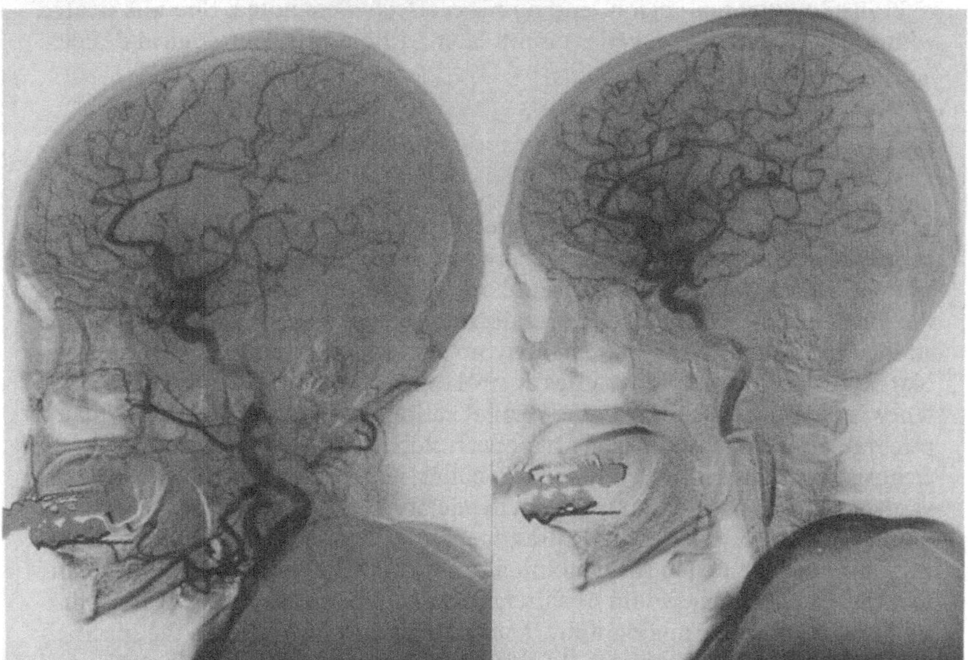

Fig. 3. CTs of Case 2. *Left*, baseline CT; *right*, 24 h later

Fig. 4. Angiograms of Case 2. *Left*, baseline right carotid angiogram; *right*, 1 h later

ty, left homonymous hemianopia, left-sided hemiparesis of mild degree, mild decrease of sensation of the left side of the body, and an extensor plantar response. The HSS score was 44 points. Systolic and diastolic murmurs were noted at the cardiac apex. A brain CT on admission was normal (Fig. 3). Right carotid angiography performed 167 h after symptom onset demonstrated MCA branch occlusions (Fig. 4). The superior division of the MCA was occluded at its origin, and flow in the angular artery was delayed and stagnant, consistent with distal occlusion. Treatment with the assigned regimen (placebo) was initiated 23 min after the angiography, and carotid angiograms were repeated 53 and 83 min after the first angiography (220 and 250 min after symptom onset). The second (30-min) angiogram showed no changes. A substantial improvement of perfusion was noted in the third (1-h) angiogram, although fragments of thrombi were present in the superior division of the MCA and in the angular artery occluding a few cortical branches (Fig. 4). The patient showed a considerable clinical improvement after the procedures. The HSS performed immediately after the procedures was 21 points. A hypodense area with a few hyperdense spots appeared on a brain CT 24 h after the procedure, consistent with hemorrhagic infarction (Fig. 3). The lesion was restricted to the right insuloputaminal region, and no mass effects were noted. She was treated with warfarin and discharged 1 month later without any neurological deficits.

Discussion

While the recanalization frequency directly represents the incidence of spontaneous recanalization in the interval between two or more separate angiographic studies, arterial patency on the initial angiogram does not accurately indicate the incidence of spontaneous recanalization between onset and angiographic study. Since some of the patients may not have (angiographically demonstrable) occlusions of cerebral arteries at stroke onset, overestimation occurs if patency is regarded as spontaneous recanalization. Strokes not caused by major cerebral artery occlusion, e.g., hypoperfusion due to severe cerebral artery stenosis, perforating artery lesions (lacunar infarction), venous thrombosis, vasospasm, or migraine, transient ischemic attacks, and nonischemic diseases mimicking stroke, e.g., focal seizures, metabolic disorders, or functional disorders, may be included in the denominator. Such a misdiagnosis would increase, and therefore patency would be falsely high, if time for observation and work-up of patients before angiography is short. This may be related to the specificity of the screening of subjects. In this study, patients with lacunar stroke and with hypoglycemia received angiography, and inclusion of those patients affected the observed frequency of patency. Nevertheless, spontaneous recanalization is at least partially responsible for patent cerebral arteries on angiographic studies. On the other hand, partial or branch recanalization (distal clot migrations or clot fragmentation with distal embolization), which is frequently observed in cerebral arteries, would be ignored on one-point

Table 1. Recanalization

Study	Subjects	*n*	Elapsed time[a]	Interval[b]	Recanalization (%)
Fieschie 1969 [8]	MCA	17	<3 days	weeks	59
Yamaguchi 1984 [23]	Carotid	42	<2 weeks	<4 days	67
Ito 1983 [11]	MCA	34	<3 days	<3 days	42
Bladin 1964 [3]	Carotid	40	<5 days	1–10 days	30
Irino 1977 [10]	Carotid	34	<1 day	1–7 days	41
Mori 1992 [16]	Carotid	12	<6 h (3.6 h)	1 h	17
Yamaguchi 1992 [22]	Carotid	46	<6 h (3.6 h)	1 h	20

[a] Elapsed time from onset to angiography.
[b] Interval between baseline and follow-up angiographies.

Table 2. Patency on initial angiography

Study	Subjects	*n*	Elapsed time[a]	Patency (%)
Bladin 1964 [3]	ICA/MCA	54	<3 weeks	69
Fieschi 1969 [8]	ICA/MCA	86	<3 days	43
Olsen 1985 [17]	ICA/MCA	73	1–3 days	52
Solis 1977 [20]	ICA/MCA	63	<24 hours	41
del Zoppo 1992 [6]	ICA/MCA	139	<8 hours	25
Fieschi 1989 [7]	ICA/MCA	80	<6 hours	24
Mori 1992 [16]	ICA/MCA	34	<6 hours	9

[a] Elapsed time from onset to angiograph.

angiographic examination and would not accurately reflect patency. If, in this study, angiographic examinations would have been performed 1 h later (only the third angiography is considered), the patency in the placebo-treated group would be estimated to be 0%, although the recanalization rate in 1 h was 17%.

Several studies using serial angiography spaced days or weeks apart [3, 8, 10, 11, 17, 23] indicated that the frequency of spontaneous recanalization in acute carotid artery territory thromboembolism was from 30% to 69% (Table 1). Although the time from onset to initial angiography varied in those studies (from <1 day to <2 weeks), it appears that the incidence of recanalization increases with interval between serial angiograms. Studies of angiographically defined series of patients with acute ischemic stroke have indicated that the actual incidence of cerebrovascular patency increases substantially with time to angiography, although all patency cannot be linked with spontaneous recanalization because of the above mentioned issues (Table 2).

A few anecdotal reports have suggested that spontaneous recanalization may occur very early after symptom onset. Recent prospective studies in which angiography was performed in acute carotid artery territory stroke reported patency of 23.7% within 6 h and 19% within 8 h after onset, suggesting the existence of very early spontaneous recanalization. The low patency on the baseline angiography in this study compared with those studies may be attributed to exclusion of patients having typical lacunar syndromes except sensorimotor stroke, patients showing resolution of symptoms before angiography, or earlier inclusion of patients. The present study for the first time demonstrates the incidence of spontaneous recanalization early (mean elapsed time = 3.6 h) after onset and suggests that early spontaneous recanalization is not uncommon. Similarly, in a recently completed, larger-scaled, placebo-controlled rt-PA trial, Yamaguchi and coworkers reported a similar recanalization rate in the placebo-treated group [22].

Because of the limited number of patients involved in this study, no clear conclusion may be made about the relationship between spontaneous recanalization and clinical outcome. Nevertheless, it would be noticeable that hemorrhagic transformation (intracerebral hematoma formation) or rapid, full recovery was followed. These phenomena are also observed after thrombolytic therapy [5].

In conclusion, early spontaneous recanalization is not an uncommon phenomenon. It would occur in nearly 20% of carotid artery thromboembolism at 4 h (mean) after onset, when branch recanalization is included. On assessing efficacy of thrombolytic treatment or designing thrombolysis trials, early spontaneous recanalization should be taken into consideration. Little information about spontaneous recanalization of thrombotic occlusion and of thromboembolic occlusion in the vertebrobasilar artery system [15] is available so far. Finally, when patency in one-point angiogram is applied for efficacy assessment, attention should be paid not only to the incidence of arterial occlusion but also to the sites of occlusion, because branch recanalization (clot fragmentation with distal clot embolization) frequently occurs.

References

1. Adams RJ, Meador KJ, Sethi KD, Grotta JC, Thompson DS (1987) Graded neurological scale for use in acute hemispheric stroke treatment protocols. Stroke 18:665–669
2. Allock JM (1967) Occlusion of the middle cerebral artery: Serial angiography as a guide to conservative therapy. J Neurosurg 27:353–363
3. Bladin PF (1964) A radiologic and pathologic study of embolism of the internal carotid-middle cerebral arterial axis. Radiology 82:615–625
4. Dalal PM, Shah PM, Sheth SC, Deshpande CK (1965) Cerebral embolism: Angiographic observations on spontaneous clot lysis. Lancet 1:61–64
5. del Zoppo GJ, Pessin MS, Mori E, Hacke W (1991) Thrombolytic intervention in acute thrombotic and embolic stroke. Semin Neurol 11:368– 384
6. del Zoppo GJ, Poeck K, Pessin MS, and 16 coauthors of the rt-PA Acute Stroke Study Group (1992) Recombinant tissue plasminogen activator in acute thrombotic and embolic stroke. Ann Neurol 32:78–86
7. Fieschi C, Argentino C, Lenzi GL, Sacchetti ML, Toni D, Bozzao L (1989) Clinical and instrumental evaluation of patients with ischemic stroke within the first six hours. J Neurol Sci 91:311–321

8. Fieschi C, Bozzao L (1969) Transient embolic occlusion of the middle cerebral and internal carotid arteries in cerebral apoplexy. J Neurol Neurosurg Psychiatry 32:236–240
9. Fisher M, Adams RD (1951) Observations on brain embolism with special reference to the mechanism of hemorrhagic infarction. Neuropathol Exp Neurol 10:92–94
10. Irino T, Taneda M, Takaku M (1977) Angiographic manifestations in postrecanalized cerebral infarction. Neurology 27:471–475
11. Ito Z, Suzuki A, Hen R, Menura K (1983) Prognostic factors in spontaneous recanalization of middle cerebral artery occlusion. In: Ito Z, Kutsuzawa T, Yasui N (eds) Cerebral ischemia – An update. Excerpta Medica, Amsterdam, p 159
12. Lehrer GM (1958) Arteriographic demonstration of collateral circulation in cerebrovascular disease. Neurology 8:27–32
13. Lhermitte F, Gautier JC, Derouesn C, Guiraud B (1968) Ischemic accidents in the middle cerebral artery territory. A study of the causes in 122 cases. Arch Neurol 19:248–256
14. Liebeskind A, Chinichian A, Schechter MM (1971) The moving embolus seen during serial cerebral angiography. Stroke 2:440–443
15. Little JR, Furlan AJ (1985) Resolving occlusive lesions of the basilar artery. Neurosurgery 17:811–814
16. Mori E, Yoneda Y, Tabuchi M, et al (1992) Intravenious recombinant tissue plasminogen activator in acute carotid artery territory stroke. Neurology 42:976–982
17. Olsen TS, Skiriver EB, Herning M (1985) Cause of cerebral infarction in the carotid territory. Its relation to size and the location of the infarct and to the underlying vascular lesion. Stroke 16:459–466
18. Silverstein A (1965) Arteriography of stroke. Arch Neurol 13:441–446
19. Sindermann F, Dichgans J, Bergleiter R (1969) Occlusion of the middle cerebral artery and its branches: Angiographic and clinical correlates. Brain 92:607–620
20. Solis OJ, Roberson GR, Taveras JM, Mohr J, Pessin MS (1977) Cerebral angiography in acute cerebral infarction. Revist Interam Radiol 2:19–25
21. Taneda M, Shimada N, Tsuchiya T (1985) Transient neurological deficits due to embolic and reopening of the cerebral arteries. Stroke 16:522–524
22. Yamaguchi T (1992) Intravenous tissue plasminogen activator in acute thromboembolic stroke: A placebo-controlled, double-blind trial. In: 2nd International Symposium on Thrombolytic Therapy for Acute Ischemic Stroke (this Proceeding)
23. Yamaguchi T, Minematsu K, Choki J-I, Ikeda M (1984) Clinical and neuroradiological analysis of thrombotic and embolic cerebral infarction. Jpn Circ J 48:50–58

Spectacular Shrinking Deficits in Acute Ischemic Stroke

K. Minematsu

The development of ischemic brain injury depends upon the severity and duration of ischemia [9, 13]. Compromised brain tissues may recover if blood flow is restored after a brief duration of ischemia [4, 13, 14, 17, 24, 27]. This concept has led to therapeutic attempts to restore flow in animal stroke models, and in human stroke, with thrombolytic therapy [3, 6, 29]. Successful salvage of brain tissues will likely require intervention within a few hours after interruption of the cerebral blood supply. During this time-window, however, acute ischemic stroke patients often recover spontaneously from the initial deficits [1].

Dramatic improvement may follow an initial major hemispheric syndrome within minutes to hours after stroke onset, leaving little or no deficit. This phenomenon, termed by Mohr and coworkers "a spectacular shrinking deficit (SSD)" [19], occurs more frequently than previously considered, is highly suggestive of cardiogenic brain embolism, and indicates a migratory embolus in the internal carotid artery (ICA)–middle cerebral artery (MCA) axis [18]. Acute treatment trials with thrombolytic therapy must consider the phenomenon of SSD. Patients with the sudden onset of a major hemispheric syndrome are likely to come to the hospital earlier than patients with milder or more gradual onset of symptoms, and embolic occlusion is perhaps more susceptible to thrombolytic agents than other mechanisms of arterial occlusion.

In the present study, I have analyzed only patients admitted within 6 h after stroke onset, potential candidates for most of the recent clinical trials with thrombolytic agents, to determine the frequency, time from stroke onset, historical and clinical features of SSD, and have compared them to the same characteristics in patients with similar initial deficits, but with no recovery.

Subjects and Methods

The study group consisted of a total of 64 consecutive ischemic stroke patients, with a sudden onset of a major hemispheric syndrome, admitted to our hospi-

National Cardiovascular Center Research Institute, Osaka, Japan

G. J. del Zoppo, E. Mori, W. Hacke (Eds.)
Thrombolytic Therapy in Acute Ischemic Stroke II

tal within 6 h after stroke onset. Detailed historical information in each patient was obtained. The neurological status was repeatedly examined at 1- to 2-h intervals. A major hemispheric syndrome was defined as a neurological syndrome strongly suggesting occlusion of the ICA or the main trunk of the MCA: combinations of profound sensory and motor deficits, conjugate deviation of eyes to the side of lesion, hemianopia, global aphasia, or anosognosia for hemiplegia. The diagnosis of SSD was made when patients showed sudden and distinct improvement within 24 h after stroke onset, leaving a mild or no deficit. The other patients were classified as non-SSD. Based on our diagnostic criteria [18], the patients were divided into 4 diagnostic subgroups: cardioembolic, atherothrombotic, lacunar brain infarction, and brain infarction (and TIA) of miscellaneous causes.

In the 2 groups, we compared the historical and clinical features including CT and angiographic findings. The infarct size on CT was classified and graded into the following 8 scores (infarct score): 0, no lesion; 1, small deep lesion (<20 mm in diameter); 2, small cortical lesion (<20 mm); 3, larger deep lesion; 4, medium-sized cortical lesion (< one lobe); 5, large cortical lesion (one to two lobes); 6, lesion occupying the most of MCA territory; and 7, lesion larger than Grade 6. The presence or absence of hemorrhagic transformation was determined with CT scans obtained more than 3 times during the first month. The clinical outcome was judged 2 months after stroke onset, and was graded as follows (outcome score): 0, no deficits; 1, minor motor/sensory deficits (physically independent); 2, mild deficits in higher brain function (socially independent); 3, severe motor/sensory deficits (physically dependent); 4, severe higher brain function deficits (socially dependent); 5, vegetative state; and 6, death.

Statistical analyses were performed using a Student *t*-test, Mann-Whitney U test, contingency table analysis, and Spearman test. The result was considered significant if the two-tailed probability was less than 0.05.

Results

In the 64 patients with an initial major hemispheric syndrome, 12 patients (19%) recovered rapidly within 24 h after stroke onset, allowing the diagnosis of SSD. No patient in either group was given thrombolytic agents during the first day. Patients with SSD were admitted 2.3 ± 1.1 (mean ± SD) h after stroke onset, almost the same time interval as in non-SSD patients (2.5 ± 1.4 h). All SSD and 90% of non-SSD patients had a cardiac source of emboli. Men were predominant in the SSD group (male/female ratio was 9/3 in the SSD and 23/29 in the non-SSD group). Patients with SSD were younger (58 ± 19 years versus 67 ± 13 years, $p < 0.1$) and had no diabetes mellitus (0% versus 17%), although statistically significant difference was not obtained for any single item. SSD patients had more of these factors (cardiac source of emboli, males younger than 60 years, and nondiabetic) than non-SSD patients (3.3 ± 0.6 versus 2.4 ± 0.7, $p < 0.001$).

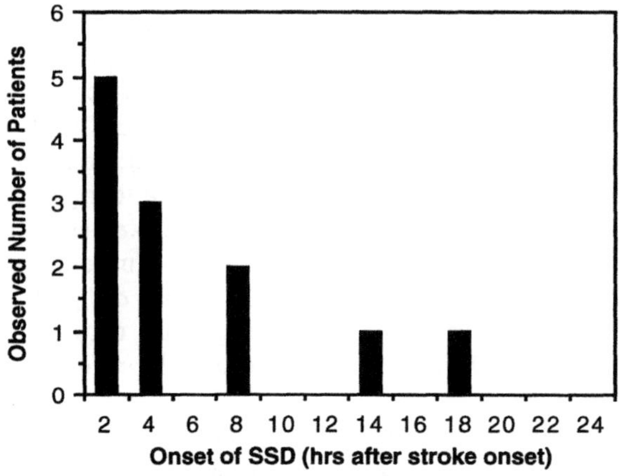

Fig. 1. Distribution of the time to onset of spectacular shrinking deficits from stroke onset. An observed number decreases exponentially over time

The onset of SSD was most frequent within the first 4 h; the first 2 h in 5 patients, the next 2 h in 3 patients, and other SSD onsets were scattered over later timepoints, making an exponential-like decline over time (Fig. 1). Angiography within 24 h after stroke onset was performed in 7 SSD patients (at 9.5 ± 6.0 h) and 31 non-SSD patients (at 8.3 ± 6.4 h). The SSD patient examined 3 h after stroke onset had an occlusion at the trunk of the MCA, which moved to distal branches when re-examined 1.5 h later. The other SSD patients, examined at a later timepoint, showed arterial occlusions of the MCA branches or no evidence of occlusion. Three patients had evidence of capillary blush or early venous filling. In all SSD patients except one, the onset of SSD preceded angiographic examination. The patient examined before the onset of SSD (18 h) had occlusions both in the upper and lower branches of the MCA at 7.5 h after stroke onset. The occlusion disappeared completely when re-examined on day 11. In all non-SSD patients, arterial occlusions were documented proximal to the MCA trunk (29 patients) or multiple MCA branches (2 patients). A difference in sites of arterial occlusion was highly significant between the two groups (Fig. 2; contingency coefficient = 0.633, $p < 0.0005$).

Patients with SSD had significantly smaller infarcts (infarct score: 1.8 ± 1.4) than non-SSD patients (5.1 ± 1.2, $p < 0.0001$). Two SSD patients had no CT lesions, 8 had a deep infarct alone or small, scattered cortical infarcts, and only 2 had medium-sized cortical infarcts. In contrast, 48 of 52 non-SSD patients had infarcts larger than one lobe. Hemorrhagic transformation was noted in only 3 SSD patients, significantly less frequent than the 67% (35/52) in the non-SSD group (contingency coefficient = 0.32, $p < 0.05$).

The 2-month outcome was significantly better in the SSD group (outcome score 0.7 ± 0.9) than in the non-SSD group (4.2 ± 1.1, $p < 0.0001$, Mann- Whitney U test). Seven of 12 SSD patients had no neurological deficits and the remaining 5 were scored as grade 1 or 2. All non-SSD patients had neurological deficits and the outcome score was greater than 3 in 49 of 52 patients (94%). In SSD patients, patient's age alone was significantly correlated with the outcome scale ($R_{Spearman} = 0.714$, $p < 0.02$). Earlier onset of SSD seemed to be

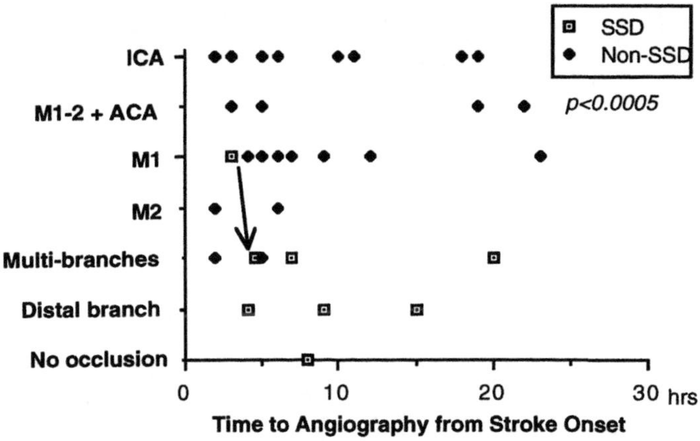

Fig. 2. Relation of time to angiography with sites of arterial occlusion in patients examined with angiography within 24 h after stroke onset. An *arrow* indicates an evolution of occlusion sites observed in an SSD patient. There is a significant difference in sites of arterial occlusion between the groups ($p < 0.0005$)

accompanied with better outcome, although the correlation was not significant ($R_{Spearman} = 0.579$, $p < 0.1$).

Case Report. Patient J.M. (07–1518–2), a 56-year-old man with hypertension and nonvalvular atrial fibrillation, had an abrupt onset of motor weakness in the left arm and leg. He paid no attention to his paralyzed extremities and denied it. At the time of admission, 2.5 h after stroke onset, neurological examination revealed a left hemiplegia, conjugate deviation of eyes to the right, unilateral spatial neglect and anosognosia. He was drowsy, and reliable assessment of the sensory, visual and cerebellar systems was impossible. At this time, he was diagnosed as having a cardioembolic stroke, probably with occlusion of the right ICA or MCA trunk. His deficits improved suddenly 1.5 h later, leaving minimal motor weakness. Angiographic examination performed 9 h after stroke onset demonstrated an occlusion of a distal branch of the right MCA, with early venous filling. He had no neurological deficits on Day 3. Contrast CT and MRI studies revealed a deep infarct with scattered cortical lesions (Fig. 3).

Discussion

The present study demonstrates that approximately 20% of patients who were admitted within 6 h of stroke onset with an initial major hemispheric syndrome improve. The SSD phenomenon seems to occur most frequently in the earliest timepoint after stroke onset, decreasing in frequency exponentially over time. Mohr and colleagues [19] presumed that SSD indicated a migratory

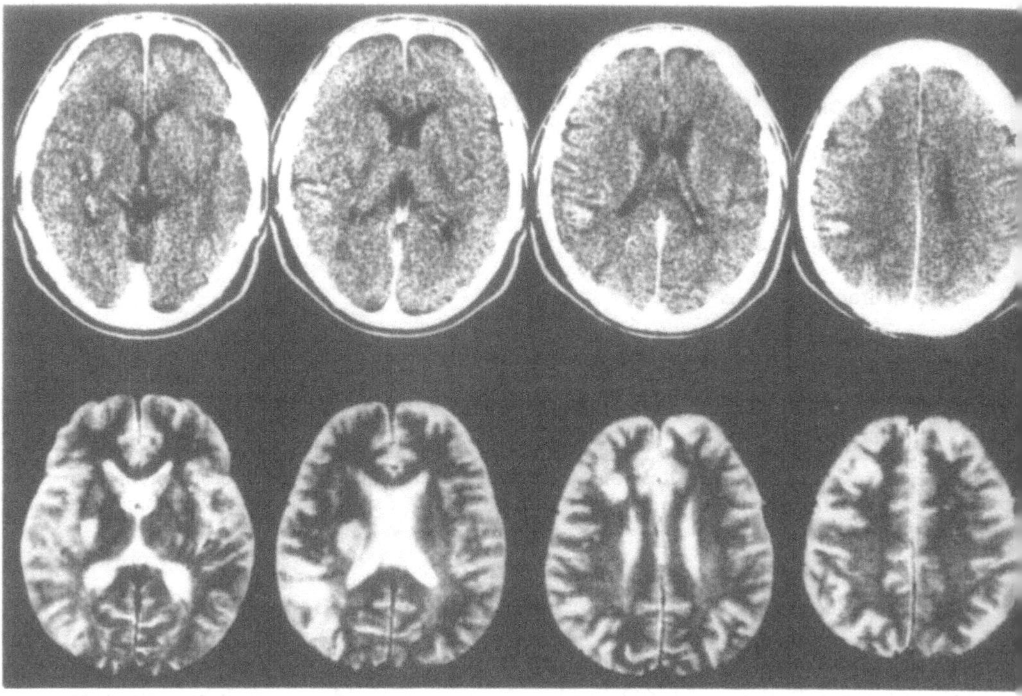

Fig. 3. Contrast CT and MRI studies in the patient J.M., indicating scattered infarcts in the basal ganglia and over the cortices

embolus in the ICA–MCA axis. The present angiographic and CT studies support this suggestion. Early, spontaneous, embolic migration from the initial occlusion site in the ICA or MCA trunk may cause no or small, scattered infarcts and less frequent hemorrhagic transformation, resulting in a favorable outcome.

In cardioembolic stroke, vanishing occlusion, or reopening of the occluded artery, occurs commonly in up to 90% of cases within days or weeks [5, 7, 28]. The reopening phenomenon, proven angiographically, usually causes no improvement but is occasionally accompanied by hemorrhagic transformation and brain edema [5, 8, 11, 12, 20]. These angiographic studies analyzed only delayed arterial reopening which occurs days after stroke onset. Early reopening within minutes or hours after stroke onset may lead to good recovery, as suggested by previous experimental studies and the present study. Taneda and coworkers [25] reported two patients with immediate embolic migration resulting in rapid recovery. Ringelstein and colleagues [21] analyzed effects of early recanalization by using initial cerebral arteriography, followed by repetitive studies with transcranial Doppler ultrasonography. They demonstrated that very early development of sufficient collaterals linked to rapid recanalization within the first 8 h may have a favorable impact on infarct size and outcome in agreement with the present results.

The location and size of infarcts on CT also suggested migratory embolism in SSD patients. Infarcts in deep structures without evidence of MCA occlusion indicated that embolic material initially occluded the MCA trunk at the site where the lenticulostriate arteries branch off [2, 15, 22, 23, 26], then migrated distally with or without scattered cortical infarcts. Hemorrhagic transformation occurred less frequently in SSD patients than in non-SSD patients, probably related to the smaller infarct size, shorter duration of ischemia and younger age of the SSD group [10, 16, 20].

The mechanism of early reopening (or recanalization) causing SSD is not yet known. Our previous study suggested that several factors, including sex, patient's age and diabetes mellitus, may influence the frequency of SSD [18]. Biller and colleagues [1] also reported a similar result that younger patients, men, and those without a history of arterial hypertension or diabetes mellitus improved to a greater degree within 6 h. In their 29 patients, at least 18 had an embolic mechanism according to their criteria. Therefore, these common factors may be linked to rapid improvement in embolic stroke patients. These factors are probably reflections of other direct mechanisms, such as nature and size of embolic materials, concomitant atherosclerotic arterial lesions, systemic coagulability, local fibrinolytic activity, or collateral blood supply, which may affect rapid clot lysis and timely embolic migration.

The phenomenon of SSD is typical of migratory embolism, but does not include all types of recovery following cardioembolic stroke. Patients with milder initial deficits and with slower improvement are excluded from this category. The present results support in part therapeutic attempts with thrombolytic therapy for acute ischemic stroke. There is no data, however, regarding whether thrombolysis causes improvements without risk. Dramatic recovery after administration of thrombolytic agents cannot always be attributable to the therapeutic effect. The earlier patients are given the agents, the more patients will recover independently from treatment effect. It is obvious that a clinical trial with thrombolytic therapy should carefully control for this spontaneous improvement.

Acknowledgment. The author thanks Dr. Marc Fisher for reviewing the manuscript.

References

1. Biller J, Love BB, Marsch EE, III, et al (1990) Spontaneous improvement after acute ischemic stroke. A pilot study. Stroke 21:1008–1012
2. Bladin PF, Berkovic SF (1984) Striatocapsular infarction: Large infarcts in the lenticulostriate arterial territory. Neurology 34:1423–1430
3. Brott T (1991) Thrombolytic therapy for stroke. Cerebrovasc Brain Metab Rev 3:91–113
4. Crowell RM, Olsson Y, Klatzo I, Ommaya A (1970) Temporary occlusion of the middle cerebral artery in the monkey. Clinical and pathological observations. Stroke 1:439–448
5. Dalal PM, Shah PM, Sheth SC, Deshpande CK (1965) Cerebral embolism: Angiographic observations on spontaneous clot lysis. Lancet 1:61–64

6. del Zoppo G, Zeumer H, Harker L (1986) Thrombolytic therapy in stroke: Possibilities and hazards. Stroke 17:595–609
7. Fieschi C, Bozzao L (1969) Transient embolic occlusion of the middle cerebral and internal carotid arteries in cerebral apoplexy. J Neurol Neurosurg Psychiatry 32:236–240
8. Fisher CM, Adams RD (1951) Observations on brain embolism with special reference to the mechanism of hemorrhagic infarction. J Neuropathol Exp Neurol 10:92–94
9. Heiss WD, Rosner G (1983) Functional recovery of cortical neurons as related to degree and duration of ischemia. Ann Neurol 14:294–301
10. Hornig CR, Dorndorf W, Agnoli AL (1986) Hemorrhagic cerebral infarction: A prospective study. Stroke 17:179–185
11. Irino T, Taneda M, Minami T (1977) Sanguineous cerebrospinal fluid in recanalized cerebral infarction. Stroke 8:50–58
12. Irino T, Taneda M, Minami T (1977) Angiographic manifestations in postrecanalized cerebral infarction. Neurology 27:471–475
13. Jones TH, Morawetz RB, Growell RM, et al (1981) Thresholds of focal cerebral ischemia in awake monkeys. J Neurosurg 54:773–782
14. Kaplan B, Brint S, Tanabe J, Jacewicz M, Wang X–J, Pulsinelli W (1991) Temporal thresholds for neocortical infarction in rats subjected to reversible focal cerebral ischemia. Stroke 22:1032–1039
15. Levine RL, Lagreze HL, Dobkin JA, Turski PA (1988) Large subcortical hemispheric infarctions. Presentation and prognosis. Arch Neurol 45:1074– 1077
16. Lodder J, Krijne-Kubat B, Broekman J (1986) Cerebral hemorrhagic infarction at autopsy: Cardiac embolic cause and the relationship to the cause of death. Stroke 17:626–629
17. Minematsu K, Li L, Fisher M, Sotak CH, Davis MA, Fisher M (1992) Reversible focal ischemic injury demonstrated by diffusion-weighted magnetic resonance imaging in rats. Stroke 23:1304–1311
18. Minematsu K, Yamaguchi T, Omae T (1992) Spectacular shrinking deficit: Rapid recovery from a major hemispheric syndrome by migration of an embolus. Neurology 42:157–162
19. Mohr JP, Barnett HJM (1986) Classification of ischemic stroke. In: Barnett HJM, Stein BM, Mohr JP, Yatsu FM (eds) Stroke: Pathophysiology, diagnosis and management. Churchill Livingstone, New York, p 281
20. Okada Y, Yamaguchi T, Minematsu K, et al (1989) Hemorrhagic transformation in cerebral embolism. Stroke 20:598–603
21. Ringelstein EB, Biniek R, Weiller C, Ammeling B, Nolte PN, Thron A (1992) Type and extent of hemispheric brain infarctions and clinical outcome in early and delayed middle cerebral artery recanalization. Neurology 42:289–298
22. Ringelstein EB, Koschorke S, Holling A, Thron A, Lambertz H, Minale C (1989) Computed tomographic patterns of proven embolic brain infarctions. Ann Neurol 26:759–765
23. Santamaria J, Graus F, Rubio F, Arbizu T, Peres J (1983) Cerebral infarction of the basal ganglia due to embolism from the heart. Stroke 14:911–914
24. Sundt TM, Jr., Grant WC, Garcia JH (1969) Restoration of middle cerebral artery flow in experimental infarction. J Neurosurg 31:311–322
25. Taneda M, Shimada N, Tsuchiya T (1985) Transient neurological deficits due to embolic occlusion and immediate reopening of the cerebral arteries. Stroke 16:522–524
26. Weiller C, Ringelstein EB, Reiche W, Thron A, Buelle U (1990) The large striatecapsular infarct. A clinical and pathophysiological entity. Arch Neurol 47:1085–1091
27. Weinstein PR, Anderson GG, Telles DA (1986) Neurological deficit and cerebral infarction after temporary middle cerebral artery occlusion in unanesthetized cats. Stroke 17:318–324
28. Yamaguchi T, Minematsu K, Choki J, Ikeda M (1984) Clinical and neuroradiological analysis of thrombotic and embolic cerebral infarction. Jpn Circ J 48:50–58
29. Zivin J, Fisher M, DeGirolami U, Hemenway CC, Stashak JA (1985) Tissue plasminogen activator reduces neurological damage after cerebral embolism. Science 230:1289–1292

The Significance of Various Factors Associated with Hemorrhagic Transformation in Patients Treated with Recombinant Tissue Plasminogen Activator for Acute Stroke

M.S. Pessin[1] and S.M. Wolpert[2] for The rt-PA Acute Stroke Study Group

Intracranial bleeding is the principal safety concern and use-limiting factor related to the application of thrombolytic agents in acute stroke. Several recent studies, using intravenously administered recombinant tissue plasminogen activator (rt-PA) for carotid and vertebrobasilar territory stroke, have documented intracranial bleeding in the form of hemorrhagic infarction (HI) and parenchymatous hematoma (PH) [2, 4, 11, 16, 19]. That intracranial bleeding is not limited to the use of thrombolytic agents in stroke patients has been amply documented in studies of patients with acute myocardial infarction treated with these agents where a small but consistent incidence has been noted in the range of approximately 0.5% (Table 1) [6, 7, 9, 10, 14, 15, 18]. The purpose of this discussion is to examine several factors presumed to be associated with intracranial bleeding in stroke patients treated with thrombolytic agents using data from the rt-PA Acute Stroke Study Group trial [4] and other recent trials [2, 8, 11, 16, 19]. A preview of this analysis suggests that many of the long and firmly held views regarding influences and effects of hemorrhagic transformation (HT) are not supported by recent information.

Table 1. Intracranial hemorrhage (ICH) in trials of rt-PA in acute myocardial infarction (modified from [14])

Study	ICH	*n*	%
ASSET [18]	7	2516	0.28
TAMI [15]	13	1696	0.77
BW [10]	9	1700	0.53
TIMI II [6]			
150 mg	14	908	1.5
100 mg	13	3016	0.43
GISSI 2 [7]	19	6182	0.31
ISG [10]	25	4190	0.60
Totals	100[a]	20208	0.49

[a] Includes five subdural hematomas.

Department of [1]Neurology and [2]Radiology (Division of Neuroradiology), Tufts University School of Medicine, New England Medical Center, Boston, MA, USA

G.J. del Zoppo, E. Mori, W. Hacke (Eds.)
Thrombolytic Therapy in Acute Ischemic Stroke II

The rt-PA Acute Stroke Study [4] served as the principal basis for this analysis. This study was a dose-escalation and safety analysis of two-chain rt-PA (duteplase) in patients with acute ischemic stroke in the carotid or vertebrobasilar territories. A negative CT for blood and angiographic documentation of an arterial occlusion (not stenosis) consistent with the clinical picture were the principal requirements. In addition, patients had to begin receiving a 60-min intravenous infusion of a pre-assigned dose of rt-PA within 8 h from stroke onset. Efficacy was defined as post-rt-PA angiographic evidence of recanalization of a previously occluded artery, and safety referred to the absence of intracranial bleeding. One-hundred four patients received rt-PA and were available for safety analyses, but only 93 patients fulfilled all study criteria and were assessed for efficacy.

Classification of Hemorrhagic Transformation

The types of intracranial bleeding encountered in thrombolytic trials for acute stroke may be classified based on CT scan as hemorrhagic infarction (HI) and parenchymatous hematoma (PH). This differentiation is important since the CT patterns, clinical consequences and even the pathogeneses may differ in HI and PH. Hemorrhagic infarction is defined as an area(s) of increased density (blood) including minor speckling or a mottled appearance with indistinct margins (sometimes in a gyriform pattern) to more complete, multiple areas of *hemorrhage within a region of infarction*. Mass effect, if present, usually reflects edema related to large infarct size. The pathogenesis of bleeding in HI, based on autopsy studies of HI in embolic infarction, is thought to result from

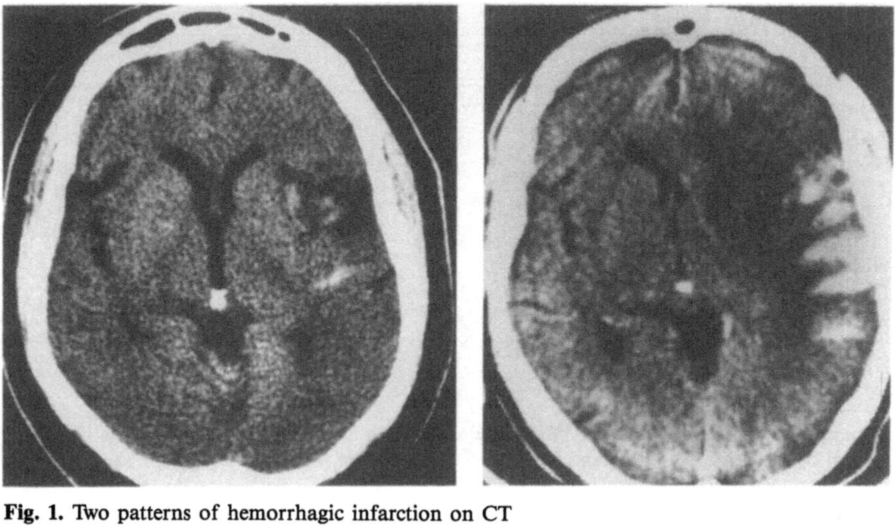

Fig. 1. Two patterns of hemorrhagic infarction on CT

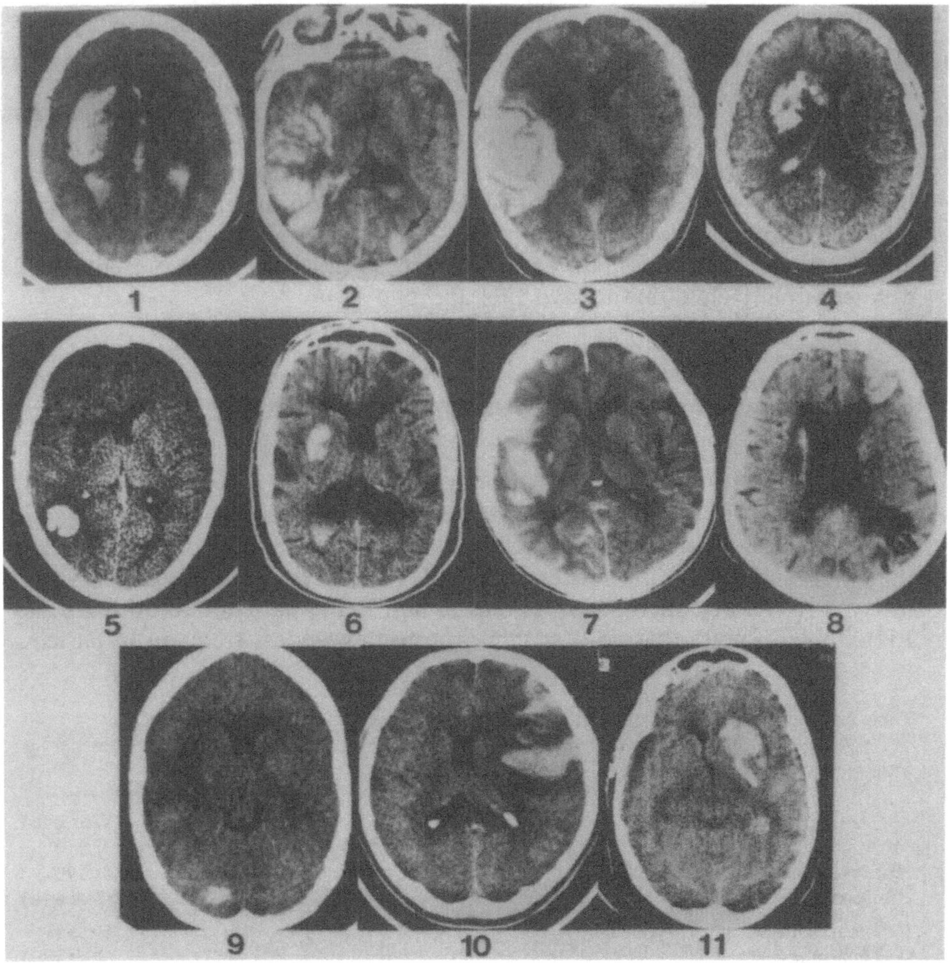

Fig. 2. Spectrum of parenchymatous hematomas. Note patient 2 has a large hemorrhagic infarct (HI) in the right hemisphere and a small discrete PH in the left occipital pole (*arrow*)

damaged and distended capillaries within the infarct with reperfusion leakage when the embolic (thrombus) material naturally lyses and clears. Alternatively, even with persistent arterial occlusion some bleeding may occur from leptomeningeal collateral blood channels [12]. Parenchymatous hematoma is defined as a more homogenous, dense area of increased density (blood) with circumscribed boundaries and mass effects, but not necessarily restricted to the area of infarction. A PH represents a solid clot of blood which displaces and destroys surrounding brain tissue. The mechanism producing PH in this setting is not clear but may represent an exaggerated form of reperfusion bleeding as in HI, or perhaps pure arteriole bleeding as in hypertensive hemorrhage. The occurrence of PH in regions remote from the infarct suggests that mechanisms other than infarction per se may be operative. It is acknowledged that in some cases the CT scan distinction between severe HI and PH may be impossible.

In the rt-PA Acute Stroke Study in which 104 patients received rt-PA, HIs and PHs varied in size and location on the 24-h post-rt-PA CT scan (Figs. 1, 2). One patient had both an HI and a PH, the latter in an area remote from the infarct. One other patient had a PH in a location distant from the bland infarct. In four patients the assignment of hemorrhagic transformation was "indeterminate" because features of both types of bleeding were present; these were eventually classified as two HIs and two PHs.

Hemorrhagic Transformation and Clinical Effects

The occurrence of hemorrhagic transformation on CT, either HI or PH, has generally been viewed as a poor prognostic sign. However, our data suggests that there was considerable variability in the clinical effects of HT and that there were significant differences between HI and PH. In the 104 patients who received rt-PA, 21 patients had HI and 11 had PH (1 patient had both HI and PH). Table 2 shows that adverse clinical effects were less frequent in patients

Table 2. Hemorrhagic transformation and clincial effects

		Clinical		
		Improved	Unchanged	Worsened
Hemorrhagic Infarct	21/104	12	5	4 (19%) (2 deaths)
Parenchymatous Hematoma	11/104	4	1	6 (55%) (2 deaths)

Table 3. Hemorrhagic transformation in recent intravenous rt-PA studies[a]

Study	b	Angio	HI	PH	Deterioration	
					(*n*)	(%)
del Zoppo et al. [4]	104	+	21	11	10	(9.6)
Mori et al. [11]	19	+	8	2	2	(10.5)
	12 controls	+	4	1	0	0
von Kummer et al. [16]	32	+	9	3	3	(9)
Yamaguchi et al. [19]	58	+	12	–	–	(–)
Brott et al. [2]	74	–	3	2	3	(4)
Haley et al. [8]	20	–	4	2	2	(10)

[a] Treatment time ⩽8 h

with HI (19%) as compared to PH (55%) ($2p = 0.056$). Many patients remained clinically stable or were improving when hemorrhagic transformation was noted on CT, including 5 of 11 patients with PH. Overall, only 10 of 104 (9.6%) patients had clinical neurologic deterioration attributed to the HT. This finding is similar to other studies in which intravenous rt-PA was administered to patients with acute stroke (Table 3). While all forms of intracranial bleeding are unwanted, the incidence of clinically significant bleeding is approximately 10%, an incidence significantly lower than might have been anticipated but one which may unalterably reflect the risks of such treatment.

Time to Treatment

In this trial, an 8-h treatment window from stroke onset was allowed with the full realization that early treatment was desirable to reduce ischemic brain tissue damage. Many factors prevent patients and doctors from timely assessment and treatment when a patient suffers a stroke. Some of these factors will be discussed in later papers. In all patients, the average time to rt-PA treatment was 5.4 h ± 1.7 h.

Table 4. Association of time to rt-PA treatment and hemorrhagic transformation in 93 subjects (HT = HI + PH)

Δ(T − 0)	HT	No HT
⩽6 h	15	46
>6 h	17	15

$2p = 0.0108$ (Fisher's Exact Test).

Hemorrhagic transformation occurred significantly more frequently in patients treated later than 6 h than those treated within 6 h from symptom onset (Table 4). Furthermore, the mean time to treatment of patients who developed HT was significantly later than those who did not demonstrate either HI or PH [4]. The explanation for this observation is not entirely clear, but it is likely that ischemic damage to the occluded vessel(s) and surrounding tissue is greater with the passage of time and that reperfusion leakage of red blood cells into the infarct is enhanced the later the treatment commences. The actual mechanism(s) underlying this observation remains unsettled.

CT Features and Hemorrhagic Transformation

Reports have suggested that signs of early ischemia on CT (sulcal effacement, loss of gray/white demarcation) [1] or large infarct size [3, 13] correlated with the occurrence of HT. Our data does not support these conclusions. CT signs of early ischemia were present in 13 of 32 (41%) patients with HI or PH ($\chi^2 = 1.412$, df 1, $2p = 0.235$), and mean infarct volume was 76.3 cm^3 in patients with HT as compared to 78.6 cm^3 in patients with no HT (9 patients with PH were excluded from this analysis since infarct size could not be accurately measured in the presence of the PH).

rt-PA Dose, Recanalization, and Hemorrhagic Transformation

This was an open dose-escalation trial which was prematurely terminated because of a patent suit. However, there was no association between the various dose groups, recanalization, and HT (Fig. 3).

Recanalization of an occluded artery might be expected to promote HT as a consequence of reperfusion bleeding based on the hypothesis of "migratory embolism" proposed by Fisher and Adams [5]. In the rt-PA Acute Stroke Study Group study HT was not associated with recanalization; however, here recanalization was assessed by repeat angiography immediately following the 60-min rt-PA infusion, while HT was identified by CT in the interval between completion of rt-PA treatment and a 24-h CT. It is possible that recanalization

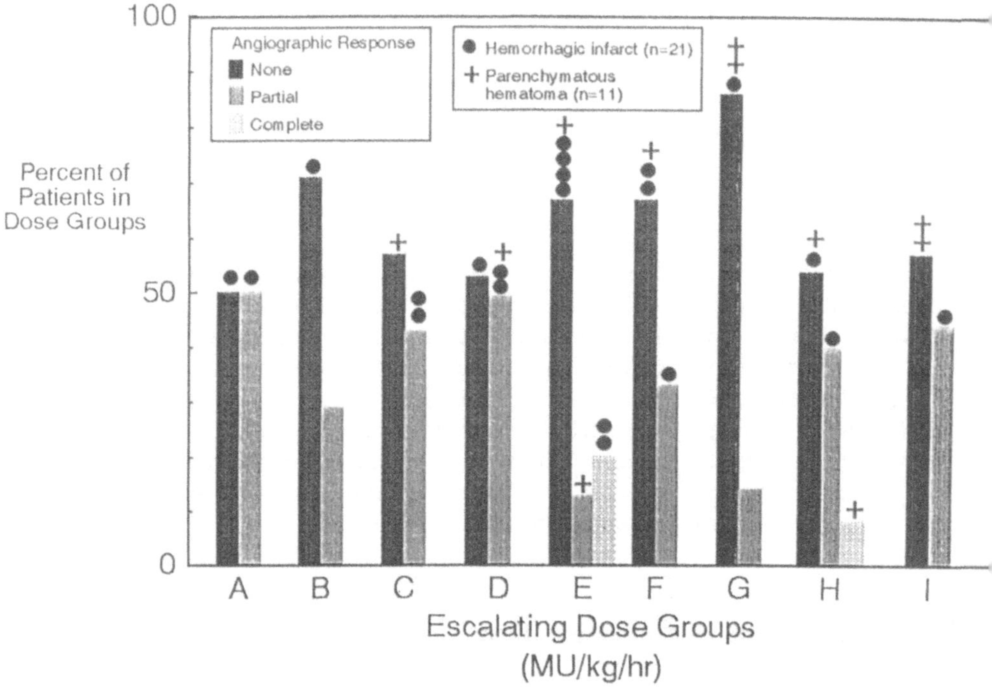

Fig. 3. The relationship between hemorrhagic transformation, rt-PA dose, and arterial recanalization

did occur after the post-rt-PA angiogram and before the hemorrhagic transformation, but was unrecognized by the limitations of the study design.

Age

Some reports have suggested a relationship between the patient's age and the development of HT in embolic stroke [13]. We analyzed age and found no relationship to HT.

Other Factors

Several other factors were analyzed and found to bear no relationship to HT. These included history of hypertension, diabetes mellitus, past stroke, presence of a hyperdense MCA sign on CT, and previous use of aspirin or dipyridamole. Heparin and warfarin were not permitted for the first 24 h (heparin) or 72 h (warfarin) following rt-PA treatment so could not have influenced HT on the 24-h CT. Finally, although fibrinogen levels were not routinely measured in these patients following rt-PA administration, hypofibrinogenemia has not been consistently associated with intracranial bleeding in myocardial infarction studies [6, 10].

Conclusions

The data from this recent rt-PA stroke trial shows that the clinical effects of HT are highly variable, with important differences between HI and PH in the risks of clinical deterioration. Overall, however, approximately 10% of patients will have clinical worsening associated with both forms of intracranial bleeding. The time to treatment from stroke onset was the only factor which influenced the occurrence of HT. The other variables discussed had no significant influence on HT. It is feasible that combinations of various factors (for example, age, infarct size, and recanalization) might act in concert to produce HT, but the number of patients was too small to make this type of analysis statistically meaningful. To date, then, the accurate prediction of HT, in the setting of thrombolytic treatment for acute stroke, is not possible and must await further study. Evolving magnetic resonance imaging technology, such as diffusion-weighted imaging, offers the hope of identifying very early tissue changes following ischemic injury and may allow the accurate prediction of later HT [17].

Acknowledgements. The authors wish to thank the members of the rt-PA Acute Stroke Study Group and the sponsor as indicated in the Appendices of del Zoppo and colleagues [4] and Alberts and colleagues (this volume).

References

1. Bozzao L, Angeloni U, Bastianello S, Fantozzi LM, Pierallini A, Fieschi C (1991) Early angiographic and CT findings in patients with hemorrhagic infarction in the distribution of the middle cerebral artery. AJNR 12:1115–1121
2. Brott TG, Haley EC, Levy DE, et al (1992) Urgent therapy for stroke. Part I. Pilot study of tissue plaminogen activator administered within 90 minutes. Stroke 23:632–640
3. Cerebral Embolism Study Group (1984) Immediate anticoagulation of embolic stroke: Brain hemorrhage and management options. Stroke 15:779–789
4. del Zoppo GJ, Poeck K, Pessin MS, and 16 coauthors of the rt-PA Acute Stroke Study Group (1992) Recombinant tissue plasminogen activator in acute thrombotic and embolic stroke. Ann Neurol 32:78–86
5. Fisher CM, Adams RD (1951) Observations on brain embolism with special reference to the mechanism of hemorrhagic infarction. J Neuropathol Exp Neurol 10:92–94
6. Gore JM, Sloan M, Price TR, et al (1991) Intracerebral hemorrhage, cerebral infarction, and subdural hematoma after acute myocardial infarction and thrombolytic therapy in the thrombolysis in myocardial infarction study. Thrombolysis in myocardial infarction, Phase II, pilot and clinical trial. Circulation 83:448–459
7. Gruppo Italiano per lo Studio della Sopravvivenza nell'Infarto Miocardico (1990) GISSI-2: A factorial randomised trial of alteplace versus streptokinase and heparin versus no heparin among 12, 490 patients with acute myocardial infarction. Lancet 336:65–71
8. Haley EC, Levy DE, Brott TG, et al (1992) Urgent therapy for stroke. Part II. Pilot study of tissue plasminogen activator administered 91–180 minutes from onset. Stroke 23:641–645
9. International Study Group (1992) In-hospital mortality and clinical course of 20, 891 patients with suspected acute myocardial infarction randomized between alteplase and streptokinase with or without heparin. Lancet 536:71–75
10. Kase CS, Pessin MS, Zivin JA, et al (1992) Intracranial hemorrhage following coronary thrombolysis with tissue plasminogen activator. Am J Med 92:384–390
11. Mori E, Yoneda Y, Tabuchi M, et al (1992) Intravenous recombinant tissue plasminogen activator in acute carotid artery territory stroke. Neurology 42:976–982
12. Ogata J, Yutani C, Imakita M, et al (1989) Hemorrhagic infarct of the brain without a reopening of the occluded arteries in cardioembolic stroke. Stroke 20:876–883
13. Okada Y, Yamaguchi T, Minematsu K, et al (1989) Hemorrhagic transformation in cerebral embolism. Stroke 20:598–603
14. Sloan MA, Price TR (1991) Intracranial hemorrhage following thrombolytic therapy for acute myocardial infarction. Semin Neurol 11:385–399
15. Uglietta JP, O'Connor CM, Boyko OB, Aldrich H, Massey EW, Heinz ER (1991) CT patterns of intracranial hemorrhage complicating thrombolytic therapy for acute myocardial infarction. Radiology 181:555–559
16. von Kummer R, Hacke W (1992) Safety and efficacy of intravenous tissue plasminogen activator and heparin in acute middle cerebral artery. Stroke 23:646–652
17. Warach S, Chien D, Li W, Ronthal M, Edelman RR (1992) Fast magnetic resonance diffusion-weighted imaging of acute human stroke. Neurology 42:1717–1723
18. Wilcox RG, Olsson CG, Skene AM, et al (1988) Trial of tissue plasminogen activator for mortality reduction in acute myocardial infarction. Anglo-Scandinavian Study of Early Thrombolysis (ASSET). Lancet 2:525–530
19. Yamaguchi T, Hayakawa T, Kikuchi H, Abe T (1991) Thrombolytic therapy in embolic and thrombotic cerebral infarction: A cooperative study. In: Hacke W, del Zoppo GJ, Hirschberg M (eds) Thrombolytic therapy in acute stroke. Springer-Verlag, Berlin Heidelberg New York, p 168

Thrombolysis: Stroke Subtype and Embolus Type

W. Hacke

The use of thrombolytic agents in acute ischemic stroke is still experimental [5, 8, 9]. It requires clear hypotheses and strict definitions concerning the group of patients considered possible candidates for this treatment. On the other hand, the decision to treat or not to treat a patient must be made under considerable time constraints prohibiting extensive diagnostic evaluation of the individual patient [2, 6]. It is nearly impossible to perform sufficient cardiac tests in case cardiac embolism is suspected. Angiography is not anymore a prerequisite for thrombolysis in ongoing major controlled studies. Routine Doppler ultrasound, both extra- and intracranially, has only rarely been performed in pretreatment diagnostic evaluation. In the majority of studies the subtype of stroke was not reported and only rarely was information on the embolus origin given. If cardiac or arterial embolus sources have been suspected, it remains unclear how they have been identified. In the majority of cases the distinction between cardiac and cervical source embolus or local thrombotic disease has been made arbitrarily. In consequence, most statements in this paper are not based upon sound scientific data. In recent angiographic open thrombolysis studies, a gross distinction of the occlusion sites often has been reported. In most studies, the distinction was made between the carotid and the vertebrobasilar (VB) territory, in some reports the distinction extracranial internal carotid artery (ecICA), intracranial ICA (icICA), and middle cerebral artery (MCA) is mentioned. Only rarely were distal MCA occlusion sites further differentiated.

The identification of stroke subtype also addresses small vessel disease and extensive arteriosclerotic disease, both at the level of the carotid bifurcation and intracranially. Although in all previous studies multiple CT scans were performed, concurrent small vessel disease was never mentioned. Only rarely was the status of the extracranial brain-supplying arteries reported.

Department of Neurology, University of Heidelberg, Heidelberg, Federal Republic of Germany

G. J. del Zoppo, E. Mori, W. Hacke (Eds.)
Thrombolytic Therapy in Acute Ischemic Stroke II

Stroke Subtype

Small Vessel Disease and Extracranial Carotid Disease

Thrombolytic therapy in patients with significant cerebral small vessel disease with multiple lesions of lacunar size and ischemic demyelination has not been performed, presumably because the investigators fear a high incidence of hemorrhagic complications. Yamaguchi [22] reported 122 patients with "thrombotic" stroke as opposed to embolic stroke who were treated within 3 days after onset of stroke. Although the study was an angiographic one, it is possible that some patients with small vessel disease were included.

Only a few investigators have studied thrombolytic therapy in extracranial carotid disease [12, 19]. Theron [19] discussed hemodynamically induced infarction in 3 patients with pure ecICA occlusion. Six patients reported by Matsumoto and Satoh [12] had ecICA occlusion, 4 of them showing good recovery.

Embolic Stroke Versus Intracranial Thrombolytic Disease

The majority of patients treated with thrombolytic therapy suffered from embolic or thrombotic cerebral branch occlusion leading to territorial infarction. In the carotid territory, the great majority of patients is considered to suffer from embolic occlusions [4, 11, 12, 14, 20, 22]. If reported, suspected cardiac sources were much more frequent than cervical sources [12, 15, 20]. del Zoppo and coworkers [4] reported 6 patients with cardiac embolism and 2 patients with arterio-arterial embolism. The origin of occlusion remained unclear in 4 patients while 4 patients had iatrogenic stroke. The remaining one suffered from MCA stenosis. Yamaguchi [22] studied a subset of patients with presumed intracranial thrombotic stroke (109 patients) in whom the occlusions were demonstrated angiographically. Among these patients 28.4% (31 of 109) had ICA occlusions, 29.4% had MCA trunk, and 8.3% MCA branch. The remainder were in various locations.

In VB territory stroke [basilar artery (BA) and vertebral artery (VA)], local thrombotic disease is common in the intracranial VA and in the mid- basilar segment, but the majority of patients suffer from embolic "top" of the BA or distal VA occlusion [10, 16, 23]. The majority of patients treated suffered from embolic occlusions at different levels.

Occlusion Site

Occlusion Sites in the Carotid Territory. The distribution of occlusion sites in the carotid territory is given as follows in some major studies: Matsumato and Satoh (1990) only distinguished ICA ($n = 11$), MCA ($n = 20$), and VB ($n = 11$) occlusion. del Zoppo and colleagues [4] reported icICA + carotid T ($n = 5$),

ICA+MCA ($n = 3$), isolated M1 ($n = 6$), M2 segments ($n = 5$) and one posterior cerebral artery occlusion among their 20 patients. They did not find a difference in recanalization rates.

Among the 44 patients in Mori's paper [14], 39 patients had carotid territory occlusion. Eight patients had intracranial ICA occlusion, 16 M1 segment occlusions and 11 M2 segment occlusions. Four suffered from multiple occlusions. Low recanalization rates were reported for ICA and multiple occlusions. For M1 and M2 occlusions the recanalization rates were 45% and 50%, respectively.

Theron [19] distinguished two MCA occlusion sites proximal ($n = 5$) and distal ($n = 5$) to the origin of the lenticulostriatal branches. In Mori's recent placebo-controlled study [15], the distribution of occlusion sites was comparable in the treatment groups.

In the study by von Kummer and Hacke [20], the principal clinical inclusion criterion was severe hemispheric stroke presenting with hemiplegia, forced eye deviation and clouding of consciousness. With this clinical inclusion criterion it is not surprising that the majority of patients had occlusions of the intracranial ICA or MCA trunk, and only 3 patients displayed distal branch occlusions. In studies which allow the inclusion of patients with less severe strokes, it is likely that the number of patients suffering from distally located occlusions will increase. This might be true in several ongoing double-blind studies, such as the NIH-sponsored trials or ECASS. Unfortunately, nonangiographic studies will not be able to define the exact site of occlusion.

The hyperdense middle cerebral artery (HMCA) sign [1] is supposed to be an indicator of proximal MCA occlusion and to allow the identification of patients with a clearly defined occlusion site. Unfortunately, the sign is not always visible in patients with documented corresponding lesions. Wolpert and colleagues showed that in all patients exhibiting a HMCA sign, MCA occlusion was documented angiographically, representing a specificity of 100% (Wolpert and colleagues, 1992; in preparation). On the other hand, the sensitivity was very low. In two studies, only 27% [21] or 50% [1] of patients with proven M1 segment occlusion revealed this sign. The presence of the sign allows one to diagnose an M1 segment occlusion, but the absence of the HMCA sign does not rule out M1 occlusion.

It is possible that the occlusion site influences the recanalization rate. Smaller clots in more distally located vessels show early and complete recanalization [20], whereas patients with extended ICA+MCA occlusions only rarely (3 out of 11; 16) or never (0 out of 6; 13) show recanalization. In the forthcoming paper by Wolpert and colleagues [21] the neuroradiological data from the rt-PA Acute Stroke Study Group trial was analyzed. They reported higher recanalization frequency in the more distally located vessels ($p=0.056$). The question remains whether this is caused by the localization or the composition of the thrombus, which will be discussed in the second part of this paper.

Occlusion Sites in the VB Territory. Hacke and coworkers [10] distinguished 4 almost equally distributed occlusion sites (caudal VB, mid-basilar, "top" of the basilar, and extended, multilevel occlusion) among their 43 patients. They identified prognostic conditions based upon both occlusion site and level of consciousness. In basilar artery occlusion, stroke subtypes can be identified who are most likely to benefit from thrombolytic therapy. Patients with "top" of the basilar artery embolism and caudal vertebrobasilar occlusion or embolism showed high recanalization rates and significantly better outcome.

Möbius and colleagues [16] had a much higher percentage of top of the basilar occlusions ($n = 8$) among their 12 patients. Again, as in the study of Zeumer and coworkers [23], recanalization was associated with improved outcome.

Collaterals

A very important feature of stroke subtype seems to be the presence or absence of leptomeningeal collaterals. During this conference, two papers by Forsting and coworkers [7] and Brucker and colleagues [3] will underline the importance of the presence of collateral flow in acute cerebral vascular occlusion. They have shown a significant correlation between the presence of collaterals prior to treatment and good outcome [3, 18, 20]. In a recent paper by Ringelstein and coworkers [18], the significance of good leptomeningeal collateral blood flow for the reduction of infarct size and improved clinical outcome was reported. In his series, as in ours, the great majority of patients had proximal MCA occlusion.

For the purpose of this paper, the following summary concerning stroke subtype can be given:

There is widespread consensus that patients suffering from small vessel disease are not candidates for thrombolytic therapy. The number of reports on thrombolysis in extracranial carotid disease is small. I would only consider treating those patients if they have additional intracranial embolic occlusions. Patients with hemodynamically induced infarctions only rarely have been treated with thrombolytic therapy.

About 70%–80% of patients with carotid circulation occlusion suffer from embolic stroke. The majority is considered to have cardiac source emboli, although the identification of cardiac sources is not always convincing. The recanalization rate is very low in intracranial embolic ICA occlusion, disappointing in proximal MCA occlusion and higher in distal MCA branch embolism. Good leptomeningeal collateral flow prior to recanalization is a predictor of good outcome. In the vertebrobasilar system, embolic and thrombotic stroke are both common. In vertebrobasilar territory occlusion stroke, subtypes can be identified which are most likely to benefit from thrombolytic therapy.

Embolus Subtype

Differences in thrombus composition between cardiac source emboli and emboli from atherothrombotic disease at the cervical level may be important for recanalization efficacy. Unfortunately, there is only a little information about thrombus composition and the susceptibility of the thrombi to dissolute with various thrombolytic agents. Only rarely has information about the thrombus composition in patients unsuccessfully undergoing thrombolytic therapy been reported. Recently Pilz and coworkers reported 2 patients who showed persistent occlusions of the vertebrobasilar artery [17]. The thrombi had low fibrin content and were in close connection to atheromas. Little information is available about the amount of plasminogen present in the embolus. One might speculate that emboli poor in plasminogen content are not very likely to be resolved by plasminogen activators. Most authors believe that cardiac emboli are usually "fresh" and more likely to dissolve than emboli coming from atheromatous plaques. Ringelstein and colleagues [18] nicely showed that cardiac source emboli reveal earlier recanalization compared with arterio-arterial emboli, and spontaneous recanalization of cardiac emboli can be accelerated by the use of thrombolytic substances. On the other hand, cardiac source emboli arising from a rheumatic valve can be old and organized. Not all cardiac source emboli are easy to recanalize. The low recanalization frequency in embolic proximal MCA occlusion underlines this statement.

There is no doubt that the volume and location of the thrombus may influence recanalization rates following thrombolytic therapy. We have already mentioned the bad prognosis of extended ICA emboli. There are good reasons to believe that extended atheroma-based thrombi, particularly from the carotid bifurcation, are unlikely to undergo recanalization. Those thrombi are large, old, platelet-rich, and may contain cholesterol and include atheromatous material [8, 9]. They tend to lodge in proximal vessels, especially in the carotid T, sometimes extending into the anterior and middle cerebral artery. Large, fresh, cardiac source emboli can occlude the ICA. In this situation, despite a favorable thrombus composition, the results are very poor [15, 20].

To summarize, three aspects of the embolus subtypes may be important for recanalization: 1) the size, 2) the origin, and 3) the composition of the thrombus.

It seems that cardiac source emboli may be associated with high recanalization rates, a fact which can be supported by some reports on immediate thrombolytic therapy after cerebral embolism during cardiac catheterization. Large thrombi, independent of their source, have a lower tendency to recanalize compared with smaller, more distally located emboli. The composition of the thrombus seems to be of great importance: fresh, fibrin- and plasminogen-rich thrombi are probably easier to recanalize than organized atheromatous plasminogen-depleted and cholesterol-rich thrombi [13]. On the other hand, many investigators consider all cardiac source emboli fresh, which is not true.

Summary

There is some evidence that the subtype of stroke, the site of occlusion, the origin of the embolus and the composition of the thrombus are important predictors of outcome. The ideal patient seems to be the one who has a fibrin-rich, fresh venous thrombus passing through an open foramen ovale lodging in the distal part of the MCA trunk or MCA branches, has good leptomeningeal flow, and receives the thrombolytic substances quite early. A patient who probably will not benefit from the therapy can be described as having a large, organized and plasminogen-depleted, cholesterol-containing embolus in the carotid with additional occlusion of the proximal MCA and poor collateral flow.

Unfortunately, it is impossible to have all this information at the time the decision is made for or against thrombolytic therapy. Maybe in the future advanced imaging technologies will allow rapid and reliable decisions on who to treat and who not to treat.

References

1. Bastionalo P, Pierallini A, Colonnese C (1991) Hyperdense middle cerebral artery CT scan. Comparison with angiography in the acute phase of ischemic supratentorial infarction. Neuroradiology 33:207–211
2. Brott T, Haley EC, Levy DE, et al (1988) The investigational use of t-PA for stroke. Ann Emerg Med 17:1202–1205
3. Brucker B, Potuschak H, Laich E, et al (1992) Relation of thrombolytic reperfusion and of collateral circulation to outcome in patients suffering cerebral main artery occlusion. In: 2nd International Symposium on Thrombolytic Therapy in Acute Ischemic Stroke (this Proceeding)
4. del Zoppo GJ, Ferbert A, Otis S, et al (1988) Local intra-arterial therapy in acute carotid territory stroke: A pilot study. Stroke 19:307–313
5. del Zoppo GJ, Pessin MS, Mori E, Hacke W (1991) Thrombolytic intervention in acute thrombotic and embolic stroke. Semin Neurol 11:368–384
6. Fieschi C, Argentino C, Lenzi GL, Sacchetti ML, Toni D, Bozzao L (1989) Clinical and instrumental evaluation of patients with ischemic stroke within the first six hours. J Neurol Sci 91:311–321
7. Forsting M, Krieger D, von Kummer R, et al (1992) The prognostic value of collateral blood flow in acute middle cerebral artery occlusion. In: 2nd International Symposium on Thrombolytic Therapy for Acute Ischemic Stroke (this Proceeding)
8. Hacke W, Hirschberg M (1990) Thrombolytic therapy in acute ischemic stroke – an update. Stroke 1:17–20
9. Hacke W, Hirschberg M, Krieger D (1990) General treatment of acute stroke. J Cerebrovasc Dis 1:93–99
10. Hacke W, Zeumer H, Ferbert A, Bruckmann H, del Zoppo GJ (1988) Intraarterial thrombolytic therapy improves outcome in patients with acute vertebrobasilar occlusive disease. Stroke 19:1216–1222
11. Hennerici M, Hacke W, von Kummer R, Hornig C, Zangemeister W (1991) Intravenous tissue plasminogen activator for the treatment of acute thromboembolic ischemia. J Cerebrovasc Dis 1 (Suppl.):124–128

12. Matsumoto K, Satoh K (1991) Topical intra-arterial urokinase infusion for acute stroke. In: Hacke W, del Zoppo GJ, Hirschberg M (eds) Thrombolytic therapy in acute ischemic stroke. Springer-Verlag, Berlin Heidelberg New York, p 207
13. Matsumoto K, Satoh K (1991) In vitro thrombus lysis by urokinase in preparation for patient studies. In: Hacke W, del Zoppo GJ, Hirschberg M (eds) Thrombolytic therapy in acute ischemic stroke. Springer-Verlag, Berlin Heidelberg New York, p 236
14. Mori E (1991) Fibrinolytic recanalization therpay in acute cerebrovascular thromboembolism. In. Hacke W, de Zoppo GJ, Hirschberg M (eds) Thrombolytic Therapy in Acute Ischemic Stroke, Springer Verlag, Berlin, p 137
15. Mori E, Yoneda Y, Tabuchi M et al (1992) Intravenious recombinant tissue plasminogen activator in acute carotid artery territory stroke. Neurology 42:976–982
16. Möbius E, Berg-Dammer E, Kühne D, et al (1989) Lokale intraarterielle fibrinolyse bei A. basilaris-Verschluß mit progredientem Hirnstamminfarkt. Akt Neurol 16:184–190
17. Pilz P, Ladurner G, Griebnitz E (1991) Neuropathological findings after thrombolytic therapy in acute ischemic stroke. In: Hacke W, del Zoppo GJ, Hirschberg M (eds) Thrombolytic therapy in acute ischemic stroke. Springer-Verlag, Berlin Heidelberg New York, p 224
18. Ringelstein EB, Biniek R, Weiller C, Ammeling B, Nolte PN, Thron A (1992) Type and extent of hemispheric brain infarctions and clinical outcome in early and delayed middle cerebral artery recanalization. Neurology 42:289–298
19. Theron J, Courtheoux P, Casco A, et al (1989) Local intra-arterial fibrinolysis in the carotid territory. AJNR 10:753–765
20. von Kummer R, Hacke W (1992) Safety and efficacy of intravenous tissue plasminogen activator and heparin in acute middle cerebral artery. Stroke 23:646–652
21. Wolpert S, Bruckmann H, Greenlee R, et al (1992) The neuroradiologic evaluation of patients with acute stroke treated with recombinant tissue plasminogen activator. Am J Neuroradiol (In Press)
22. Yamaguchi T, Minematsu K, Choki J, Ikeda M (1984) Clinical and neuroradiological analysis of thrombotic and embolic cerebral infarction. Jpn Circ J 48:50–58
23. Zeumer H, Frietag H-J, Grzyska M, Neunzig H-P (1989) Local intraarterial fibrinolysis in acute vertebrobasilar occlusion. Neurology 31:336–340

The Prognostic Value of Collateral Blood Flow in Acute Middle Cerebral Artery Occlusion

M. Forsting[1], D. Krieger[2], R. von Kummer[1], W. Hacke[2], and K. Sartor[1]

Recent clinical studies of thrombolysis in acute cerebral ischemia emphasize mostly the efficacy and safety of this kind of treatment [5–7, 11]. The main objective in these studies, designed to find the optimal dose/application form and the best thrombolytic agent in acute stroke, is recanalization. Another important objective is to determine the therapeutic efficacy by correlating infarction size with recanalization. We doubt that the infarction size depends only on the degree of recanalization achieved by thrombolysis. While vascular collateral systems in the cerebral circulation other than the circle of Willis have long been known [4], their role in maintaining the blood supply to the brain in occlusion of cerebral arteries is not entirely clear [2, 12, 13, 15]. The pial anastomoses among the anterior, posterior, and middle cerebral arteries responsible for leptomeningeal collateral blood supply (LCBS) are known as the "circulus arteriosus intrahemisphaericus," or intrahemispheric arterial circle, and can be shown angiographically.

The purpose of our study was to determine the prognostic role of the LCBS in patients with acute occlusion of the M1 segment of the middle cerebral artery (MCA).

Subjects and Methods

We both retrospectively and (in part) prospectively analyzed a subgroup of patients with acute stroke who were referred to us for thrombolytic therapy. Further details of this thrombolytic study are described by von Kummer and coauthors in this issue.

Intra-arterial digital subtraction angiography was performed in all 28 patients within 6 h after onset of stroke symptoms. In all patients the presumably diseased carotid artery and one vertebral artery were injected. Vertebral angiography was considered necessary to fully evaluate the leptomeningeal collaterals of the symptomatic hemisphere.

Department of [1]Neuroradiology and [2]Neurology, University of Heidelberg, Heidelberg, Federal Republic of Germany

G. J. del Zoppo, E. Mori, W. Hacke (Eds.)
Thrombolytic Therapy in Acute Ischemic Stroke II

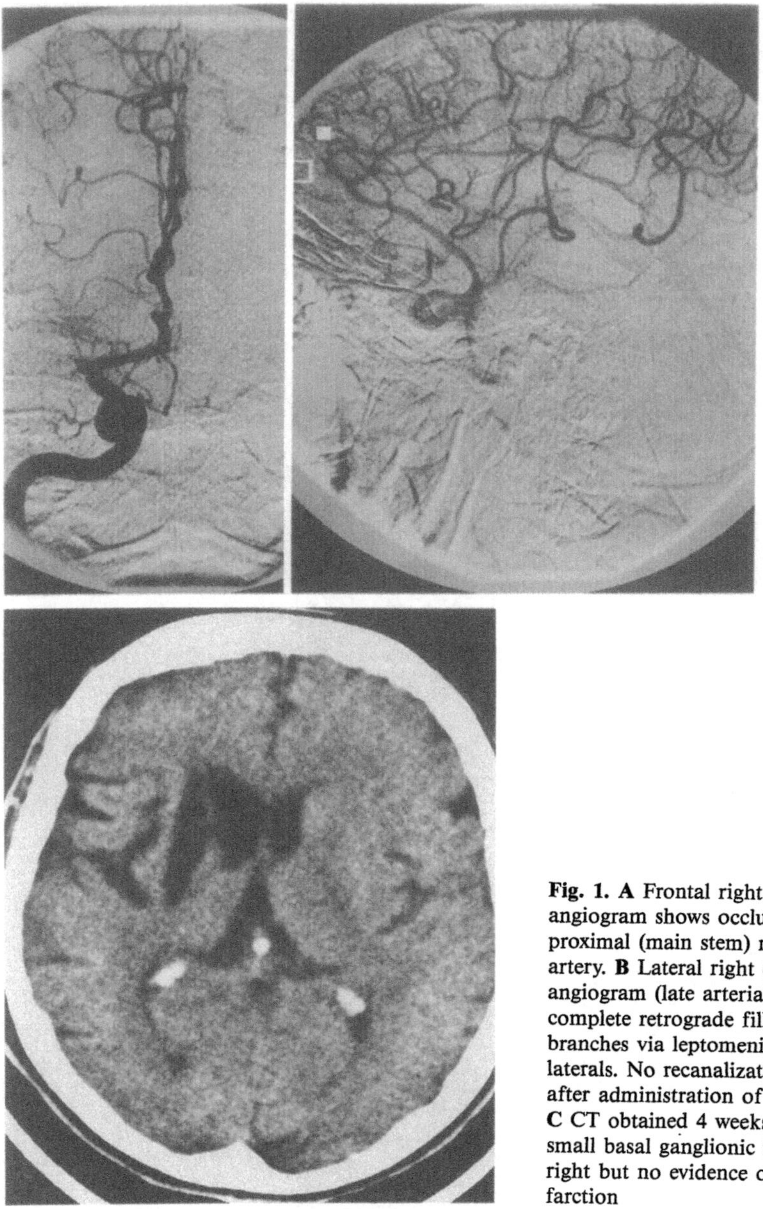

A B C

Fig. 1. A Frontal right carotid angiogram shows occlusion of the proximal (main stem) middle cerebral artery. **B** Lateral right carotid angiogram (late arterial phase) shows complete retrograde filling of MCA branches via leptomeningeal collaterals. No recanalization is visible after administration of 100 mg rt-PA. **C** CT obtained 4 weeks later reveals small basal ganglionic infarct on the right but no evidence of cortical infarction

We included only patients with proximal, or stem, occlusions of the MCA (M1 occlusions) and excluded those with occlusions distal to the origin of the temporal branches.

The degree of leptomeningeal collateral blood supply from the anterior and posterior cerebral arteries was graded according to how complete retrograde filling of the MCA branches was: grade 0 represented complete absence of lep-

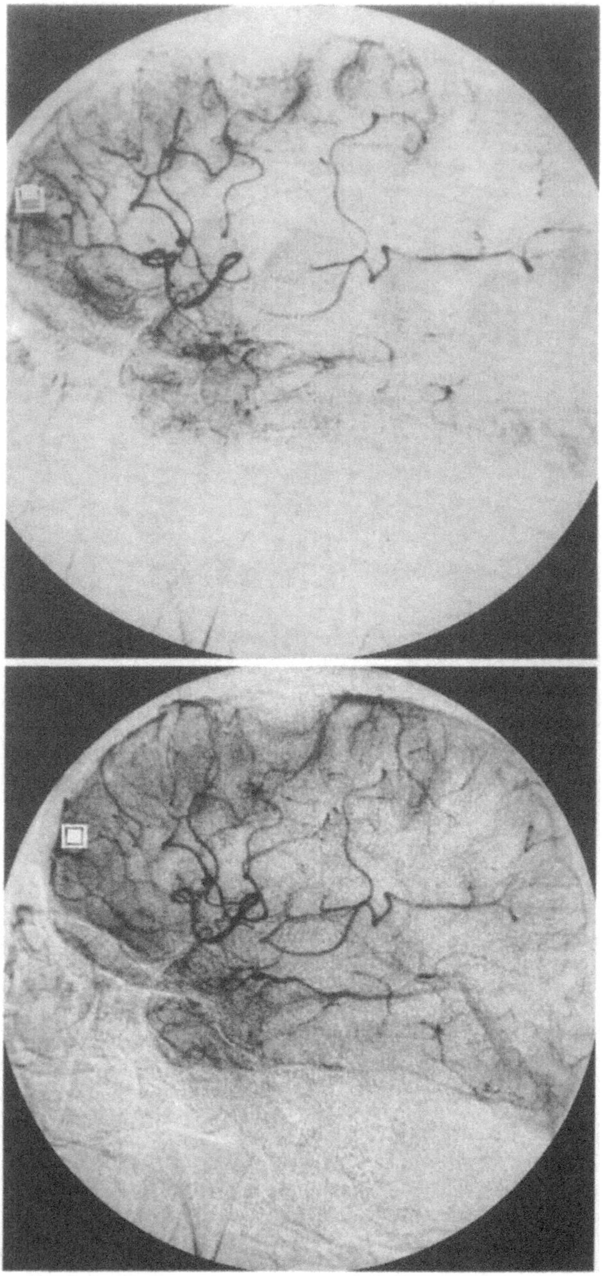

A

B

tomeningeal collaterals; grade 1 represented partial retrograde filling of MCA branches; and grade 2 represented complete retrograde filling of all MCA branches (Figs. 1–3). The final size of the infarcted area was determined by CT or MR about 1 month after the stroke.

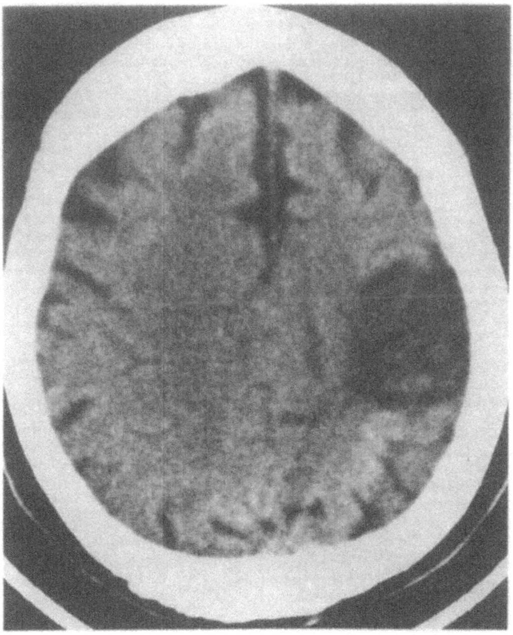

C

Fig. 2A–C. A, B Early (**A**) and late (**B**) phase of a left carotid angiogram in patient with acute occlusion of proximal (main stem) MCA show incomplete retrograde filling of MCA branches via leptomeningeal collaterals; note avascular posterior parietal region. **C** CT obtained 4 weeks later reveals small territorial infarct corresponding to poor leptomeningeal collateral blood supply

Results

The mean age of our 28 patients with acute M1 occlusion (13 men, 15 women) was 56.4 years. Complete recanalization was achieved in 3 patients (11%); partial recanalization in 9 patients (32%); in the remaining 16 patients (57%) the M1 occlusion persisted despite thrombolytic therapy with tissue plasminogen activator (rt-PA). CT or MR eventually showed basal ganglia infarction in 11 patients. Five patients had additional partial hemispheric infarctions, and 12 patients had large territorial infarctions in the supply area of the MCA. Table 1 illustrates the relation between infarction size and LCBS.

Basal ganglia infarctions, the minimal variant of cerebral infarction in MCA occlusion, occurred only in patients who before treatment with rt-PA were

Table 1. Relationship between infarction size nad leptomeningeal collateral blood supply (LCBS) in acute M1 occlusion ($n = 28$)

	Basal ganglionic infarction only	Partial hemispheric infarct	Complete hemispheric infarct
Total	11	5	12
Complete LCBS	11	2	2
Partial LCBS	0	3	4
Absent LCBS	0	0	6

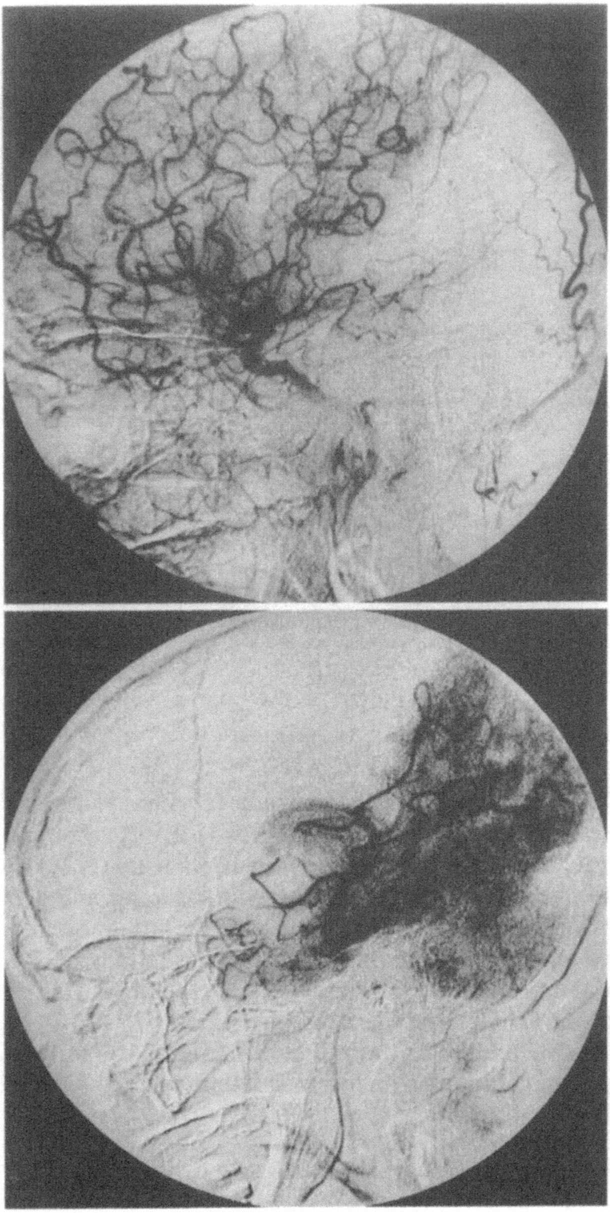

A

B

Fig. 3 A, B. Late arterial phase in left lateral carotid (**A**) and left vertebral (**B**) angiogram in patient with acute occlusion of proximal (main stem) MCA. Reliable determination of degree of leptomeningeal collateral blood supply depends on angiography of both anterior and posterior cerebral circulation. Retrograde filling of posterior parietal MCA branches is visible only on vertebral angiogram

found to have a complete LCBS as manifested on angiography by retrograde filling of MCA branches. Nevertheless, 2 patients out of this group with excellent LCBS developed additional partial infarction, and 2 others developed complete hemispheric infarction. Partial LCBS was associated with partial hemispheric infarction in 3 patients and with complete hemispheric infarction in 4. All patients without any visible LCBS in acute MCA occlusion developed complete hemispheric cerebral infarction. In none of the patients in the latter two groups was the infarction limited to the basal ganglia.

Discussion

The goal of thrombolytic therapy is to promote recanalization of the occluded vessel in order to improve the prognosis of cerebral ischemia. Although recent electrophysiologic findings suggest that ischemic injury to cerebral tissue may be tolerated for longer periods than previously thought [9, 10], thrombolytic therapy may only preserve tissue within the ischemic penumbra. The term "penumbra" designates a region of viable but nonfunctioning cerebral tissue that surrounds a core zone of completed infarction [1, 8]. In a given individual the size of the penumbra may be related to the amount of collateral blood flow. Assuming this to be true, it is still doubtful whether the definitive area of infarction depends *mainly* on the degree of recanalization achieved within a few hours by thrombolytic therapy. Unfortunately, in most previous studies the role of the leptomeningeal collateral anastomoses for the compromised brain area was ignored [5–7, 11]. The purpose of our study was to determine the prognostic value of LCBS in patients with acute occlusion of the MCA main stem. The basal ganglia of the occluded MCA were damaged in all of our patients. Our data confirm the conclusion of Ringelstein and coauthors [12] that infarction of the basal ganglia is unavoidable in proximal MCA occlusion: lenticulostriate vessels are endarteries, and there are thus no available anastomoses for collateral blood supply; correspondingly, "giant lacunes" in the basal ganglia are really territorial infarctions of the lenticulostriate endarteries [3, 13]. In our study cerebral infarction limited to the basal ganglia occurred only in those patients who at early angiography had complete retrograde filling of MCA branches via a functioning LCBS; this type of collateral supply is apparently necessary to limit infarction extent. However, 4 out of 15 patients with pre-therapeutic complete collateral blood supply developed additional partial or complete hemispheric infarctions in the MCA territory despite such a good collateral supply. An explanation for this somewhat surprising observation was recently given by Ringelstein and coauthors [12], who found that the presence of good LCBS does not limit the size of the infarct in every patient but seems to constitute only one of several key factors in the natural history of MCA occlusion. In their opinion LCBS has a powerful but sometimes only temporarily protective effect. Such collateral flow elevates cerebral cortical perfusion from that associated with irreversible cell death to that of the ischemic penumbra, in which the brain parenchyma has a chance of surviving. It is still not known, though, how long functionally paralyzed brain tissue can survive under such conditions [14]. Possibly, the degree of LCBS determines the temporal width of the therapeutic window; in patients with a satisfactory LCBS, thrombolysis may thus be useful even later than 4–6 h after the onset of symptoms.

All patients without angiographically visible LCBS developed large hemispheric infarction. In this situation, according to the above hypothesis, there is probably no ischemic penumbra present. Without an ischemic penumbra, any type of treatment designed to promote recanalization of the occluded artery is useless. Patients with no apparent LCBS may even be harmed by thrombolytic therapy because recanalization increases the likelihood of reperfusion injury, the most important factor for edema formation and hemorrhagic transformation.

In conclusion, our data suggest that the initial degree of LCBS in acute MCA occlusion is an important factor because it modifies the size of cerebral infarction. In patients without angiographically visible LCBS, thrombolytic therapy is probably useless; with or without treatment, these patients are likely to develop large hemispheric infarctions. Thrombolytic therapy may be useful, though, in patients who have visible LCBS, as both hemodynamic decompensation and secondary enlargement of the area of infarction may be avoided. Thus far we have analyzed only a small number of patients. A confirmation of our preliminary results would require that a detailed angiographic analysis of LCBS and recanalization rates be performed both pre- and post-therapeutically in a larger number of patients undergoing treatment with rt-PA for acute ischemic stroke. This systemic angiographic approach may be one way of defining a subgroup of stroke patients who might benefit from thrombolytic therapy.

References

1. Astrup J, Siesjoe BK, Symon L (1981) Thresholds in cerebral ischemia – the ischemic penumbra. Stroke 12(6):723–725
2. Bozzao L, Fantozzi LM, Bastianello S, Bozzao A, Fieschi C (1989) Early collateral blood supply and late parenchymal brain damage in patients with middle cerebral artery occlusion. Stroke 20:735–740
3. Caplan L, Babikian V, Helgason C, et al (1985) Occlusive disease of the middle cerebral artery. Neurology 35:975–982
4. Cobb S (1931) The cerebral circulation: The question of end-arteries of the brain and the mechanism of infarction. Arch Neurol Psychiatr 25:273–284
5. del Zoppo G, Zeumer H, Harker L (1986) Thrombolytic therapy in stroke: Possibilities and hazards. Stroke 17:595–609
6. del Zoppo GJ, Ferbert A, Otis S, et al (1988) Local intra-arterial therapy in acute carotid territory stroke: A pilot study. Stroke 19:307–313
7. del Zoppo GJ, Poeck K, Pessin MS, and 16 coauthors of the rt-PA Acute Stroke Study Group (1992) Recombinant tissue plasminogen activator in acute thrombotic and embolic stroke. Ann Neurol 32:78–86

8. Heiss WD, Rosner G (1983) Functional recovery of cortical neurons as related to degree and duration of ischemia. Ann Neurol 14:294–301
9. Hossmann K-A, Bodsch W, Grosse Ophoff B (1985) Recovery of electrophysiological function and protein synthesis in monkey brain after prolonged ischemia. In: Plum F, Pulsinelli W (eds) Cerebrovascular diseases. Fourteenth Research Conference. Raven Press, New York, p 173
10. Kleihues P, Hossmann K-A, Pegg AE, Kobayashi K, Zimmerman V (1975) Resuscitation of the monkey brain after one hour complete ischemia. III. Indications of metabolic recovery. Brain Res 95:61–73
11. Mori E (1991) Fibrinolytic recanalization therapy in acute cerebrovascular thromboembolism. In: Hacke W, del Zoppo GJ, Hirschberg M (eds) Thrombolytic therapy in acute ischemic stroke. Springer-Verlag, Berlin Heidelberg New York, p 137
12. Ringelstein EB, Biniek R, Weiller C, Ammeling B, Nolte PN, Thron A (1992) Type and extent of hemispheric brain infarctions and clinical outcome in early and delayed middle cerebral artery recanalization. Neurology 42:289–298
13. Saito I, Segawa H, Shiokawa Y, Taniguchi M, Tsutsumi K (1987) Middle cerebral artery occlusion. Correlation of computed tomography with clinical outcome. Stroke 18:863–868
14. Sindermann F, Dichgans J, Bergleiter R (1969) Occlusion of the middle cerebral artery and its branches: Angiographic and clinical correlates. Brain 92:607–620
15. Zülch KJ, Behrend CH (1961) Pathogenesis and topography of anoxia, hypoxia and ischemia of the brain in men. In: Meyer JS, Gastaut H (eds) Cerebral anoxia and electroencephalogram. Charles C Thomas, Springfield, p 144

Morphological Evidence of Progressive Microvascular Impairment in Middle Cerebral Artery Occlusion-Reperfusion *

G. J. del Zoppo [1] and J. H. Garcia [2]

Approximately 80% of patients with focal cerebral ischemia, manifest as acute stroke, have either atherothrombotic or thromboembolic occlusions when examined within 6 h from symptom onset [4, 9]. Recent experience with the intra-arterial and intravenous infusions of fibrinolytic agents in patients with acute focal cerebral ischemia has demonstrated both the feasibility of effecting cerebral arterial reperfusion [3, 4, 13, 20, 21, 25, 27] and the clinical benefit of the procedure [13, 21]. However, residual CT scan abnormalities and neurological deficits have been observed in all studies. Particularly vulnerable is the territory of the lenticulostriate arteries where persistent occlusions exist following M_1 segment middle cerebral artery (MCA) occlusion and reperfusion [29]. This phenomenon is most commonly attributed to the absence of functional collaterals. The status and responses of the downstream microvascular bed to ischemia and reperfusion in this territory are unknown, but both ischemia and reperfusion may contribute to the radiographic and clinical defects detected in the lenticulostriatal territory. Furthermore, it is unknown if microvascular alterations following ischemia/reperfusion might be analogous to those developing in the microvascular beds of other organ systems following similar types of injury.

Since the initial description of the "no-reflow" phenomenon following experimental global cerebral ischemia and reperfusion [1], the pathogenesis of this phenomenon has remained unresolved. Microvascular perfusion defects in other organ systems may develop secondary to perivascular edema [10] or hemorrhage, in situ thrombosis, endothelial tags [7], erythrocyte aggregation, platelet aggregation, polymorphonuclear (PMN) leukocyte– endothelial cell adherence [8, 16, 23], endothelial cell edema [17], and other mechanisms. Recent work in skeletal and cardiac muscle ischemia preparations demonstrated the presence of PMN leukocytes in capillaries and postcapillary venules during

* Supported in part by grant number 1 RO1 NS26945 from the National Institutes of Health. This is publication number 7506-MEM from Scripps Clinic & Research Foundation, La Jolla, California.
[1] Department of Molecular and Experimental Medicine, Scripps Clinic & Research Foundation, La Jolla, CA, USA
[2] Department of Neuropathology, Henry Ford Hospital, Detroit, MI, USA

G. J. del Zoppo, E. Mori, W. Hacke (Eds.)
Thrombolytic Therapy in Acute Ischemic Stroke II

the post-reperfusion period [8, 11, 23, 24]. The potential role of PMN leukocytes in aggravating a cerebral ischemia has been suggested by studies of global ischemia employing either hypotension or air embolism [14], and by at least one intervention study [26]. The participation of PMN leukocytes in the microvascular events initiated by focal cerebral ischemia and reperfusion has not been directly demonstrated until recently [5]. Leukocytes may interact with the vasculature by i) occluding microvessels, and ii) direct contact with endothelial cells via well-defined regulatable adherence complexes (integrins/selectins). Vascular injury and changes in endothelial cell permeability may be partly mediated by these processes. PMN leukocytes and monocytes are known to be involved in the maturation of cerebral infarctions. The parenchymal events attending focal ischemic damage include i) invasion and ii) tissue injury by leukocytes. The timing and the topography of PMN leukocytes into or through the microvasculature and ultimately into the surrounding parenchyma during focal ischemia/reperfusion and focal ischemia is the subject of studies in baboon (MCA : O/R) and rat (MCA : O) models of MCA occlusion. In preparation for therapeutic intervention trials, which may modify PMN leukocytic function and, ultimately, after microvascular patency and parenchymal events, systematic studies of PMN leukocyte function and migration during focal cerebral ischemia have been undertaken.

Leukocytes in Microvascular Occlusions Following MCA Occlusion-Reperfusion (MCA : O/R)

The presence of PMN leukocytes in microvascular obstructions in the periischemic zone following 3-h flow interruption and subsequent 1-h re-establishment of the MCA flow has been evaluated in an established awake nonhuman primate (baboon) model of focal ischemia/reperfusion [5]. With this experimental paradigm, obstructions of the microvasculature by erythrocytes, degranulated platelets, and PMN leukocytes were noted in the periphery of the MCA ischemic zone upon reperfusion, but not within the contralateral nonischemic territory [2]. The relationship of microvascular perfusion defects, consistent with the "no-reflow" phenomenon, and their constituents have been subsequently examined in 4 adolescent male baboons (*Papio anubis/cynocephalus*) [5]. All procedures in the above experiments and those that follow were undertaken after receiving approval of the Institutional Animal Research Committee. All experiments were performed in accordance with guidelines of the National Research Council, the National Institutes of Health Policy in the Humane Care and use of Laboratory Animals, and the USDA Animal Welfare Act.

Quantitation of Microvascular Perfusion Defects

Two groups of 2 animals each were studied to determine the presence of perfusion defects by carbon tracer – fixation technique (patency), and the presence and status of PMN leukocytes by colloidal gold–fixation (occlusion). The surgical preparation of the primate, characteristics and placement of the MCA device, and the details of the experimental procedure have been presented previously [2, 5]. MCA occlusion was performed and maintained for 180 min in the awake animal without use of analeptic agents or compounds with known neuronal protective potential. Each experiment was terminated, under general anesthesia, by pressure perfusion–fixation at 160–220 torr 60 min after MCA balloon deflation and initiation of reperfusion. The 2 perfusion-fixation schemes employed were developed for optimal demonstration of microvascular occlusions (scheme 1: colloidal gold suspension in 2% paraformaldehyde/ 0.5% glutaraldehyde) and microvascular patency (scheme 2: filtered india ink in 2% paraformaldehyde/0.5% glutaraldehyde) under isosmotic conditions [5]. The former strategy was developed for high quality definition of PMN leukocyte and endothelial cell morphology by light and transmission electron microscopy, and the latter to define vascular patency in optimally fixed microvessels. A pre-fixation perfusion flush with isosmotic fluid containing heparin (2 IU/ml) was performed to inhibit thrombosis during perfusion and to remove blood elements prior to fixation. Sections prepared for light microscopy were analyzed with a computer-based video-imaging system comprised of an image-processing unit connected in-line with a Hamamatsu C2400–07 Newvicon NTSC video camera vertically staged on an Axioskop 20 light microscope (Carl Zeiss, Munich). Microvascular occlusions (scheme 1) were readily identified by the presence of packed intravascular erythrocytes. The minimum diameter of occluded leukocyte-containing and patent microvessels was computed by video-image processing. Reconstruction of 10 randomly chosen occluded capillaries from serial 1 μm sections, along a 110 μm length was performed for each vessel. Microvascular patency was tabulated relative to vessel minimum transverse diameter by automatic acquisition from up to 637 fields (526 μm × 491 μm each) at 200x from stereoanatomically identical sites from the ischemic and the nonischemic basal ganglia. Data were plotted in histogram form for vessel diameter frequency distribution, and as "percent reflow," which was defined as the normalized ratio:

$$\left(\frac{\text{patent vessels, ischemic zone}}{\text{patent vessels, non-ischemic zone}}\right) \times 100$$

for each vessel diameter class.

Microvascular Occlusions

Among the experiments conducted to assess microvascular occlusion characteristics, no occlusions were seen in the lenticulostriatal microvascular bed of the nonischemic basal ganglia or temporal cortex. In contrast, PMN leukocyte-containing obstructions were documented in microvessels of capillary diameter (4.0–7.5 μm) and in postcapillary venules (7.5–30 μm) within the ischemic basal ganglia. Among 425 microvessels ⩽10 μm transverse diameter, 8.2%

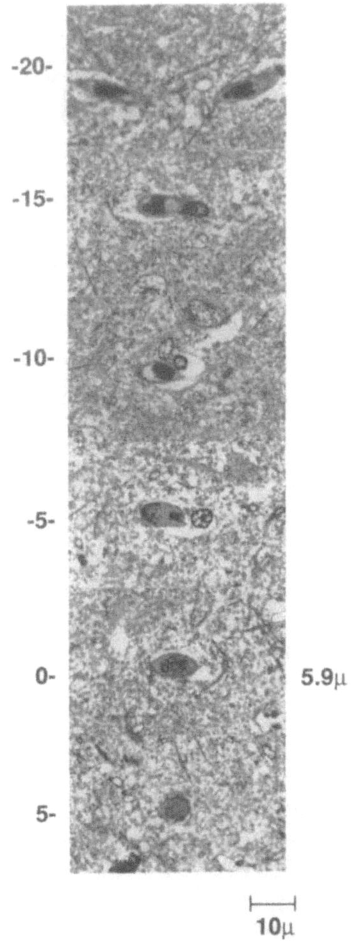

Fig. 1. Reconstruction of occluded capillary (baboon) in postischemia/reperfusion bed of middle cerebral artery from serial transverse sections (light microscopy). The location of a capillary-occluding leukocyte is noted by the reference 0 (*left margin*), and the relative distance of successive sections (in μm) is also shown

contained single PMN leukocytes, completely obstructing 4.7% microvessels of 6.9 ± 1.3 μm diameter and partially obstructing 3.5% microvessels of 10.2 ± 2.0 μm diameter. Among 10 occluded microvessels of capillary diameter reconstructed at 1 μm intervals along a 110 μm length, single PMN leukocytes were seen completely occluding 40% of microvessels 6.4 ± 0.8 μm diameter.

Microvascular obstructions were comprised of individual leukocytes and packed, deformed erythrocytes (Fig. 1). Platelets were not discernible by light microscopy. Electron microscopic evaluation of individual PMN leukocytes and their endothelial contact provided additional insights (Fig. 2). Degranulation of isolated leukocytes was not evident. Extended leukocyte–endothelial cell contact surfaces were apparent with an intercellular gap which ranged from 0 to 160 nm. No endothelial cell swelling or "endothelial tags" were seen in these preparations. In postcapillary venules, a number of PMN leukocytes could be found in direct apposition to the endothelium, none of which alone

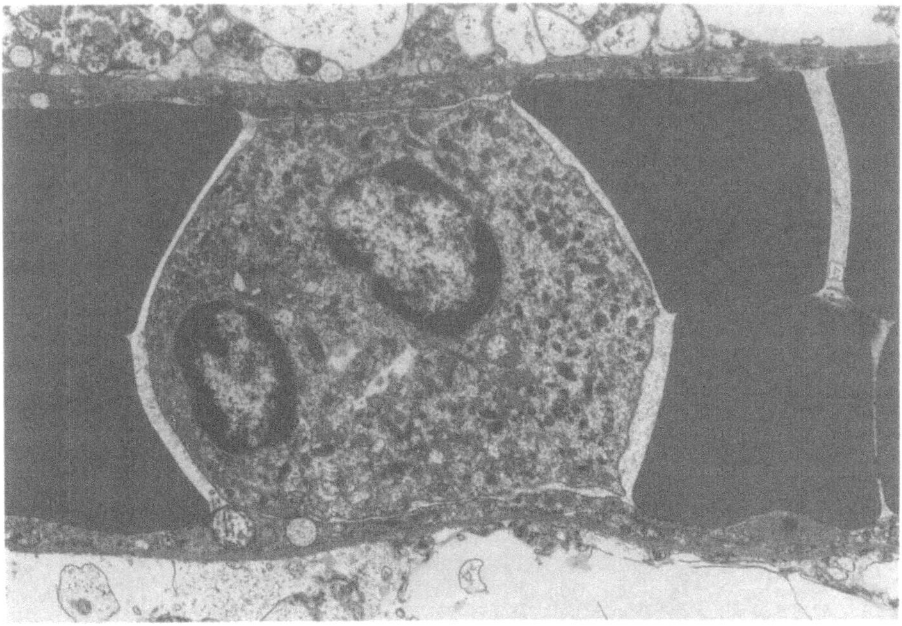

Fig. 2. Longitudinal section of LSA capillary with occluding PMN leukocyte. Capillary diameter = 6.0 μm; leukocyte–endothelial cell contact length = 6.0 μm and 3.6 μm; and leukocyte–endothelial gap = 0–160 nm. Note the three attachment points

completely obstructed the vascular lumen in fields examined (see G.W. Schmid-Schönbein, G. J. del Zoppo, this volume). In other portions of the microvasculature, degranulated platelets associated with fibrin were found in close juxtaposition to PMN leukocytes, which apparently occluded capillaries (Fig. 3). Fibrin was found unusually in other portions of the microvasculature, but not in association with PMN leukocyte-endothelial cell contact. In capillaries where fibrin was seen, it was apparently nonobstructing, but was oriented next to endothelial cells along the axis of the vessel, on either the luminal or the abluminal side (Fig. 4).

Microvascular Patency

Under the identical experimental conditions which demonstrated obstructing PMN leukocytes, microvascular patency was examined. A significant reduction in the numbers of microvessels (all diameter classes ⩽100 μm) was observed after ischemia/reperfusion (Fig. 5). This included vessels of capillary diameter, in which the "percent reflow" was 26.5% and 38.5% of that measured in the contralateral normal basal ganglia in the 2 subjects.

These studies indicate that following MCA occlusion/reperfusion under conditions which produce "no-reflow," as defined by carbon tracer studies,

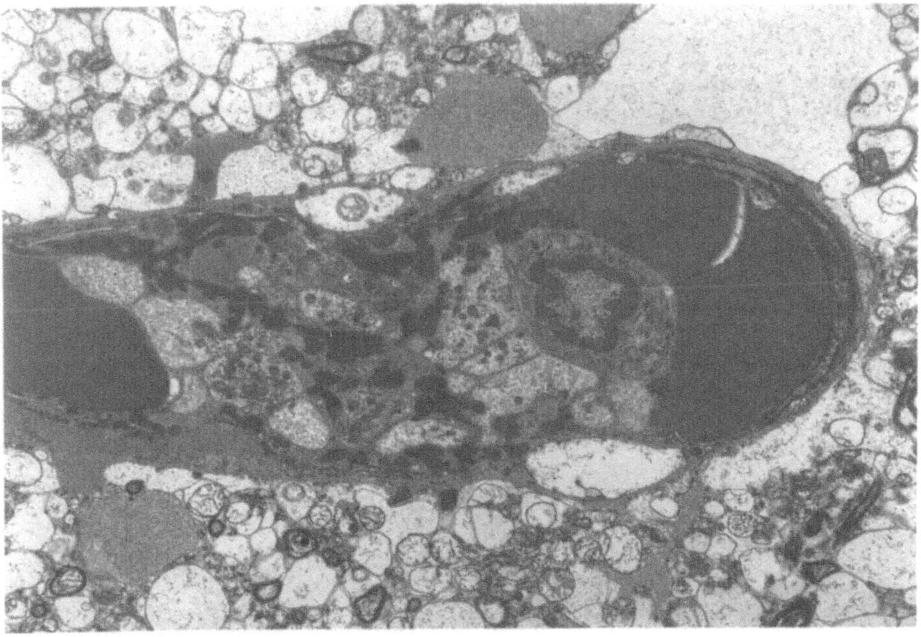

Fig. 3. Longitudinal section of LSA capillary following MCA occlusion/reperfusion, with PMN leukocyte, degranulated platelets, and interposed fibrin. Maximum microvessel diameter = 6.5 μm. No PMN leukocyte attachment in this field. Note lack of endothelial swelling

PMN leukocytes are present in microvessels <100 μm diameter and obstruct capillaries in the focal ischemic zone. Here, PMN leukocytes were observed within 1 h of reperfusion in several configurations: i) as single cells completely obstructing the lumen of a capillary, ii) as single cells partially occluding either postcapillary venules (or precapillary arterioles), iii) as multiple cells attached to the endothelial surface in postcapillary venules, and iv) in association with degranulated platelets and interposed fibrin in microvessels of various diameter. Platelets were not observed as thrombi or in masses, except as noted above. However, a formal electron microscopic reconstruction was not performed. Fibrin, in addition to the above, was seen inconsistently along the luminal endothelial surface, and occasionally along the abluminal side, but not as a part of a platelet thrombus.

The finding of PMN leukocytes in capillaries and microvessels in the ischemic zone only during reperfusion fulfills an essential requirement for postulating their involvement in early microvascular injury following focal cerebral ischemia. These findings are consistent with the observations of PMN leukocytes following ischemia/reperfusion in other organ systems [8, 11, 23, 24]. Capillary obstruction most probably results from the size and specific rheologic properties of PMN leukocytes, whereas the finding of cells in postcapillary venules suggests the interplay of specific leukocyte integrins (e.g., CD11/CD18, Mac 1 adherence complex), and endothelial cell selectins (e.g.,

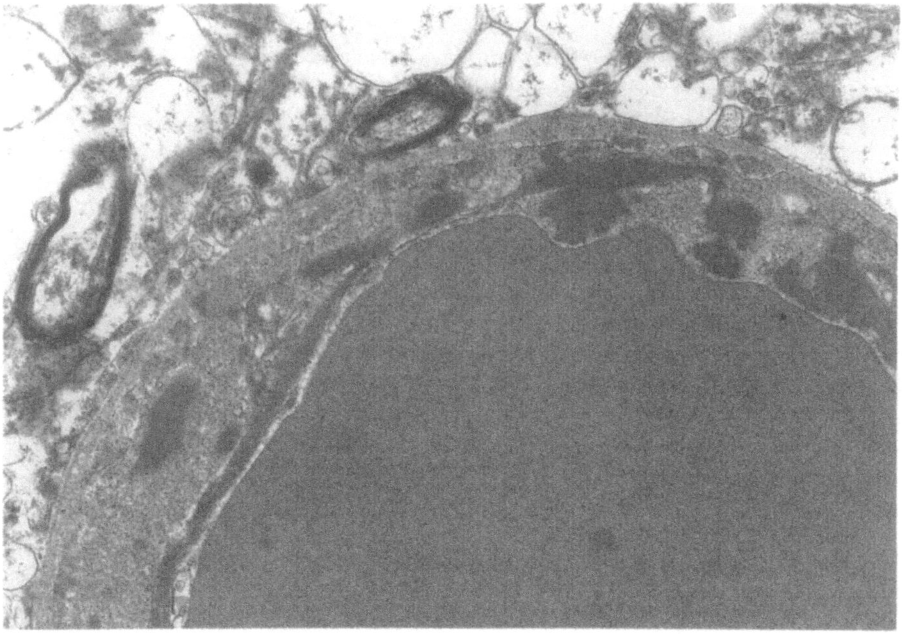

Fig. 4. Transverse section of LSA capillary demonstrating fibrin within the plasma space and in apposition to the endothelium. Lumen contains a distorted erythrocyte. Capillary diameter = 4.8 μm

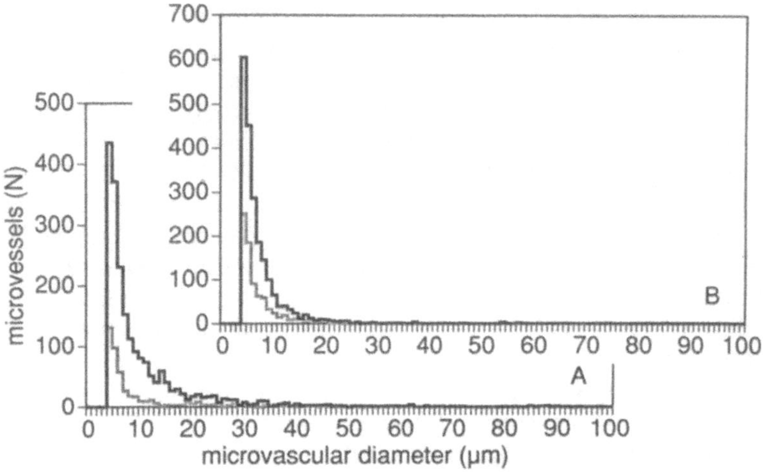

Fig. 5. Relative distribution of microvascular occlusion in two microvascular patency experiments (*A* and *B*)

GMP-140) under conditions of reperfusion [18]. The microvascular configuration of PMN leukocyte involvement in early reperfusion events during focal ischemia suggests approaches which may further define their role in microvascular injury. For this, further studies of PMN leukocyte activation/adherence in focal cerebral ischemia in the setting of MCA : O/R are necessary. Additional basic investigations into the movement of the PMN leukocyte from the microvascular compartment to the parenchyma during the focal cerebral ischemia of MCA occlusion (MCA : O) and MCA occlusion/reperfusion are required to begin defining the consequences of such microvascular events.

PMN Leukocytes in the Development of Focal Infarction Following Permanent MCA Occlusion (MCA O)

The timing, the topographic distribution, and the nature of the cellular inflammatory events in focal ischemia *without* reperfusion has been studied in two groups of adult rats by Dereski and coworkers [6], and Garcia and colleagues [12]. Here, we summarize observations made in a "closed" model of experimental focal ischemia, utilizing laboratory methods that occlude an intracranial artery in the absence of craniotomy or other procedures that may significantly alter the intracranial pressure.

Background

The rodent model of focal brain ischemia used in these studies was described and validated by Zea-Longa and colleagues [28]. The validity of this single vessel occlusion model as a useful paradigm of focal cerebral ischemia rested upon i) the existence of unilateral neurologic deficits in all 70 animals subjected to the experimental procedure, ii) the demonstration of a brain infarct (or area of coagulation necrosis) in 11 animals 72 h after completion of the experimental procedure, and iii) correspondence of the brain infarct to the territory normally supplied by the occluded artery.

Using an identical method of MCA occlusion in the rat, Minematsu and colleagues demonstrated that within 30 min of completing the procedure, brain changes were detectable by magnetic resonance imaging in the MCA territory, and that these changes were reversible upon removal of the arterial occlusion [19].

Additional validation of this model as one that indeed causes focal brain ischemia was obtained by Nagasawa and Kogure [22]. Utilizing ^{14}C-iodoantipyrine autoradiographic methods, the occlusion of the MCA with a nylon monofilament inserted into the right carotid artery caused local CBF to fall below the thresholds of nerve cell injury. Moreover, these authors reported that the local CBF values (within the territory of the occluded artery) were lower

6 h after MCA occlusion than after 3 h. This suggests that in the absence of either additional intracranial manipulations or demonstrable systemic changes, there is a progressive worsening of the circulatory conditions within the area supplied by the occluded artery.

Hossmann [15] suggested that several factors may be responsible for the development of "no-reflow" in previously ischemic tissues. Potential contributors to the "no-reflow" phenomenon include vasospasm (especially affecting arterioles) and occlusion of the vascular lumen by various circulating elements, including erythrocytes, leukocytes, platelets, fibrin, and fragments of endothelial cells that may become detached from the vascular lining. The same factors may be responsible for the progression of the microcirculatory impairment. We agree with Hossmann's observation that there are very few morphologic studies documenting the time-dependent reactions that involve circulating elements in various models of focal brain ischemia.

Middle Cerebral Artery Occlusion

Fifty-eight experimental and 10 control animals were prepared for a study that aimed to define the morphological condition of the microvasculature. The selected subject was the adult Wistar rat (body weight 250–290 g). Focal brain ischemia was induced, under general anesthesia, with halothane by inserting a nylon monofilament (4–0 caliber) into the right carotid artery for a distance sufficient to just reach the exact point of origin of the ipsilateral anterior cerebral artery. The experimental procedure followed the method described by Zea-Longa and coinvestigators [28]. A detailed description of the methods of fixation, tissue preparation, and statistical analysis are provided in a separate publication [12]. Among experimental subjects, the time interval of complete MCA occlusion spanned the period between 30 min and 7 days after MCA occlusion. Control animals were subjected to sham operations. All subjects received an intravenous injection of the 48 kDa macromolecule, horseradish peroxidase (Sigma, St. Louis, MO), to allow assessment of vascular permeability.

Two-thirds of the brains were fixed by cardiovascular perfusion; the remainder by immersion into aldehyde fixatives. Each brain specimen was cut into 7 coronal sections that were embedded in paraffin for light microscopy, except for one section (adjacent to the coronal section showing the lesion) which was used to embed tissue samples in araldite for subsequent electronmicroscopy. Among the brains fixed by immersion, one slab was cut in a vibratome to 50 μm thickness for demonstration of the distribution of horseradish peroxidase that had been infused prior to perfusion fixation.

After locating and measuring the brain lesion by light microscopy, the adjoining brain surface (prepared in 1.0 μm thick sections) was used to identify the topographic location and the number of obstructed microvessels (<50 μm in diameter) in various regions of the ischemic hemisphere. Subsequent electron microscopic evaluation of selected areas defined the nature of the intravascular occlusion and corroborated the data derived from the light microscopic studies.

Focal Ischemic Lesion

We have observed and reported separately [12] that i) the lesioned (injured) brain area grows as a function of time, especially during the period 6 to 24 h after complete MCA occlusion, and ii) coagulation necrosis involving large numbers of neurons does not occur in this model before 12 h.

The cellular inflammatory response that is initiated by occluding an intracranial artery develops as early as 30 min in regions that may be considered the core of the lesion. The numbers of obstructed microvessels, within the area of focal brain ischemia, increases as a function of time (Fig. 6). The topographic distribution of plugged vessels spreads from the pre-optic area to the striatum and, finally, to the cerebral neocortex. In some regions, the number of plugged microvessels reaches 100% as early as 4 h after the occlusion of the parent artery. Erythrocytes, leukocytes, and platelets are all components of the intravascular plugs; the most commonly found type of leukocyte is the PMN leukocyte (Fig. 7), and the vessel type most commonly plugged by these circulating cells is either a capillary or postcapillary venule (Fig. 8). Very few microvessels containing either platelets or fibrin were observed during the initial 6 h.

Finally, the phenomenon of extravasation of circulating macromolecules was limited to the supraoptic region of the ischemic hemisphere and was observed only during the interval 3 to 6 h after MCA occlusion.

These observations further validate this experimental model of focal brain ischemia and begin to clarify some of the morphological alterations occurring in areas of focal ischemia as a function of time. Of interest, a pattern of PMN

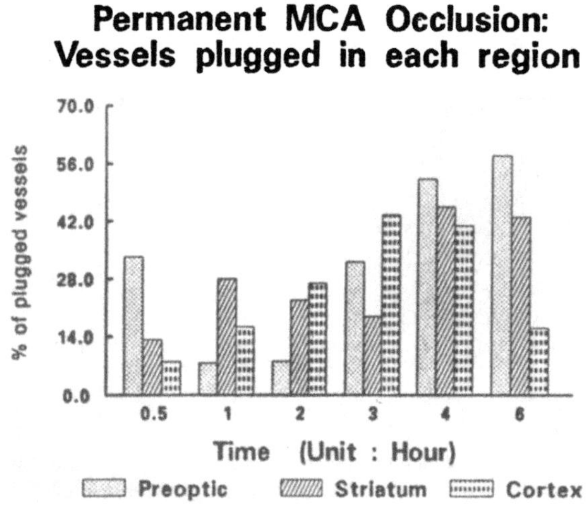

Fig. 6. Histogram depicting the progressive impairment of the microvasculature both as a function of time and location in the hemisphere

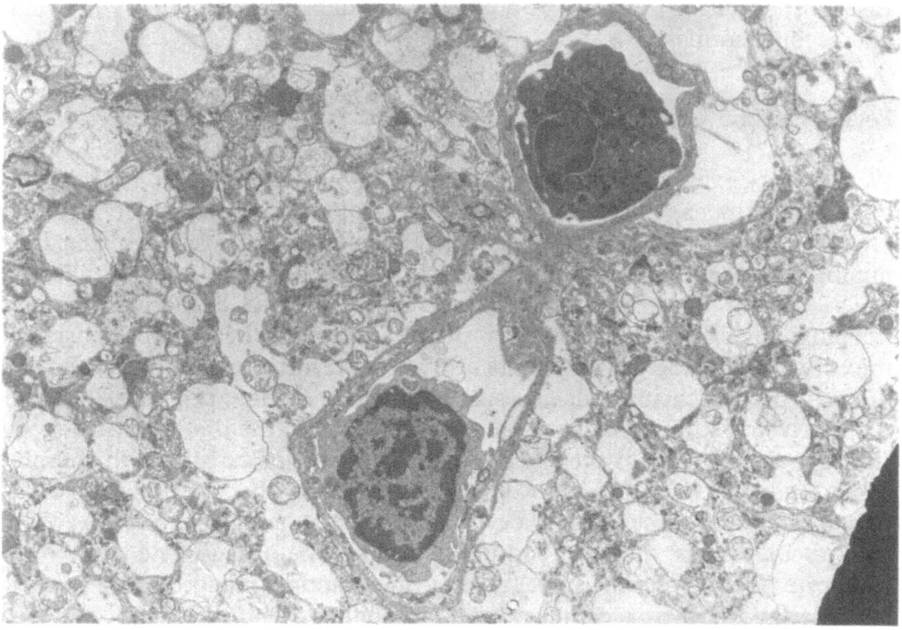

Fig. 7. Striatum (rat), 6 h after permanent occlusion of the MCA. Numerous microvessels ($\leqslant$50 µm diameter) are plugged by leukocytes (original magnification·4500)

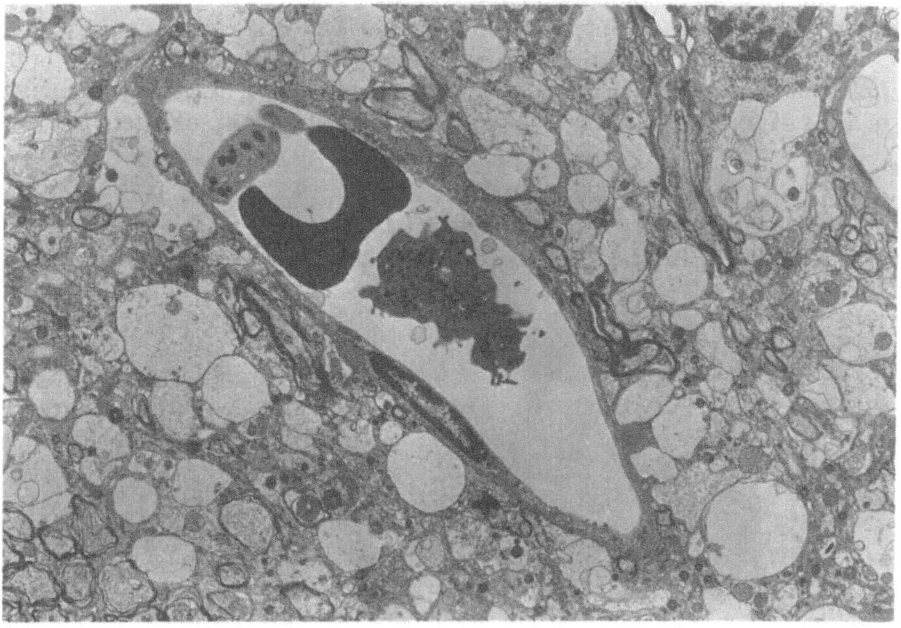

Fig. 8. Preoptic area (rat), 3 h after permanent occlusion of the MCA. A postcapillary venule appears plugged by platelets, erythrocytes, and PMN leukocytes (original magnification·7000)

leukocyte transit emerges which extends from the microvasculature into the injured parenchyma.

Summary

In two animal models of MCA occlusion (reperfusion), the awake nonhuman primate (MCA:O/R) and the anesthetized rat (MCA : O), PMN leukocytes have been observed within microvessels of the ischemic zone very early (30 min) following the onset of ischemia (rat) and early following reperfusion (primates). In the latter, the finding of PMN leukocytes within microvascular obstructions under conditions which produce microvascular perfusion defects suggests a potentially fundamental contribution to "no- reflow" in focal cerebral ischemia. The involvement of leukocytes in capillary obstructions and in postcapillary venules is similar to findings within other organ systems. By example this involves different properties of leukocyte-endothelial cell adherence, which may be differentially amenable to therapeutic abrogation or modulation. The aim of such approaches would be timely reduction of microvascular injury upon reperfusion.

Investigations of the migration of leukocytes into the ischemic parenchyma during MCA : O suggest that the chemoattractant may originate from endothelial cells, and that the progressive parenchymal injury may be related to the increasing numbers of PMN leukocytes that arrive into the area of focal ischemia.

References

1. Ames A, Wright LW, Kowade M, Thurston JM, Majors G (1968) Cerebral ischemia: II. The no-reflow phenomenon. Am J Pathol 52:437–453
2. del Zoppo GJ, Copeland BR, Harker LA, et al (1986) Experimental acute thrombotic stroke in baboons. Stroke 17:1254–1265
3. del Zoppo GJ, Ferbert A, Otis S, et al (1988) Local intra-arterial fibrinolytic therapy in acute carotid territory stroke: A pilot study. Stroke 19:307–313
4. del Zoppo GJ, Poeck K, Pessin MS, and 16 coauthors of the rt-PA Acute Stroke Study Group (1992) Recombinant tissue plasminogen activator in acute thrombotic and embolic stroke. Ann Neurol 32:76–87
5. del Zoppo GJ, Schmid-Schönbein GW, Mori E, Copeland BR, Chang C-M (1991) Polymorphonuclear leukocytes occlude capillaries following middle cerebral artery occlusion and reperfusion in baboons. Stroke 22:1276–1283
6. Deresk MO, Chopp M, Knight RA, Garcia JH (1992) Focal cerebral ischemia in the rat: Evolution and distribution of histopathologic abnormalities. Stroke 23:138 (Abstract)
7. Dietrich WD, Bush R, Yoshida S, Ginsberg MD (1987) Histopathological and hemodynamic consequences of complete versus incomplete ischemia in the rat. J Cereb Blood Flow Metab 7:300–308
8. Engler RE, Schmid-Schönbein GW, Pavelec RS (1987) Leukocyte capillary plugging in myocardial ischemia and reperfusion in the dog. Am J Pathol 111:98–111

9. Fieschi C, Argentino C, Lenzi GL, Sacchetti ML, Toni D, Bozzao L (1989) Clinical and instrumental evaluation of patients with ischemic stroke within the first six hours. J Neurol Sci 91:311–321
10. Fischer EG, Ames A, Hedley-White ET, O'Gorman S (1977) Reassessment of cerebral capillary changes in acute global ischemia and their relationship to the "no-reflow phenomenon". Stroke 8:36–39
11. Gairn JB, Humphrey SM, Kerdson PB (1983) The no-reflow phenomenon in ischemic myocardium. Int Rev Exp Pathol 25:361–383
12. Garcia JH, Yoshida Y, Chen H, Li Y, Zhang AG, Chopp M (1992) Eosinophilic (red) and ghost neurons are delayed effects of focal brain ischemia. J Neuropathol Exp Neurol 51:In Press (Abstract)
13. Hacke W, Zeumer H, Ferbert A, Bruckmann H, del Zoppo GJ (1988) Intraarterial thrombolytic therapy improves outcome in patients with acute vertebrobasilar occlusive disease. Stroke 19:1216–1222
14. Hallenbeck JM, Dutka AJ, Tanishima T, et al (1986) Polymorphonuclear leukocyte accumulation in brain regions with low blood flow during the early postischemic period. Stroke 17:246–253
15. Hossmann KA (1990) Hemodynamics of post ischemic reperfusion of the brain. In: Weinstein PR, Faden AI (eds) Protection of the brain from ischemia. Williams and Wilkins, Baltimore, p 21
16. Kloner RA, Ganote CE, Jennings RB (1974) The "no-reflow" phenomenon after temporary coronary occlusion in the dog. J Clin Invest 54:1496–1508
17. Leaf A (1973) Cell swelling: A factor in ischemic tissue injury. Circulation 48:455–458
18. McEver RP (1991) Selectins: Novel receptors that mediate leukocyte adhesion during inflammation. Thromb Haemost 65:223–228
19. Minematsu K, Yamaguchi T, Omae T (1992) "Spectacular shrinking deficit:" Rapid recovery from a major hemispheric syndrome by migration of an embolus. Neurology 42:157–162
20. Mori E, Tabuchi M, Yoshida T, Yamadori A (1988) Intracarotid urokinase with thromboembolic occlusion of the middle cerebral artery. Stroke 19:802–812
21. Mori E, Yoneda Y, Tabuchi M, et al (1992) Intravenous recombinant tissue plasminogen activator in acute carotid artery territory stroke. Neurology 42:976–982
22. Nagasawa H, Kogene K (1989) Correlation between cerebral blood flow and histologic changes in a new rat model of middle cerebral artery occlusion. Stroke 20:1037–1043
23. Schmid-Schönbein GW (1987) Capillary plugging by granulocytes and the no-reflow phenomenon in the microcirculation. Fed Proc 46:2397–2401
24. Schmid-Schönbein GW, Engler RL (1987) Granulocytes as active participants in acute myocardial ischemia and infarction. Am J Cardiovasc Pathol 1:15–30
25. Theron J, Courtheoux P, Casaseo A, et al (1989) Local intra-arterial fibrinolysis in the carotid territory. Am J Neuroradiol 10:753–765
26. Vasthare US, Heinel LA, Rosenwasser RH, Tuma RF (1990) Leukocyte involvement in cerebral ischemia and reperfusion injury. Surg Neurol 33:261–265
27. von Kummer R, Hutschenreuter M, Wildemann B, Hacke W (1991) Thrombolytic therapy with intravenous recombinant tissue plasminogen activator in acute occlusions of intracranial arteries. J Cereb Blood Flow Metab 9(Suppl):5721
28. Zea-Longa E, Weinstein PR, Carlson S, Cummins R (1989) Reversible middle cerebral artery occlusion without cranectomy in rats. Stroke 20:84–91
29. Zulch K-J (1985) The cerebral infarct: Pathology, pathogenesis, and computed tomography. Springer-Verlag, Berlin Heidelberg New York, p 23

Discussion Summary: Insights into the Pathogenesis of Cerebral Ischemia Relevant to Fibrinolysis

Chaired by J. Toole[1] and T. Yamaguchi[2]

Dr. Asplund reported that artery to artery embolism is increasingly being recognized as a cause of many strokes. In such cases, there is often evidence of microemboli around the zone of infarction, which may cause extension of brain infarct and further clinical deterioration. These microthrombi are best demonstrated in patients who die soon after the onset of stroke and are much more common in patients with large than with small infarcts.

In addition to embolic plugging, there is local vascular reaction from the endothelium caused by thromboxane A2 and other byproducts which results in a further increase of the ischemic area. With occlusion, there is cerebral acidosis with formation of lactate, edema, toxic-oxygen metabolites, and neutrophil activation with release of neurolytic enzymes which contribute to spreading neuronal death. Davalos and colleagues (ref), published in *NEUROLOGY* in 1990, showed a sustained mass effect of the same proportion in 8 h and again in 7 days following a cerebral infarction. In experimental stroke, hypoglycemic animals developed larger infarcts than those maintained at normo-glycemic levels, presumably due to formation of excessive quantities of lactate by anaerobic metabolism.

Dr. Asplund further noted observed a marked reduction in the number of patients who showed early progression of neural deficit following stroke from 35% to 19% for 1980–1990. One explanation for this improvement is increased use of aspirin. Comparison of patients taking and not taking aspirin at the time of entry showed a marked difference, with those using aspirin doing better than those who were not.

Dr. Fieschi, inquiring about the decline in the number of progressive strokes over the years, asked whether the same quantitative examination was performed over the time span. Dr. Asplund replied that the examination protocol was identical so that this was not the variable which accounted for the change.

Dr. Mori then discussed *spontaneous* recanalization of ICA and MCA occlusions. An understanding of this mechanism of spontaneous recanalization is necessary before one can draw conclusions regarding the putative effects of

[1] Department of Neurology, Bowman Gray School of Medicine, Winston-Salem, NC, USA
[2] Cerebrovascular Division, Department of Internal Medicine, National Cardiovascular Center, Suita, Osaka, Japan

G. J. del Zoppo, E. Mori, W. Hacke (Eds.)
Thrombolytic Therapy in Acute Ischemic Stroke II

thrombolytic agents. In a publication in Neurology, 1992, of 34 patients suspected to have acute cardioembolic embolism, 12 satisfied the entry criteria and were randomly assigned to 1 of 3 regimens: high and medium dose-rates of rt-PA or placebo. All were less than 6 h following onset of clinical phenomena, had arteriographic evidence of carotid or MCA occlusion. rt-TPA was given intravenously over the course of 1 h. Antiplatelet treatment was delayed for 24 h. Baseline angiography was performed 1.5 – 6 h after the onset and repeated 30 and 60 min following the start of rt-PA.

In the placebo group, partial recanalization was observed in 1/3 of patients. A review of the literature reveals spontaneous recanalization in from 20% – 70%, a percentage which increases with the interval between baseline and repeat angiogram. Therefore, early spontaneous recanalization must be taken into consideration in the design of all trials regarding the efficacy of thrombolytic agents. Dr. Mori thinks that hemorrhagic transformation may be augmented by fragmentation of the embolus and its lodgement in small distal arteries.

Dr. Hacke discussed embolus subtypes about which there is a limited knowledge. In the literature, only rarely is the stroke subtype, the origin of embolism, or its composition identified. In many studies, emboli are attributed to a cardiac source without any proof.

Among factors influencing the rate of embolism lysis are clot consistency, age, composition, size, location, presence of collaterals, thrombolytic substances and stroke subtype. Many reports identify only the location of the arterial occlusion as ICA or MCA. In the vertebrobasilar system, only two occlusion sites are identified in most reports and the source of emboli has seldom been identified. Isolated extracranial ICA lesions have only rarely been treated. Of the 5 to 6 cases in the literature, in three, the lesion was considered to be hemodynamic in etiology.

Dr. Hacke observed that there are reports of attempts at recanalization of patients suffering with lacunar stroke. He believes that between 60% and 90% of patients in the carotid territory have cardiogenic embolism, whereas in the vertebrobasilar territory, about 60% are embolic and 40% local thrombosis. Detailed cardiac examinations have not routinely been performed but it has been commonly believed that if the patient has atrial fibrillation, the stroke is the result of embolism. This is probable, but it has not yet been proved.

Dr. Ringelstein suggested that cardiac emboli are associated with earlier recanalization compared with artery-to-artery embolism so that the source of the embolus is of importance in designing studies to determine the efficacy of rt-PA. Most distally located emboli and occlusions are more easily lysed than those that are proximal. Smaller clots are more easily recanalized than larger ones because the thrombolytic substance can perfuse it more easily.

Of the patients in Dr. Hacke's study, even those who have spontaneous recanalization do poorly with regard to clinical outcome. The question is whether cardiac emboli are all of the same age or whether some are fresh and some are old. The same may also be true of artery-to-artery embolism from the carotid bifurcation.

Dr. Minamatsu presented data regarding the spectacular shrinking deficit (SSD). Some patients have an extreme deficit which improves remarkably rapidly, perhaps the result of migration of embolism through the vascular system, particularly the carotid system. In an analysis of patients admitted within 6 h of stroke onset, patients who had a rapid recovery were compared with those who had no recovery. This recovery was durable over time, in contrast with that of the patients who had fixed deficits in the first 24 h after onset. The present studies suggested that young nondiabetic men have the potential for SSD. Those emboli depend upon the nature and size of the atherosclerotic material, concomitant atherosclerosis, coagulability, and the size of the vessel involved.

Dr. Pessin described hemorrhagic transformation of ischemic infarction which is the principal concern in thrombolytic therapy for acute stroke. Hemorrhagic transformation of the infarction was classified as: 1) hemorrhagic infarction or 2) parenchymatous hematoma. This is an important differentiation because the CT pattern, clinical consequences, and pathogenesis may differ.

In the rt-PA Acute Stroke Study Group study, 10 of 104 (9.6%) patients receiving rt-PA showed clinical and neurological deterioration. Among the hemorrhagic infarction patients, 19% worsened, while among the hematoma patients, 55% worsened. In the NIH-sponsored rt-PA trial, the complication rate was 3.6%, perhaps related to the abbreviated time to treatment. In the aggregate, the incidence of hemorrhagic complications are about 10% which may represent the ultimate risk of treatment in this time frame. Patients treated at or after 6 h have a higher incidence of hemorrhagic transformation than those treated more rapidly.

Dr. Forsting discussed the prognostic value of collateral blood supply for determination of the therapeutic window. All patients without angiographic evidence of collateral blood supply at the time of MCA occlusion suffered with complete MCA infarction despite the use of rt-PA. It may well be that such patients are harmed by fibrinolysis so that a criterion for its utilization could be the presence of collateral circulation which maintains a certain degree of cortical perfusion protecting the ischemic penumbra from terminal cell death.

Dr. del Zoppo presented the morphologic evidence of progressive microvascular impairment during ischemia and discussed the effect of recanalization on the downstream microvasculature and the effect of vascular injury upon infarct size. There is evidence that activated polymorphonuclear (PMN) leukocytes play a role in plugging the microvasculature or the extracellular space when they are activated by ischemia. This, therefore, leads to the theoretical possibility that PMN leukocytes may contribute to the infarction size by blocking reperfusion. Heretofore, most attention has been paid to the large vessels, whereas the microvasculature constitutes 90% of the total vasculature of the body and has been largely ignored because of the emphasis on arteriographic visualization. Using carbon black to measure the degree of vascular reperfusion, a binary model for computer analysis can be used to produce a vascular profile for the degree of vascular patency. In animals with 3 h ischemia followed by 1 h perfusion, there is a 30% – 40% reflow with 60% – 70% no-reflow in the area previously occluded. What prevents reperfusion? Often it is

PMN leukocytes, typically 10–12 μ in diameter which cannot traverse through slow flowing capillaries. Furthermore, multiple PMN leukocytes are found attached to the post-capillary venules which, in addition to fibrin and degranulated platelets, may form an obstructing mass.

Dr. Garcia described a rat model with a monofilament threaded through the carotid into the intracranial arteries. There PMN leukocytes remain as long as 7 days after the onset of the infarction. They contain large amounts of glycogen as if they were preparing themselves for sustaining metabolism at the neurons. These occur only in capillaries and venules, never in arteries or arterioles and appear as early as 30 min after the onset of ischemia.

During the discussion, Dr. Toole observed that many patients who have clinical embolic events have preceding microemboli which can be detected by Doppler ultrasonography (which can differentiate whether emboli are coming from a cardiac or arterial source). Some of these may result in asymptomatic (silent) cerebral infarctions.

Dr. Ferraro (Mexico City) asked whether hemorrhagic transformation of infarcts differs in its frequency with intravenous versus intra-arterial rt-PA, and whether the presence of collateral circulation indicated by angiography has a prognostic value for neurological outcome. Dr. Pessin replied that the difference between the intra-arterial and the intravenous routes is that the recanalization frequency is greater with intra-arterial delivery, but the incidence of hemorrhagic events between the two is about the same.

Dr. Verstraete observed that spontaneous recanalization in the carotid artery appears to occur within the first 48 h after the occlusion, whereas in the coronary arteries it occurs after the first week. He wonders if this is, in fact, the case. Dr. Mori replied that it may be due to selection bias because patients for inclusion very early in the course of stroke are more likely to recanalize. It also depends upon the etiology of the occlusion which, in the case of embolism, may be more easily recanalized than thrombus. Dr. Fieschi suggested further that it is the rapidity with which angiography is performed: if performed within 3 h, there is more recanalization [in the carotid arteries] than at 6 h.

Dr. Fieschi asked Dr. Forsting whether SPECT, instead of angiography, would not be the procedure of choice to determine whether collaterals existed so that patients could be selected for rt-PA. Whereupon Dr. Williams inquired whether methods to improve collateral flow with either hypervolemic therapy or vasodilators would be useful.

The possibility of cerebral arterial reperfusion raised the possibility that microvascular events may be important. Dr. Grotta asked if the PMN leukocyte plugging of capillaries, or cytotoxicity from these cells, might play a role in the breakdown of the blood/brain barrier and deterioration of the patient. Dr. Garcia replied that the PMN leukocytes occlude the vessels so there is no flow. At present there is no direct information or method for testing this question in the cerebral microvasculature.

Regarding the appearance of hemorrhagic transformation, Dr. Molinari asked Dr. Pessin what the latency between the onset of ischemia and the appearance of life-threatening parenchymatous hematoma was in the rt-PA Acute

Stroke Study Group study. Dr. Pessin replied that it was 4.5 h. Within 30 min of receiving the rt-PA, the patient sneezed, and subsequently deteriorated. In another case, it was 4 to 5 h. Dr. Molinari then inquired whether the homogeneous consistency of hematoma observed on CT scan was due to hemorrhage of the deep gray matter, whereas in the cortex it was more stippled because of diapedesis. Dr. Pessin suggested that the bleeding in the deep gray matter in the one instance that he showed was due to a ruptured artery, rather than capillary extravasation.

Diagnosis and Assessment of Outcomes in Acute Cerebral Ischemia

The Relevance of CT Scanning and Angiography for Patients with Acute Stroke Treated with Recombinant Tissue Plasminogen Activator

S.M. Wolpert[1] and M.S. Pessin[2] for The rt-PA Acute Stroke Study Group

We recently carried out a multicenter dose-escalation study to evaluate the efficacy of intravenous recombinant tissue plasminogen activator (rt-PA; duteplase) administered within 8 h of the onset of symptoms in patients without CT signs of cerebral hemorrhage and with angiographically demonstrated acute thrombotic or embolic arterial occlusion [1, 2]. All patients had CT scans prior to entry into the study, pre- and posttreatment angiograms, and CT scans at 24 h following therapy. The significance of the appearance on the CT scans and angiograms of signs of early ischemia, the presence of a hyperdense middle cerebral artery sign (HMCAS), the site of the occluded arteries, the incidence and site of the recanalization, and the size of infarcts following therapy forms the substance of this report.

Subjects and Methods

One hundred twelve of 139 patients (80%) with symptoms of acute focal cerebral or brain stem ischemia within 8 h of the anticipated time of commencing the rt-PA infusion, and with normal cranial CT scans, had occluded extra- or intracranial arteries. Eight patients were excluded from further study because of arterial dissections ($n = 6$) or incidental aneurysms ($n = 2$), and 11 patients were excluded because of suspected drug allergy, angiographic complications, and other reasons [1]. Thus, 93 patients fulfilled all study criteria, completed the rt-PA infusion, and were available for final analysis.

Two abnormalities were evaluated retrospectively on the initial CT scans taken prior to initiation of therapy: 1) signs of early ischemia (i.e., sulcal effacement with loss of the gray-white matter differentiation), and 2) a HMCAS indicative of a presumed thrombotic occlusion within the middle cerebral artery (MCA) stem. The size of the infarcts were also assessed on CT scans obtained 24 h following initiation of the fibrinolytic therapy. The angiograms were examined for the extent of angiographic perfusion before and after rt-PA therapy.

Department of [1]Radiology and [2]Neurology, Tufts University School of Medicine, New England Medical Center Hospitals, Boston, MA, USA

G.J. del Zoppo, E. Mori, W. Hacke (Eds.)
Thrombolytic Therapy in Acute Ischemic Stroke II

The following were examined:

1. The relationship between early signs of ischemia and size of the infarct;
2. The relationship between the presence of a HMCAS indicating the angiographic occlusion site and the size of the infarct;
3. The relationship between recanalization and site of occlusion; and
4. The relationship between recanalization and the size of the infarct.

The comparisons for the nominal data sets were made with the Yates corrected chi-square test, two-tailed. Comparisons for the continuous data sets were made using Student's *t*-test, two-tailed. For both, significance was set at $2p < 0.05$.

Results

Early Signs of Ischemia and Size of Infarct. The mean size of the infarcts in the patients with the early signs of ischemia was 121.5 cm^3, and 57.4 cm^3 in the patients without early signs. These differences were significant ($2p = 0.0006$).

HMCAS, Angiographic Location of Occlusion, and Size of Infarct. The sign was present in 16 of 60 patients with documented occlusion of the MCA stem or division. Patients with HMCAS had larger infarcts (mean size = 116 cm^3) than those without HMCAS (mean size = 65.6 cm^3) ($2p = 0.092$).

Recanalization and Site of Occlusion. Recanalization of arteries occurred more frequently with intracranial occlusions (30 of 70) than with extracranial occlusions (2 of 23) ($2p = 0.012$).

Recanalization and Size of Infarct. Patients with recanalized arteries had smaller infarcts (mean size = 54.4 cm^3) than patients without recanalized arteries (mean size = 90.4 cm^3) ($2p = 0.094$).

Discussion

Patients with early CT signs of ischemia had larger infarcts than those without such signs, suggesting that the presence of early ischemia indicates a relatively large area of morphological and perhaps irreversible changes in the brain.

The HMCAS has been reported as the harbinger of a large infarct in the middle cerebral artery distribution. The sign, which corresponds to the clot itself [3], was seen in 16 of 60 patients with documented occlusion of the middle cerebral artery or its divisions. As observed by others [3, 6] the sign was more frequently found in patients who subsequently developed large infarcts than in those who developed small infarcts, although we did not find this association to be significant.

Recanalization of occluded arteries occurred more frequently with distal than with proximal occlusions. Mori and coworkers [4] also reported that MCA occlusions recanalized more frequently than internal carotid artery occlusions. Conceivably, the more effective access of rt-PA to the thrombus when it was located intracranially, rather than in the extracranial carotid artery where a long segment of the artery usually is occluded, could account for those differences. Another reason may be the resistance to rt-PA therapy of large atheromatous-based extracranial thrombi compared to smaller occlusions of the intracranial arteries unrelated to an underlying atheromatous substrate.

We found that smaller infarcts were associated with recanalized arteries. This suggests either that there may be an increased tendency for distal arterial occlusions to respond to thrombolysis leading to prevention of neuronal tissue, or that infarct size reflects the limited vascular territory at risk from distal occlusions regardless of thrombolysis.

In this paper, we did not primarily address the relationship among the three variables of early signs of ischemia, the HMCAS, and the site of the angiographically documented occlusion with the site and nature of the hemorrhagic transformations (hemorrhagic infarction and hematoma). These relationships are reported elsewhere in these proceedings [5].

In conclusion, signs of early ischemia, but not the presence of a HMCAS, on CT scans in patients with acute atherothrombotic and embolic stroke are associated with relatively large infarcts. Recanalization of occluded arteries is more frequent with distal than with proximal occlusions. Finally, recanalization, probably because it occurs more frequently with distal than with proximal occlusions, may lead to relatively small infarcts.

Acknowledgements. The author wishes to thank the members of the rt-PA Acute Stroke Study Group and the sponsor as indicated in the Appendices of del Zoppo and colleagues [1] and Alberts (this volume).

References

1. del Zoppo GJ, Poeck K, Pessin MS, and 16 coauthors of the rt-PA Acute Stroke Study Group (1992) Recombinant tissue plasminogen activator in acute thrombotic and embolic stroke. Ann Neurol 32:78–86
2. Wolpert SM, Bruckmann H, Greenlee R, Wechsler L, Pessin MS, del Zoppo GJ, and the rt-PA Acute Stroke Study Group (1993) Neuroradiologic evaluation of patients with acute stroke treated with recombinant tissue plasminogen activator. AJNR 14:2–13
3. Leys D, Pruvo JP, Godefroy O, Rondepierre P, Leclerc X (1992) Prevalence and significance of hyperdense middle cerebral artery in acute stroke. Stroke 23:317–324
4. Mori E (1991) Fibrinolytic recanalization therapy in acute cerebrovascular thromboembolism. In: Hacke W, del Zoppo GJ, Hirschberg M (eds) Thrombolytic therapy in acute ischemic stroke. Springer-Verlag, Berlin Heidelberg New York, p 137
5. in MS, Wolpert SM (1992) The significance of various factors associated with hemorrhagic transformation in patients treated with tissue plasminogen activator for acute stroke. In: 2nd International Symposium on Thrombolytic Therapy in Acute Ischemic Stroke (these Proceedings)
6. Tomsick T, Brott T, Barsan W, Broderick J, Haley EC, Spiller J (1992) Thrombus localization with emergency cerebral CT. Am J Neuroradiol 13:257–263

Recanalization of the Embolically Occluded Middle Cerebral Artery in Acute Stroke Patients: Noninvasive Assessment and Outcome

E. B. Ringelstein, R. Biniek, B. Ammeling, and P. N. Nolte

The timing of spontaneous recanalization of an embolically occluded intracerebral artery is unknown, as is modification of the size of the infarction and the clinical course by the rapidity and degree of reperfusion. Most recanalized middle cerebral arteries (MCAs), after arterioarterial or cardiogenic embolic occlusions, occur within the first days [3, 5, 7, 12]. Even under favorable conditions, however, severely ischemic brain tissue can not survive longer than several hours [1, 6], and rapid recanalization of the embolically occluded brain arteries at an early time would be expected to be decisive for recovery. The quality of the leptomeningeal anastomoses, particularly during the first hours, is another important factor modifying both the size of infarction and clinical outcome [2, 11].

In evaluating the clinical role of flow renewal following acute MCA occlusion, we prospectively investigated a series of 34 patients with embolism into the main stem or major branches of the MCA by means of close-meshed transcranial Doppler (TCD) sonography studies, cerebral arteriography, brain imaging on CT, and clinical tests to analyze the precise time course and effect of MCA recanalization and its impact on infarct size and prognosis. We tried to estimate the time window within which recanalization of the MCA would be beneficial for the patient. Such knowledge would have relevance to any acute treatment in ischemic hemispheric strokes.

Subjects and Methods

Thirty-four consecutive patients with an acute stroke due to occlusion of the MCA were recruited. Inclusion criteria were: 1) exactly defined and witnessed time of onset of stroke, 2) complete clinical, ultrasound, and CT investigations available within 24 h after stroke onset, at the latest, 3) a visible infarction on initial or repeat CT, and 4) MCA occlusion on admission documented by either initial cerebral arteriography ($n = 21$) or TCD sonography ($n = 13$).

Department of Neurology Klinikum RWTH, University Hospital Aachen, Aachen, Federal Republic of Germany

G. J. del Zoppo, E. Mori, W. Hacke (Eds.)
Thrombolytic Therapy in Acute Ischemic Stroke II

A neurological examination was performed and was repeated subsequently in close temporal connection with each repeat TCD study (see time schedule below). Surviving patients were reexamined 10 months after the ictus. Clinical findings were scored according to a modification of the Scandinavian Stroke Assessment Scale, ranging from 13 for normal findings to 0 for death [10]. Extracranial Doppler sonography, arteriography in most cases, and echocardiography were used as diagnostic tests to relate stroke etiology to either large-vessel atherothrombosis of the ipsilateral internal carotid artery (ICA) or cardiac embolism. The cause of stroke remained undetermined if these diagnostic tests revealed normal findings.

Ultrasound Evaluations

For ultrasound evaluation of the middle cerebral artery, TCD sonography was performed via the transtemporal approach according to a technique recently described [9]. An occlusion of the MCA was diagnosed if at least two of the following criteria were fulfilled: 1) Absence of any signal in the MCA area at insonation depths of 35 to 50 mm. This criterion was an absolute prerequisite.

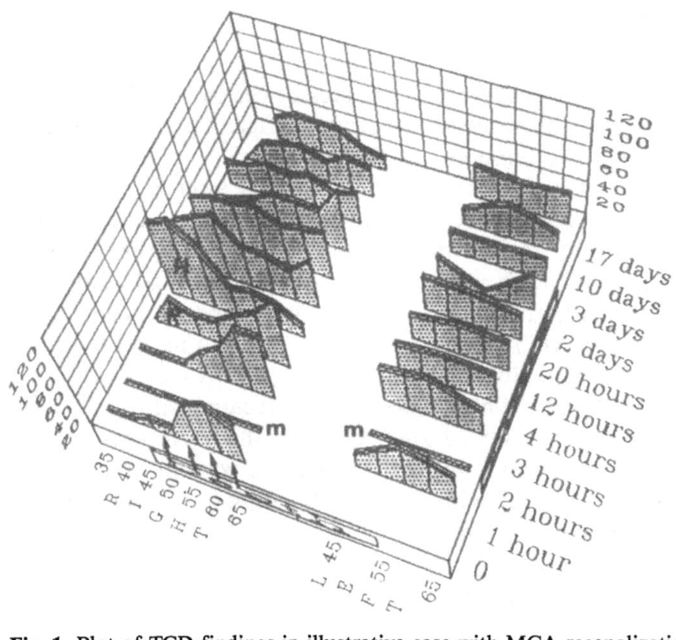

Fig. 1. Plot of TCD findings in illustrative case with MCA recanalization. At corresponding insonation depths (35 – 50 mm) on the left (*abscissa*), no MCA flow signal was available within the first 3 h. At the same time, a flow velocity signal could be derived from the carotid siphon (corresponding to 55, 60 and 65 mm insonation depths). After 4 h partial recanalization (*P*) occurred and changed to hyperperfusion (*H*) during the following 36 h (maximum at 12 h). *m*, missing values; *o*, time of onset of stroke on z axis; *ordinate* , flow velocity in cm/s; *left*, unaffected side

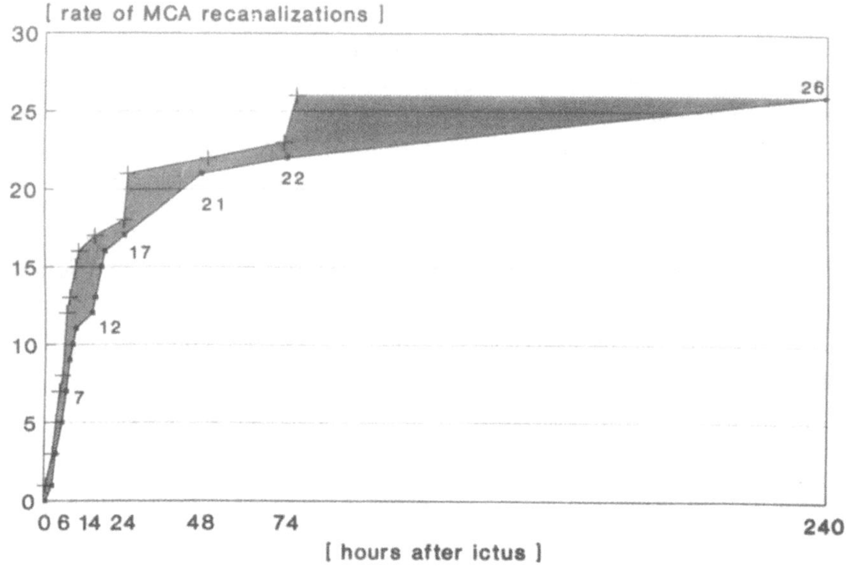

Fig. 2. Frequency of MCA recanalization versus time ($n = 34$). The *hatched zone* indicates the recanalization period, i.e., the time span within which reopening of the MCA must have occurred. The majority of cases (21/34) had MCA recanalization within the first 48 h. Only the first 240 h are plotted on *abscissa* (from [10])

2) Demonstration of a flow signal from the posterior cerebral and/or anterior cerebral arteries. The latter was necessary to prove sufficient penetration of the ultrasound beam through the temporal bone.

Repetitive TCD flow velocity studies were performed after 2, 3, 4, 12, 20, and 44 h (Fig. 1). Further checks were performed on days 3, 10, and 17. A so-called recanalization period was defined within which recanalization must have occurred. This period began with the time of the last TCD study when the MCA was still occluded, and ended with the first reappearence of a flow signal within the occluded MCA during repetitive TCD studies (Fig. 2). Accordingly, patients were arbitrarily subdivided into 3 groups with "very early" (<4 h), "early" ($\geqslant 4$ to 8 h), or "late" ($\geqslant 8$ h) MCA recanalization. Low-flow was defined as a flow velocity slower than 80% of the corresponding contralateral MCA flow velocity value. Full recanalization was specified as soon as flow velocities were identical with or slightly higher than on the contralateral side, and hyperperfusion was defined as flow velocities within a previously occluded MCA exceeding corresponding flow velocities of the nonaffected hemisphere by more than 20%.

Neuroradiological Investigations

CT was immediately performed after admission, and, if negative, was repeated the following day and 1 week later. The size of the definite final infarct was roughly quantified from 1 to 4 according to the involvement of the MCA subareas (lenticulostriate artery territory, and anterior, middle, and posterior part of the MCA-supplied cortex).

A subset of 21 patients was initially subjected to selective 2-plane intracarotid digital subtraction arteriography via the transfemoral route, including the late venous filling phase. All angiograms were done within 6 h after the acute onset of stroke. Occlusions of the origin of the MCA, or of the main trunk of the MCA distal to the lenticulostriate arteries, and of the M2 segments of the MCA were differentiated. The degree of leptomeningeal collateralization on the initial arteriograms was quantified as good, moderate or poor. "Good" means at least two or more major MCA branches showing retrograde filling, "moderate" if only one branch occurred on the venogram, and "poor" if this was not the case.

Results

Eighteen men (aged 61±8 years) and 16 women (aged 54±14 years) were recruited. Fifteen patients were treated with rt-PA (duteplase) according to a protocol described elsewhere, the remaining 19 patients underwent immediate therapeutic heparinization for at least 2 weeks with aPTT values 2 to 3 times normal control.

On admission, the initial neurological scores were 5.9±1.8 for the rt-PA group ($n = 15$) and 4.4±1.6 for the heparin group ($n = 19$), indicating a significantly worse impairment in the latter. This finding kept us from performing further comparisons between both groups in terms of infarct size and final outcome.

A large proportion of MCA occlusions (35%) were of cardiac origin. Patients had nonvalvular atrial fibrillation ($n = 6$), severe aortic and mitral valve disease ($n = 3$), intracardiac thrombi ($n = 3$), and recent myocardial infarction ($n = 1$). In these 12 cases, a cardiac source of embolism was also highly probable for clinical reasons. Fifteen patients (44%) had suffered secondary arterioarterial embolism from extracranial ICA lesions (13 ICA occlusions, 1 dissection, 1 high-grade ICA stenosis). In 7 cases, the etiology of MCA occlusions remained unknown, but in 6 out of the 7 subsequent rapid recanalization made in situ thrombosis of the MCA very improbable.

Depending on the site of occlusion within the MCA, the size and the topographic distribution of ensuing lesions varied considerably but shared certain uniform features. Patients with proximal MCA occlusion (18 of 21) always developed ischemic damage at least in the territory of the deep perforators, irrespective of the rapidity of MCA recanalization. In 5 of these patients, the "large striatocapsular infarct" was seen without cortical involvement. It became evident that proximal MCA occlusions nearly always led to infarctions involving the striatum and internal capsule, whereas more distally located emboli/thromboses (3 of 21) led to infarctions of the white matter and cortex, sparing the lenticulostriate territory.

Twenty-two patients (65%) showed recanalization of their occluded MCA within three days (Fig. 2). This proportion rose to 26 (76%) within the entire 17-day observation period.

A striking hyperperfusion after recanalization was seen in 15 cases (44%) (Fig. 1), and occurred from 95±99 h (range, 4 to 322; median, 49) to 270±132 h (range, 22 to 410; median 241) after the ictus.

If only patients with an MCA recanalization within the first 20 h ($n = 16$) were considered, a trend became evident that the more rapidly the recanalization occurred, the smaller the size of the infarct (p-value 0.06, Spearman rank correlation coefficient).

In the following, only patients in whom the MCA reopened within 3 days ($n = 22$) were considered. Four patients with so-called large striatocapsular infarctions were selectively considered and compared with the remaining 18 patients with more extended types of infarctions. In the first group, mean recanalization time was 5.4±2.2 h (range, 2 to 7.5), but was 22.9±20.6 h (range, 3 to 74) for the other patients ($n=18$). This difference just failed to be statistically significant ($p = 0.062$). Rapid recanalization of the MCA within the first 18 h preferably led to the manifestation of the prognostically relatively benign, purely subcortical, large striatocapsular infarct, leaving the cortex grossly intact.

Subgroups of patients who had a good/moderate leptomeningeal collateralization *and* an MCA recanalization within 8 h ($n = 8$), or very early recanalization within 4 h *and* good/moderate transcortical blood flow ($n = 6$) presented with relatively small infarcts, i.e., involvement of 1 or 2 MCA subareas (CT score, 1.33±0.47). This was different than those with poor or moderate leptomeningeal network *and/or* recanalization later than 8 h ($n = 10$), who mostly showed involvement of 3 or 4 MCA territory subareas (CT score 2.7±1.19). This difference was statistically significant ($p = 0.053$, Wilcoxon-Mann-Whitney U-test; $p = 0.047$, Pitman randomization test). Deaths ($n = 5$) exclusively occurred in the latter group ($p = 0.058$, one-tailed

Table 1. Comparison of neurologic score on admission and during follow-up versus recanalization time and leptomeningeal collateral flow

Subgroups	N	Neurological Scores: On Admission	On Day 17	After 10 Months
Good or moderate collateralization and recanalization ≤8 hours	8	6.5	10.9	10.5
versus				
any collateralization and recanalization >8 hours	10	4.9	5.7 (1 died)	3.9 (6 died)
p values		0.11	0.0006	0.0018

Fisher's exact test). Interestingly, no patient with very early recanalization was seen who, simultaneously, had poor leptomeningeal blood supply.

Highly significant differences were found, if both the quality of the anastomotic network *and* the recanalization time were related to the clinical outcome after 17 days or 10 months (Table 1). Patients with either early recanalization or good/moderate leptomeningeal collateralization, or both, had a highly significantly better neurological outcome score than those with late or no recanalization and/or poor leptomeningeal anastomotic network.

Discussion

The difference between reversible neuronal electrical dysfunction and membrane pump failure has led to the concept of the ischemic penumbra, which designates a region of viable but nonfunctioning cerebral tissue surrounding a core zone of definite infarction [1, 4]. This concept implies a range of reversible ischemia between the functional threshold and cell death in which jeopardized neurons may be salvaged. Such a situation may be present in MCA occlusions with marginally sufficient leptomeningeal collateral blood supply. The extent to which chronic ischemic penumbra exists in such low-pressure vascular beds, and how long functionally paralysed tissue can survive under such conditions, is unknown, or at least unproven. Studies by many investigators using various animal models have demonstrated a critical period of MCA occlusion ranging from 2 to 7 h that may be tolerated without, or with limited, infarction [8, 13, 14]. Findings in our above-mentioned subset of patients with purely subcortical striatocapsular infarctions [15] compare favorably with these figures.

There is conflicting information in the literature as to the degree of leptomeningeal anastomoses as an indicator of the prognosis of MCA occlusion. The reasons for these discrepancies might be methodologic, since in some studies angiographic evaluation of the leptomeningeal collateral blood flow was not performed within the first few hours after stroke onset, but days or weeks later. In accordance with similar findings published recently [2, 5, 10, 11], the presence of a collateral leptomeningeal circulation reduced infarct size and improved clinical outcome. The presence of a good collateral blood supply, however, does not reliably limit the extension of the infarct in every case and seems to constitute only one of several important factors in the natural history of embolic MCA occlusions. Early recanalization of an occluded MCA is obviously helpful only as long as leptomeningeal anastomoses are operating to maintain a certain blood supply to the MCA distribution. Perhaps the extent of the leptomeningeal blood supply defines the temporal width of the therapeutic window.

In conclusion, our findings show the favorable effect of good leptomeningeal circulation in conjunction with rapid recanalization of an embolically occluded MCA to produce limited infarction and benign outcome. We speculate that only the very early development of a sufficient leptomeningeal blood supply, linked to rapid recanalization of the occluded MCA within the first 8 h, may prevent large MCA territory infarctions, whereas neither factor is sufficient by itself. This interpretation would further justify trials with fibrinolytic substances, but would also explain why fibrinolysis would be efficacious only in a limited subset of acute stroke patients and only within a very narrow time window.

References

1. Astrup J, Siesjo BK, Symon L (1981) Thresholds in cerebral ischemia – the ischemic penumbra. Stroke 12:723–725
2. Bozzao L, Fantozzi LM, Bastianello S, Bozzao A, Fieschi C (1989) Early collateral blood supply and late parenchymal brain damage in patients with middle cerebral artery occlusion. Stroke 20:735–740
3. Dalal PM, Shah PM, Sheth SC, Deshpande CK (1965) Cerebral embolism: Angiographic observations on spontaneous clot lysis. Lancet 1:61–64
4. Heiss WD, Rosner G (1983) Functional recovery of cortical neurons as related to degree and duration of ischemia. Ann Neurol 14:294–301
5. Ito Z, Suzuki A, Hen R, Menura K (1983) Prognostic factors in spontaneous recanalization of middle cerebral artery occlusion. In: Ito Z, Kutsuzawa T, Yasui N (eds) Cerebral ischemia – An update. Excerpta Medica, Amsterdam, p 159
6. Jones TH, Morawetz RB, Crowell RM, et al (1981) Thresholds of focal cerebral ischemia in awake monkeys. J Neurosurg 54(6):773–782
7. Lhermitte F, Gautier JC, Derouesn C, Guiraud B (1968) Ischemic accidents in the middle cerebral artery territory. A study of the causes in 122 cases. Arch Neurol 19:248–256
8. Pulsinelli WA, Brierley JB, Plum F (1982) Temporal profile of neuronal damage in a model of transient forebrain ischemia. Ann Neurol 11:491–498
9. Ringelstein EB (1989) A practical guide to transcranial Doppler sonography. In: Weinberger J (ed) Noninvasive imaging of cerebral vascular disease. AR Liss Publishers, New York, p 75
10. Ringelstein EB, Biniek R, Weiller C, Ammeling B, Nolte PN, Thron A (1992) Type and extent of hemispheric brain infarctions and clinical outcome in early and delayed middle cerebral artery recanalization. Neurology 42:289–298
11. Saito I, Segawa H, Shiokawa Y, Taniguchi M, Tsutsumi K (1987) Middle cerebral artery occlusion. Correlation of computed tomography with clinical outcome. Stroke 18:863–868
12. Sindermann F, Dichgans J, Bergleiter R (1969) Occlusion of the middle cerebral artery and its branches: Angiographic and clinical correlates. Brain 92:607–620
13. Sundt TM, Jr., Grant WC, Garcia JH (1969) Restoration of middle cerebral artery flow in experimental infarction. J Neurosurg 31:311–322
14. Watanabe O, West CR, Bremer A (1977) Experimental regional cerebral ischemia in the middle cerebral artery territory in primates. Part II: Effects on brain water and electrolytes in the early phase of MCA stroke. Stroke 8:71–76
15. Weiller C, Ringelstein EB, Reiche W, Thron A, Buelle U (1990) The large striatecapsular infarct. A clinical and pathophysiological entity. Arch Neurol 47:1085–1091

Potential Role of Magnetic Resonance Imaging in Selecting Patients for Thrombolytic Therapy

A. J. Furlan

The emergence of very early treatment strategies for acute stroke, such as thrombolysis, raises a number of interesting questions regarding the approach to imaging in such patients. The traditional approach to imaging in acute stroke employs CT, mainly to exclude brain hemorrhage masquerading as infarction. Some early treatment strategies, including anticoagulation and, more recently, thrombolytic therapy are considered contraindicated in the presence of CT-detected brain hemorrhage.

Although more sensitive than CT for detecting brain infarction, the role of magnetic resonance imaging (MRI) in the evaluation of patients with acute stroke, and the impact of early MR imaging on the treatment decision process, has not been adequately studied [1, 2, 15]. In the early years of MR there was considerable difficulty in distinguishing an intracerebral hemorrhage from brain infarction [13]. The ability to distinguish parenchymal hematoma from infarction has become increasingly refined and is less of a problem currently. However, MR will frequently detect small hemorrhages not visible on CT within an area of infarction. The frequency of hemorrhagic infarction detected by MR in patients with very acute stroke is not known [10]. Among 46 noncontrast MR studies performed within a mean 23 days of cerebral infarction, 11 (23.9%) showed areas of increased T1 and decreased T2 signal at the periphery consistent with small hemorrhages [10]. Noncontrast CT was either isodense or slightly hyperdense in these areas. Another study found evidence of hemorrhagic infarction on CT in 2 of 31 (6.5%) patients scanned within 24 h of stroke onset, compared to 3 of 31 (9.7%) on MR. On follow-up scan 7 to 10 days after onset, hemorrhagic changes were more frequent on MR (6 of 20, 30.0%) than CT (2 of 19, 10.5%) [3]. A recent study found neither CT nor MR superior in the early detection of hematoma or infarction [8]. The clinical significance of these observations vis a vis neurologic outcome or selection of treatments such as anticoagulation or thrombolysis is unclear.

Very few patients have been imaged by MR within the first hours of stroke onset. This partly reflects logistical problems since many hospitals are not

Medical Director, Cerebrovascular Program, Section of Adult Neurology, The Cleveland Clinic Foundation, Cleveland, OH, USA

G. J. del Zoppo, E. Mori, W. Hacke (Eds.)
Thrombolytic Therapy in Acute Ischemic Stroke II

Table 1. MR findings in acute cerebral ischemia. From [3]

Mechanism	MR finding	Possible causes	Estimated time[a] (hr)
Flow kinematics	Absent flow	Slow flow; occlusion	Early
	Arterial enhancement	Accentuation of flow derangement	Early
Biophysiologic	T1 morphologic change	Cytotoxic edema (free water)	2 – 4
	T2 signal change	BBB breakdown; vasogenic edema; macromolecular binding	8
	T1 signal change	BBB breakdown; vasogenic edema; macromolecular binding	16 – 24
Combination	Delayed parenchymal enhancement[b]	Impaired delivery of significant contrast agent	>24[c]
	Early exaggerated enhancement[d]	Intract deliver of contrast agent; BBB leakage; focal hyperemia	2 – 4[d]

BBB, blood-brain barrier.
[a] Time at which findings generally could first be detected by available MR examinations; this does not necessarily imply the exact time of onset.
[b] Typical frinding in completed cortical infarctions.
[c] Usually not detected before 5 – 7 days.
[d] Found in a few cases with transient or partial occlusions and in watershed infarctions

designed to facilitate urgent MR imaging, especially in the middle of the night. Beyond logistics, MR scanning sequences and results have not been systematically studied in well-defined groups of patients with very early brain ischemia. The series reported by Yuh et al. [16] contained 16 lesions scanned within 8 h of "ischemic symptoms," although clinical details are not provided. An additional 25 lesions were scanned between 8 and 24 h of onset. Increased signal on T2 appeared *late*, i.e., after 8 h. The earliest MR changes reflected flow kinetics and included absent flow void or arterial enhancement with gadolinium within the territory of the symptomatic artery (Table 1).

Despite these problems, MR remains attractive for the study of acute stroke precisely because of its increased sensitivity to ischemia and, more recently, because of the introduction of new techniques including MR angiography (MRA) and, most recently, MR diffusion (MRD) and perfusion (MRP) techniques. MRD requires special coil gradients which can be used to image very early tissue changes, possibly related to cytotoxic edema, occurring within 1 h of stroke onset [8]. MRP techniques permit analysis of cerebral blood flow and flow metabolism coupling. MDR and MRP are still in the developmental stage and are not ready for routine clinical application [7]. However, MRA has already reached the stage of clinical application and, when combined with conventional spin-echo MR imaging, offers the potential for conjoint anatomic and vascular imaging in patients with acute stroke.

The principles of MRA have been extensively reviewed [9]. A variety of phase contrast (PC) and time of flight (TOF) techniques are under investigation. PC is sensitive to very slow flow, but is highly subject to complex flow and motion artifacts. PC also requires prolonged acquisition and processing time. For large vessel occlusive disease, 3-dimensional TOF techniques seem to hold the most promise for quick, accurate detection of stenosis or occlusion. Two- dimensional (2-D) TOF may be superior for very low flow states, especially posterior circulation studies. Currently, we are using 3-D TOF techniques to image specific vascular systems, either the extracranial carotid, Circle of Willis, extracranial vertebrals, or basilar artery. Each vessel system analyzed with MRA adds only 8–10 min to the standard T2 MR study. Hence, the spin-echo MR image combined with MRA of the suspected symptomatic vessel system should take 20–30 min in most patients.

Initial studies have shown a high degree of correlation in the degree of extracranial carotid artery stenosis when comparing 3-D TOF MRA images with intra-arterial digital subtraction angiography (IA DSA) [6, 11]. More severe degrees of stenosis (>70%) tend to slightly over-estimated by MRA. A number of potential problems, including motion artifact, have been described. Subacute (4–7 days) thrombus containing methemoglobin can give a false-positive "flow" reading, and special sequences are needed to identify dissections. The accuracy of 3-D TOF MRA for detecting intracranial vascular disease is unknown since there have been no correlative studies done with IA DSA. Accumulated experience, however, suggests a similar high degree of accuracy of 3-D TOF MRA for detecting large vessel anterior circulation occlusive disease to the level of the middle cerebral artery (MCA) bifurcation [5]. MRA also appears highly accurate for detecting vertebral and basilar artery occlusive disease and occlusion of the posterior cerebral arteries [12]. Technical limitations prohibit accurate imaging of MCA branch occlusive disease, and smaller basilar artery branches including the posterior inferior cerebellar artery (PICA), anterior inferior cerebellar artery (AICA) and superior cerebellar artery (SCA). Nonetheless, MRA appears to be highly accurate for detecting occlusion of vessels most often treated with thrombolytic therapy (Figs. 1–4).

CT combined with ultrasound [carotid duplex plus transcranial Doppler (TCD)] has been suggested as an alternative to MR/MRA for the vascular/anatomic evaluation of patients with acute brain ischemia [14]. The advantages and problems of MR imaging versus CT for anatomic imaging of very early stroke have been alluded to above. Ultrasound techniques, while in some ways less cumbersome than MRA, are highly technician-dependent and of uncertain accuracy in patients with intracranial occlusive disease, especially vertebral basilar lesions. MRA offers the advantage of direct visualization of the occlusive process and is probably more accurate than TCD for detecting vertebral basilar occlusive disease. In some situations ultrasound may compliment MRA. *The central point is, however, that if MR imaging becomes the anatom-*

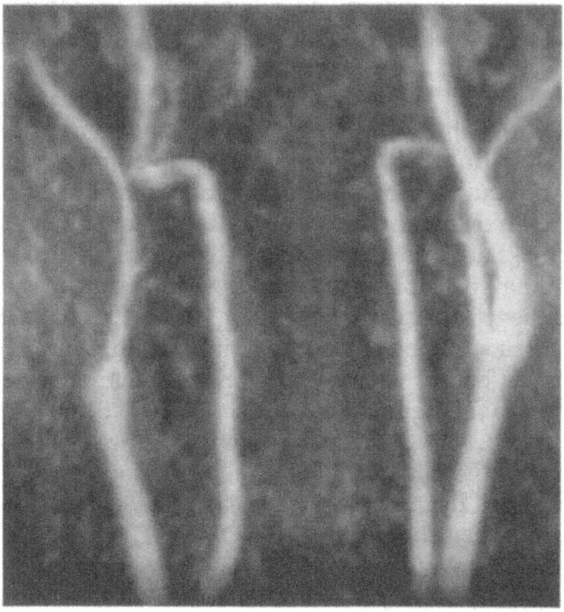

Fig. 1. 3-D TOF MRA. Occluded left internal carotid origin

Fig. 2. Occluded middle cerebral artery on 3-D TOF MRA with corresponding infarct on MR
▼

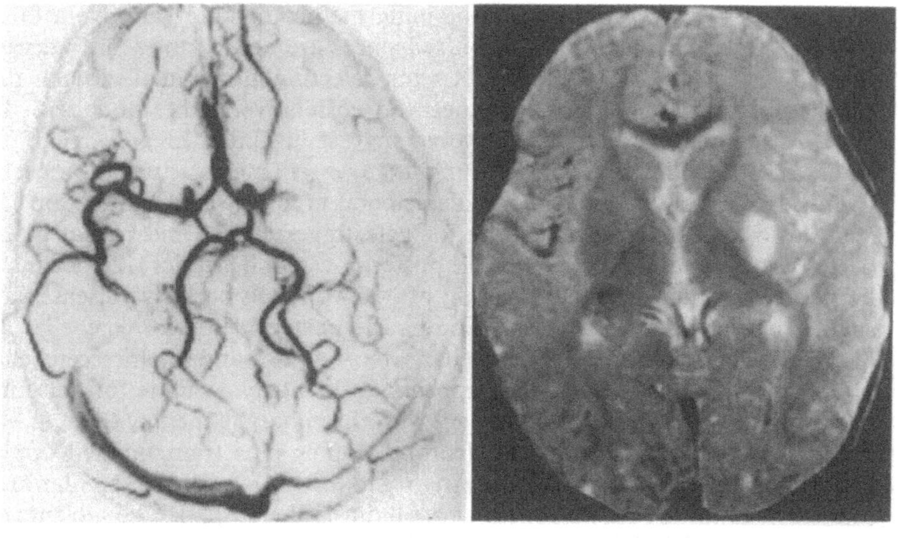

ic imaging modality of choice in patients with early brain ischemia, the additional 8–10 min required for MRA will become a standard part of the MR evaluation of patients with acute stroke.

Assuming, therefore, that anatomic imaging of patients with acute focal neurologic deficits remains necessary to exclude brain hemorrhage, the central question to be decided is whether we should continue with our traditional CT

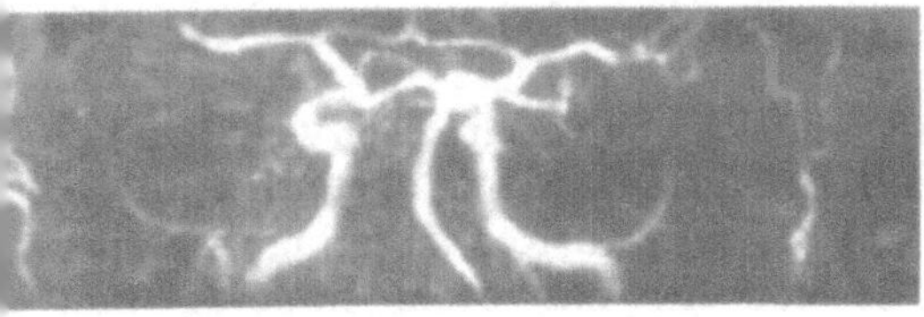

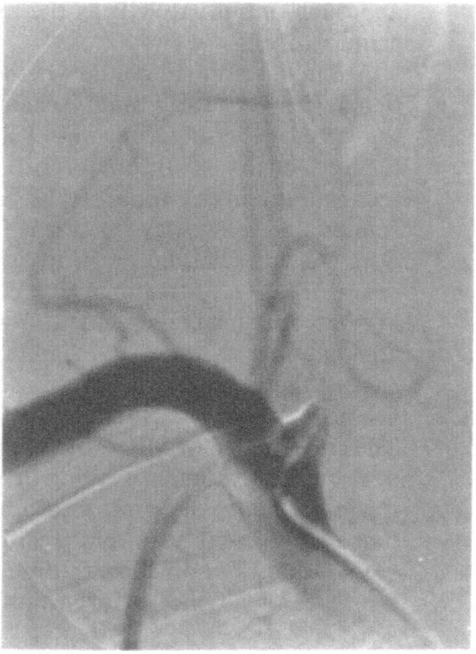

Fig. 3. Occluded right vertebral artery on 3-D TOF MRA confirmed by selective angiography

Fig. 4. 3-D TOF MRA. Occluded right posterior cerebral artery
▼

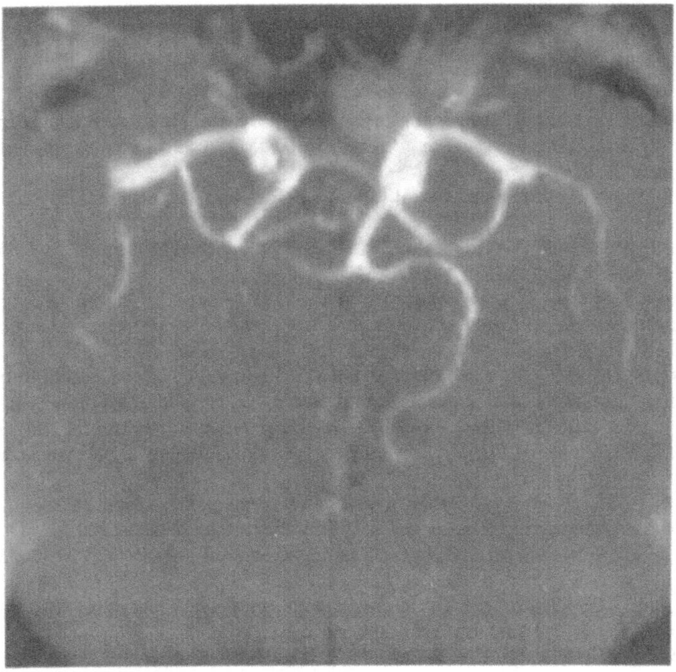

approach or shift to MR as the imaging modality of choice in patients with acute stroke.

A final question might be whether vascular imaging is necessary at all in patients with very early brain ischemia. Most, I think, would agree that ideally the state of the offending vessel should be known before initiating a specific therapy such as thrombolysis. The concern has been, however, that angiography in the acute stroke patient is not only hazardous but time consuming and may delay treatment for up to 2 h. While the rt-PA Acute Stroke Study Group trial did not find angiography in acute stroke hazardous, it did delay initiation of treatment for 1.5 h [4]. On the other hand, 25% of patients in that study were excluded from thrombolytic therapy on the basis of angiographic criteria (i.e., eligible by clinical and CT criteria). These results suggest that it will be difficult to select the best candidates for very early intravenous thrombolytic therapy on the basis of the clinical examinations only. The great appeal of MRA, therefore, is the ability to acquire not only anatomic data but also vascular imaging in a very brief period of time so that a specific treatment plan can be initiated. Finally, MRD may permit early assessment of tissue salvageability so that treatment can be selected on a more physiologic basis rather than on clinical (time from onset, severity of deficit) or anatomic (presence or absence of occlusion) criteria alone.

References

1. Bose B, Jones SC, Lorig R, et al (1988) Evolving focal cerebral ischemia in cats: Spatial correlation of nuclear magnetic resonance imaging, cerebral flood flow, tetrazolium staining, and histopathology. Stroke 19:28–37
2. Brant-Zawadzki M, Pereira B, Weinstein P, et al (1986) MRI of acute experimental ischemia in rats. AJNR 7:7–11
3. Bryan RN, Levy LM, Whitlow WD, et al (1991) Diagnosis of acute cerebral infarction: Comparison of CT and MR imaging. AJNR 12:611–620
4. del Zoppo GJ, Poeck K, Pessin MS, 16 coauthors of the rt-PA Acute Stroke Study Group (1992) Recombinant tissue plasminogen activator in acute thrombotic and embolic stroke. Ann Neurol 32:78–86
5. Masaryk AM, Ross JS, DiCello MC, et al (1991) 3DFT MR angiography of the carotid bifurcation: Potential and limitations as a screening examination. Neuroradiology 179:797–804
6. Masaryk TJ, Tkach J, Glicklich M (1991) Flow radiofrequency pulse sequences and gradient magnetic fields: Basic interactions and adoptations to angiographic imaging. Top Magn Reson Imaging 3:1–11
7. Minematsu K, Li L, Fisher M, et al (1992) Diffusion weighted magnetic resonance imaging: Rapid and quantitative detection of focal brain ischemia. Neurology 42:235–240
8. Mohr JP, Biller J, Hilal SK, et al (1992) MR vs CT imaging in acute stroke. Stroke 23:142 (Abstract)
9. Moseley ME, Wedland MF, Kuchorczyk J (1991) Magnetic resonance imaging of diffusion and perfusion. Top Magn Reson Imaging 3:50–67
10. Nabatame H, Fujimoto N, Nakamura K, et al (1990) High intensity areas of noncontrast T1-weighted MR images in cerebral infarction. J Comput Assist Tomogr 14:521–526
11. Ross JS, Masaryk TJ, Ruggieri PM (1991) Magnetic resonance angiography of the carotid bifurcation. Top Magn Reson Imaging 3:12–22

12. Ruggieri PM, Masaryk TJ, Ross JS, Modic MT (1991) Magnetic resonance angiography of the intracranial vasculature. Top Magn Reson Imaging 3:23–33
13. Salgado ED, Weinstein M, Furlan AJ, et al (1986) Proton magnetic resonance imaging in ischemic cerebrovascular disease. Ann Neurol 20:502–507
14. Schwaighofer BW, Klein MV, Lyden PD, Hesselink JR (1990) MR imaging of vertebrobasilar vascular disease. J Comput Assist Tomogr 14:895–904
15. Unger EC, Gado MH, Fulling KF, Littlefield JL (1987) Acute cerebral infarction in monkeys: An experimental study using MR imaging. Radiology 162:789–795
16. Yuh WTC, Crain MR, Loes DJ, et al (1991) MR imaging of cerebral ischemia: Findings in the first 24 hours. AJNR 12:621–629

The Role of SPECT in Acute Stroke Thrombolysis

B. Sperling[1], K. Overgaard[2], G. Boysen[2], and N.A. Lassen[1]

During recent years thrombolytic trials in cerebral ischemia have indicated that time, both from the onset of symptoms to hospitalisation and from first examination to treatment initiation, is the all-important factor on which the success of thrombolytic therapy relies, a success measured in both good recovery and in absence of excess hemorrhage. As the thrombolytic therapy is not without danger of hemorrhage, it is of considerable importance to diagnose patients accurately. For this reason, many studies have so far included a pretreatment contrast x-ray angiography to verify the vascular occlusion followed by a repeated angiography to verify recanalization. This approach, however, includes both a time delay and the risk of possible adverse effects of the contrast x-ray angiography.

Likewise, studies including a pretreatment MRI and MR angiography have been or are being conducted, but as concluded by Huk [5], only when the results can be obtained within a few minutes are the use of these techniques justified in the acute phase. Furthermore, conventional MRI is, as is CT, often negative in the hyperacute phase, although the affected areas usually are visible already at approximately 4 h from the onset of symptoms with MRI.

In order to minimize the time delay, several studies are now being conducted or are planned with a minimum of pretreatment investigations, consisting only of clinical examinations and a CT scan to exclude hemorrhage or edema formation associated with larger infarcts.

The natural history of an acute embolism is, however, extremely variable. Pretreatment verification of an occlusion and the extent of ischemia is desirable not only to confirm an indication for thrombolysis (arterial occlusion), but also to establish a pretreatment status upon which to evaluate the treatment [6].

Both Positron Emission Tomography (PET) and Single Photon Emission Computed Tomography (SPECT) will, immediately after onset of symptoms of acute embolism, show hypoperfusion in the involved cerebral region, which may ultimately develop into infarction. Although PET methodologically excels over SPECT in that it provides information about metabolic changes, and

[1]Department of Clinical Physiology, Bispebjerg Hospital and [2]Department of Neurology, Rigshospitalet, Copenhagen, Denmark

G.J. del Zoppo, E. Mori, W. Hacke (Eds.)
Thrombolytic Therapy in Acute Ischemic Stroke II

thereby possibly of tissue viability, in addition to regional cerebral blood flow (rCBF), the method has so far been too cumbersome and time-consuming for more than a few examinations of hyperacute patients to have been made worldwide over a decade. SPECT examination takes about 10 to 30 min and yields a precise image of large ischemic areas. It would, however, also introduce a delay in the application of thrombolysis.

The recent development of CBF tracers for SPECT which are retained for hours in a distribution pattern proportional to the rCBF at the time of injection does, however, offer an alternative approach to the evaluation of acute stroke thrombolysis with neuroimaging.

Subjects and Methods

Hexamethyl-propyleneamineoxime marked with ^{99m}Tc (Tc-HMPAO) is a lipophilic CBF tracer which crosses the blood–brain barrier following intravenous administration and is then converted to a hydrophilic form and retained in the same distribution for several hours [1]. This allows one to perform the actual SPECT hours after the administration of Tc-HMPAO showing the rCBF distribution at the time of the injection. It is thus possible to give Tc-HMPAO immediately before thrombolytic therapy is instituted and, with no delay of treatment, to obtain a pretreatment rCBF distribution image.

Using a brain-dedicated SPECT (e.g., TOMOMATIC 232) or rotating gamma cameras, one can atraumatically obtain images of brain slices in 5 to 20 min depending on the system [1]. Furthermore, if a low dose of Tc-HMPAO is administered initially, a repeated SPECT using image subtraction procedures is possible following administration of a second Tc-HMPAO dose twice the strength of the first dose, the so-called split-dose technique [4]. This arrangement allows one to assess whether reperfusion has occurred.

rCBF with SPECT in Acute Ischemic Stroke

The visualization of acute rCBF changes with SPECT in stroke patients within 6 h from the onset of symptoms is feasible [2, 3] and does not delay treatment [9].

By analyzing which vascular territories are hypoperfused in acute cerebral ischemia, the SPECT image provides a crude "consequence angiogram" localizing the occlusion to either the internal carotid artery (ICA), the anterior cerebral artery (ACA), the posterior cerebral artery (PCA), the middle cerebral artery (MCA), the MCA stem or an MCA branch. It might be argued that this "angiogram" is not very accurate as, for example, a distinction between an ICA and an MCA stem occlusion would depend on the presence or absence of collateral perfusion of the ACA territory via the circle of Willis. This is true, but then the "consequence" of the occlusion would only be ischemia in the MCA territory such as would follow an MCA stem occlusion. This furthermore illustrates the difference between demonstrating an occlusion and showing the actual extent of neuronal tissue hypoperfusion which might develop into infarction. In x-ray angiography this is partly overcome by estimating the collateral blood supply by contrast injection in the nonaffected side first [11] and by following the filling of vessels distal to the occlusion from cortical anastomoses [8]. But, again, these procedures introduce a time delay.

Giubilei [2] showed "that an early (<6 h) severe decrease in CBF readily detected with SPECT is highly predictive of a poor neurological outcome," suggesting that SPECT might be used not only as a quantitative diagnostic tool, but also possibly as a prognostic tool in selecting patients for treatment. The distinct diagnosis of marked hypoperfusion is of particular interest in the very early selection for a treatment which, like thrombolysis, is not without serious adverse effects, but also in the evaluation of other therapeutic approaches such as neuroprotective agents.

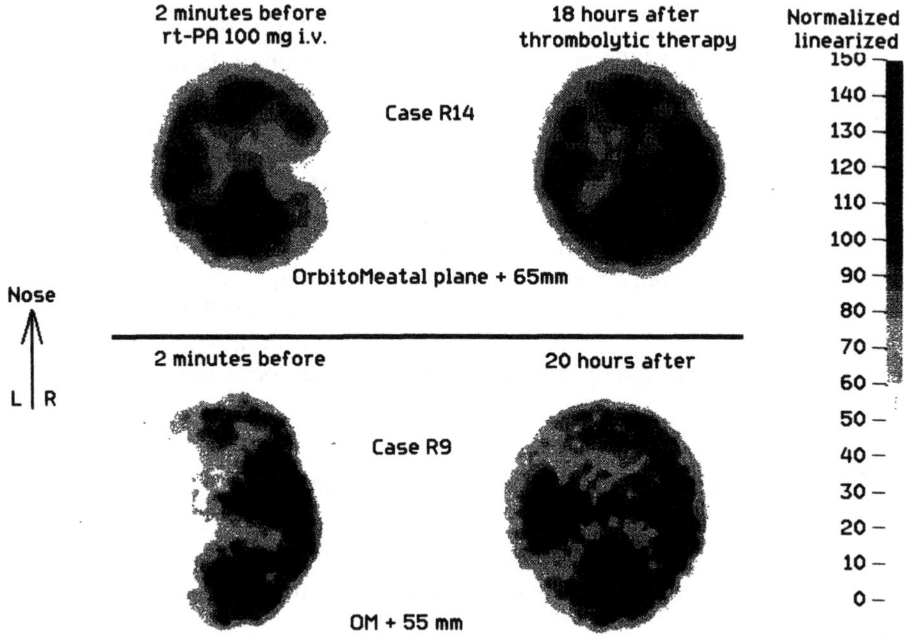

Fig. 1. SPECT flow distribution images with values in percent of the mean Tc-HMPAO uptake in the ipsilateral cerebellar hemisphere. *Above the line:* Case R14, a 31-year-old male with pretreatment hypoperfusion in the left posterior MCA branch followed by reperfusion hyperemia at 18 h after start of the rt-PA infusion. *Below the line:* Case R9, a 40-year-old male with hypoperfusion in all of the right MCA territory followed by reperfusion at 20 h

The Danish Multicenter Pilot Study

In thirteen of the 23 patients in the Danish Pilot Study of thrombolytic therapy in acute ischemic stroke, reported by Overgaard [7], pretreatment SPECT images of rCBF were obtained 2 to 5 min before infusion of 100 mg rt-PA was initiated. In one patient with suspected brain stem infarction, SPECT was normal. The remaining 12 SPECT studies showed a clinically relevant hypoperfusion of all or part of the MCA territory, including the ACA territory in 5 separate examinations. Repeated SPECT within 24 h after therapy showed complete or partial reperfusion in 10 (Fig. 1), while rCBF showed no change in 2 patients with severe MCA and ACA hypoperfusion. In these 2 patients x-ray angiography 24 h after therapy showed persistent occlusion of both ICA and MCA.

The 10 patients with reperfusion were compared with the remaining patients who did not show reperfusion or in whom repeated SPECT was not performed. The reperfused group had smaller infarcts on CT scans at 30 days than the remaining patients. However, it is important to note that although early reperfusion was obtained, the ischemic period resulted in infarction in all but one patient. Furthermore, if reperfusion was obtained, there was a greater clinical improvement the sooner from onset of symptoms treatment was initiated.

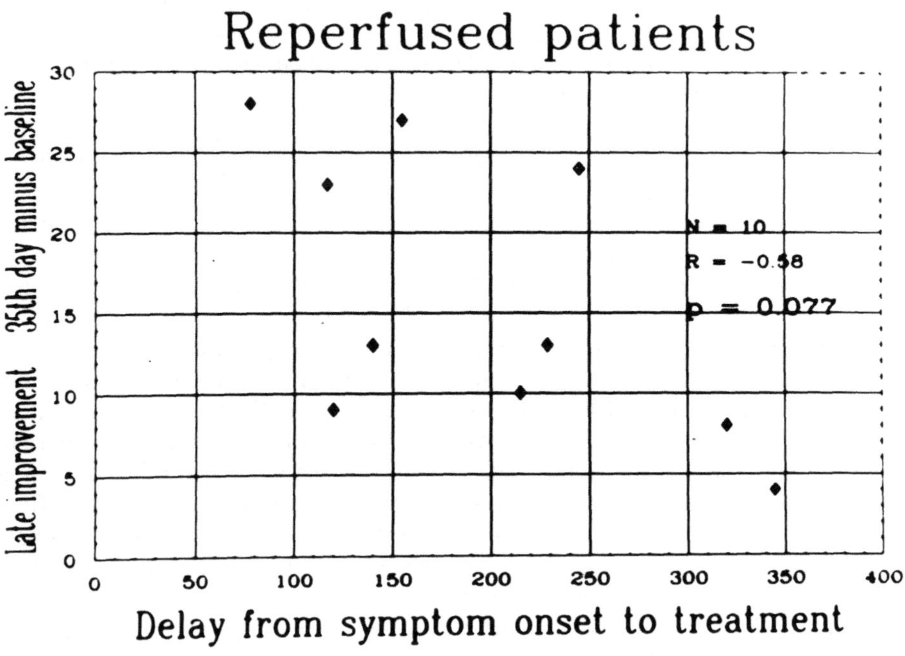

Fig. 2. Improvement evaluated with the Scandinavian Stroke Scale score before treatment and at day 35. *N*, number of patients. *R* and *p*, Spearman nonparametric correlation test coefficient (*R*) and probability value (*p*)

Furthermore, if reperfusion was obtained, there was a greater clinical improvement, although not significant, the sooner from symptom onset treatment was initiated (Fig. 2).

Future Roles of SPECT

The natural history of stroke involves in the majority of patients a considerable improvement from the initial symptoms estimated with clinical neurological scores. In the placebo-controlled ECASS study, the primary hypothesis is that the thrombolytic treatment will result in improved clinical outcome. As early thrombolysis will not occur in all patients treated with rt- PA [7, 10], the result will be "diluted" by these nonresponders. As the result will be even further "diluted" by early spontaneous reperfusion in the placebo-treated group, there is a risk of overlooking a potential beneficial effect of early reperfusion in the subset of patients where recanalization is obtained.

With SPECT and Tc-HMPAO it may be possible to divide the patients into two groups, with and without reperfusion. In the group of patients with early reperfusion consisting of arterial recanalization "responders" and early spontaneous reperfused patients, one would expect a considerably better outcome [7]. If a positive effect of early reperfusion on outcome can be established and if reperfusion occurs more often following thrombolytic therapy, which should be demonstratable in a rather small study, then this together with the safety data from large double-blinded, placebo-controlled studies could document the efficacy of the treatment.

As recanalization is not obtained in all patients, one might consider a second dose of the thrombolytic agent provided that bleeding had not occurred. Repeated SPECT with the "split dose technique" after, for example, 1 or 2 h would show whether reperfusion had occurred or indicate the need for further infusion of the thrombolytic agent.

Whether it is possible to initially exclude/select patients for thrombolytic therapy on the basis of SPECT images obtained before the start of treatment, as reported by Herderscheê [3] in 5 patients, will depend on the results from further studies of the outcome of acute stroke patients using thrombolytic agents evaluated with SPECT. However, as thrombolytic therapy is not without a danger of hemorrhage, it is of considerable importance to diagnose patients accurately prior to treatment and to select patients with embolic occlusions with a potentially good prognosis, if lysed. Alternatively, if the benefit of thrombolytic therapy is found to be very small in certain subtypes of stroke, for example, occlusions involving only the lenticulostriate arteries, then exclusion of these patients may be warranted.

In the First International Symposium on Thrombolysis in Acute Cerebral Ischemia (1990), Mohr stated that among other "Problems in Formulating Therapeutic Trials" it "would be quite desirable" to have a brain image confirming the clinical diagnosis [6]. In trials of acute thrombolytic therapy, a pretreatment image confirming the extent of marked ischemia is, in our opinion, very important for the interpretation of the findings. We, therefore, recommend that a pretreatment rCBF image be obtained with this technique. This is feasible not only with brain-dedicated SPECT scanners, but also with "ordinary" rotating gamma cameras, which are found at most hospitals. The positive CT and MRI findings within the first hours are few. As early initiation of treatment is imperative, any delay by other procedures such as x-ray angiography and MR angiography should be avoided if possible. At the present, the only method, which provides an atraumatic, practical, fast, and reliable image of acute cerebral ischemia without delaying the start of thrombolytic therapy, is SPECT.

References

1. Andersen AR (1991) Tc99m-D,L-Hexamethyl-propyleneamine oxime (Tc99m-HMPAO): Basic kinetic studies of a tracer of cerebral blood flow. Thesis. Cerebrovasc Brain Metab Rev 1:288–318
2. Giubilei F, Lenzi GL, Di Pierro V, et al (1990) Predictive value of brain perfusion single-photon emission computed tomorgraphy in acute ischemic stroke. Stroke 21:895–900
3. Herderscheê D, Limburg M, van Reyen EA, Hijdra A, Büller HR, Koster PA (1991) Thrombolysis with recombinant tissue plasminogen activator in acute ischemic stroke: Evaluation with rCBF-SPECT. Acta Neurol Scand 83:317–322
4. Holm S, Madsen PL, Rubin P, Sperling B, Friberg L, Lassen NA (1991) Tc-99m HMPAO activation studies of the split-dose, image subtraction approach. J Cereb Blood Flow Metab 11:S766
5. Huk WJ (1991) Invasive and noninvasive vascular imaging techniques and their role in clinical stroke trials. In: Hacke W, del Zoppo GJ, Hirschberg M (eds) Thrombolytic therapy in acute ischemic stroke. Springer-Verlag, Berlin Heidelberg New York, p 186
6. Mohr JP (1991) Problems in formulating therapeutic trials. In: Hacke W, del Zoppo GJ, Hirschberg M (eds) Thrombolytic therapy in acute ischemic stroke. Springer-Verlag, Berlin Heidelberg New York, p 177
7. Overgaard K, Sperling B, Boysen G, et al (1992) Thrombolytic therapy in acute ischemic stroke: A Danish pilot study. (Submitted for publication)
8. Saito I, Segawa H, Shiokawa S, Taniguchi M, Tsutsumi K (1987) Middle cerebral artery occlusion: Correlation of computed tomography and angiography with clinical outcome. Stroke 18:863–868
9. Sperling B, Boysen G, Overgaard K, Lassen NA (1991) The expectations of rCBF measurements in thrombolytic therapy of acute ischemic stroke. J Neurol 238:S124
10. von Kummer R, Forsting M, Sartor K, Hacke W (1991) Intravenous recombinant tissue plasminogen activator in acute stroke. In: Hacke W, del Zoppo GJ, Hirschberg M (eds) Thrombolytic therapy in acute ischemic stroke. Springer-Verlag, Berlin Heidelberg New York, p 161
11. Zeumer H, Siepmann G, Müller-Jensen M, Goossens-Merkt H (1991) Invasive imaging techniques in the evaluation of patient selection and cerebrovascular recanalization. In: Hacke W, del Zoppo GJ, Hirschberg M (eds) Thrombolytic therapy in acute ischemic stroke. Springer-Verlag, Berlin Heidelberg New York, p 91

Clinical and Brain Hemodynamic Evaluations of Thrombolytic Therapy in Acute Ischemic Stroke: SPECT Study

Y. Okada[1], S. Sadoshima[4], M. Katsuragi[2], K. Irie[1], H. Utsunomiya[3], and M. Fujishima[4]

Thrombolytic therapy has been proposed as a promising therapy for acute ischemic stroke when it is initiated very early after the onset of stroke symptoms [2, 6, 7]. However, thrombolytic therapy may not be reliably applied when the patients are evaluated based on clinical signs only. The absence of early CT hypodensity before the therapy may be one implication for safe and effective thrombolysis [7]. Recently, single photon emission tomography (SPECT) has been used in the examination of emergency patients. It may also be useful for the early diagnosis of ischemic stroke, and especially reperfusion after thrombolytic therapy in acute ischemic stroke [4]. In the present study, we describe preliminary results of regional cerebral blood flow (rCBF) SPECT imaging at fixed intervals before and after thrombolytic therapy with recombinant tissue plasminogen activator (rt-PA), and correlate them with the clinical and angiographic outcomes.

Subjects and Methods

We studied 6 patients with acute ischemic stroke, aged 54 to 78 years (mean 63), admitted to St. Mary's Hospital during the period 1 January to 31 December, 1991. Informed consent was obtained from the patients or their families before the therapy (Table 1). The inclusion criteria for the thrombolytic therapy were: 1) abrupt onset of symptoms in the internal carotid artery territory, 2) age <80 years, 3) arterial fibrillation or other heart diseases, 4) occlusion of the cerebral artery on angiogram, and 5) rt-PA infusion initiated within 6 h from the onset of stroke. In this study, all the patients were examined by serial SPECT and angiographies mentioned below. Neurological examination, computed tomography (CT), and SPECT were examined before and at 24 to 48 h, 14 days, and 2 months after thrombolytic therapy. Soon after the initial CT and SPECT examination, the first cerebral angiography was performed to

Department of [1]Cerebrovascular Disease and Divisions of [2]Nuclear Medicine and [3]Neuroradiology, St. Mary's Hospital, Kurume, and the [4]Second Department of Internal Medicine, Faculty of Medicine, Kyushu University, Fukuoka, Japan

G. J. del Zoppo, E. Mori, W. Hacke (Eds.)
Thrombolytic Therapy in Acute Ischemic Stroke II

Table 1. Clinical and angiographical characteristics of 6 patients

Clinical manifestation	Case 1	Case 2	Case 3	Case 4	Case 5	Case 6
Age/Sex	54/M	63/F	60/M	78/F	54/M	58/M
Underlying Disease	HT, Dissection?	Af, MSR	Af, HT	Af, HT	Af	Af
rt-PA (dose; MIU)	0	10 i.v.	20 i.a.	20 i.v.	30 i.v.	20 i.a.
Clinical Recovery at 24 hours	–	–	–	+ + +	+	–
2 Months Outcome	Fair	Fair	Fair	Fair	Good	Fair
Infarct Size on CT	Medium	Medium	Large	Medium	Large	Large
(Infarct Index; %)	28.2	27.6	57.6	22.5	44.1	33.7
Angiography						
Site of Occlusion (1st)	LICA M2	LICA M1,A1	RM1	RM2	RM1	RICA M1
Reopening (2nd)	None	Partial 2a	Partial 2a	Partial 2a	None	None
Reopening (3rd)	Partial 2a	Partial 2b	Complete	Partial 2b	Complete	Complete
(Follow-up Day)	(10)	(8)	(3)	(8)	(7)	(7)

M, male; F, female; HT, hypertension; Af, atrial fibrillation; Dissection, dissection of common carotid artery; MSR, mitral stenosis and regurgitation; rt-PA, recombinant tissue plasminogen activator; MIU, million international units; i.v./i.a., intravenously/intra-arterially; ICA, internal carotid artery; M1/M2, M1/M2 portion of middle cerebral artery; A1, A1 portion of anterior cerebral artery; Partial 2a/2b, partial reopening of less/more than half of the occluded arteries

assess the site of occluded arteries. Then, recombinant tissue plasminogen activator (rt-PA) was intravenously or intra-arterially administered for 1 h. The second angiography just after the end of rt-PA administration and the third angiography about 1 week after the onset of stroke were examined to assess the reopening of the occluded arteries. We estimated the severity of neurological deficits by means of the Hemispheric Stroke Scale [1]. The changes in clinical features at 24 h and the outcome of reopening/occlusion on the second angiography were regarded as acute effect of thrombolysis. The neurological state at 2 months was considered as the clinical outcome. The size of the infarcted lesion on day 3 was expressed as the maximum hypodense area/ipsilateral hemisphere × 100% [8] and was classified as either small (<10%), medium (10%–30%), or large (>30%).

The initial SPECT was examined within 5 h after the onset of stroke. Imaging was obtained 5–10 min after intravenous injection of 740–925 MBq ^{99m}Tc hexamethylpropyleneamine oxime (Tc-HMPAO), using a ring-type rotating gamma camera (Headtome SET070, Shimazu, Kyoto, Japan) equipped with high resolution collimator. A complete set of axial tomographic 16 slices were obtained from the posterior fossa up to the vertex. The slices were 1.0 cm thick and the spatial resolution was 0.7 cm full-width half-maximum. The SPECT slice demonstrating the greatest asymmetry of perfusion was selected for analysis of the severity of brain ischemia. The interhemispheric asymmetry index was calculated by dividing the mean hemispheric cerebral blood flow value of the [affected-unaffected side] by half the value of the [affected+unaffected sides].

Results

The patients were treated with 10, 20, or 30 MIU of rt-PA (duteplase), except one (case 1), who was suggested to have carotid artery occlusion by dissection and received conventional treatment. Neurological improvement after 24 h was seen in 2 of the 6 patients (cases 4 and 5), and one (case 4) had 27 points reduction in Hemispheric Stroke Scale. Neurological symptoms of the other patients also gradually improved during 2 months (Fig. 1A). One patient (case 5) achieved good outcome and the others had fair outcome at 2 months after stroke onset. The initial CT was performed at 60–231 min (mean 123) after the onset of stroke. All except one (case 5) did not show any early hypodensity on CT. The size of infarcted lesion on day 3 was medium in 4 and large in 2. Hemorrhagic transformation was not significant in all patients. Partial reopening of the occluded arteries immediately after the thrombolytic therapy was seen in 3 patients (cases 2, 3 and 4), and 4 patients (cases 3, 4, 5 and 6) also showed complete reopening on the third angiography at 3 to 10 days after the onset (Table 1). The initial SPECT of the 6 patients showed a wide hypoperfusion area in the affected middle cerebral artery or internal carotid artery territory. Their interhemispheric asymmetry indexes were −13% to −24% (−20±5, mean±2 S.D.) and significant low values compared with those of normal subjects (1.4±1.4, mean±2 S.D., unpublished data). After 24 h from the thrombolytic therapy, cerebral blood flow increased around the

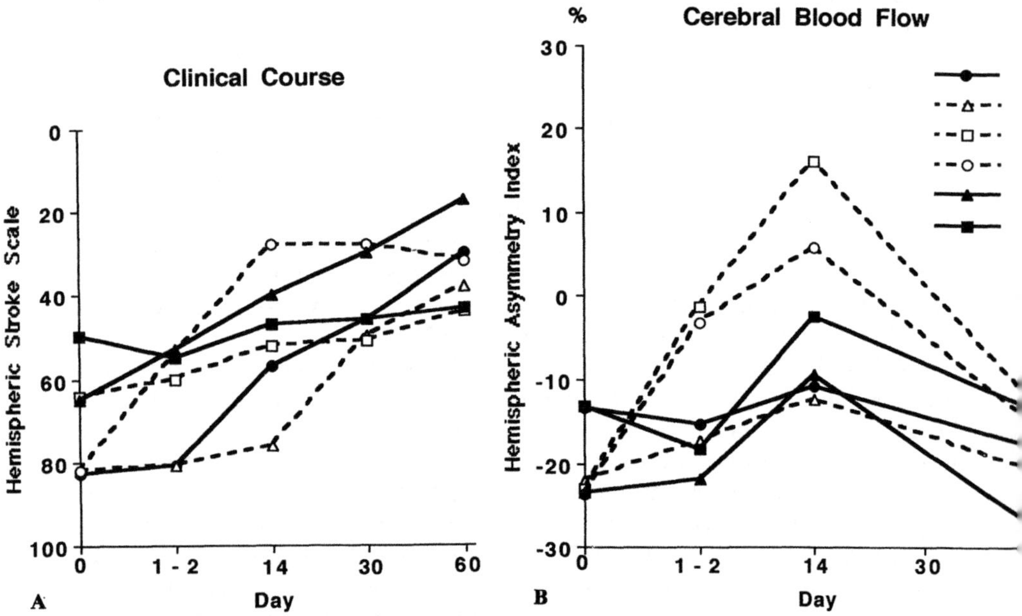

Fig. 1. A Serial neurological scores (Hemispheric Stroke Scale) of 6 cases during 2 months. **B** The pattern of cerebral blood flow change of SPECT presented by the interhemispheric asymmetry index

ischemic area, particularly in 3 patients who obtained partial reopening of the occluded arteries. All the patients had the greatest asymmetry index at 14 days, and these areas with hyperperfusion area again turned into wide hypoperfusion at 2 months, almost the same as the initial SPECT image (Fig. 1B).

Discussion

In the present study, we evaluated the usefulness of SPECT for thrombolytic therapy in acute ischemic stroke patients who had angiographically proven large arterial occlusions. Although the pattern of the changes in rCBF in the affected hemisphere was significantly different from that in neurological scores, SPECT in the acute stage revealed some useful implications for clinical and angiographic outcomes. The initial SPECT showed distinct, vascular territory-matched hypoperfusion areas in the affected hemisphere before the CT hypodensity appeared. Significant low values (−13% to −24%) of the asymmetry index also strongly suggested large arterial occlusion. Thus, SPECT may be useful in the decision to initiate thrombolytic therapy if it is used at a very early stage of stroke. The second SPECT at 24 to 48 h showed an increase in blood flow around the ischemic area, particularly in 3 cases with partial reopening just after rt-PA infusion. Furthermore, the SPECT at 14 days showed maximal increase in rCBF in all cases after the third angiogram had demonstrated complete or partial reopening of the occluded arteries. This evidence suggested that SPECT examined early after thrombolytic therapy may well reflect the angiographic outcome of the occlusion/reopening status in the ischemic area. However, the redistribution of blood flow was not parallel with the patients' clinical course. This discrepancy may be explained by reopening of the occluded arteries beyond the therapeutic window (several hours or less after the onset) or the possibility that the reopened vessel had no effect on clinical outcome. In addition, this may be partly explained by factors affecting SPECT images, such as luxury perfusion, membrane permeability changes, and increased blood volume in the ischemic area [9]. Hyperperfusion on SPECT at 14 days may more generally reflect such changes. SPECT at 2 months showed a marked decrease in rCBF again, and rCBF by SPECT in the chronic stage was not consistent with the clinical status at that time. These discrepancies have also been observed in other SPECT studies for acute ischemic stroke with [4] or without thrombolytic therapy [3, 5]. To explore further the relationship between SPECT-rCBF and the clinical outcome, we should examine the best timing of SPECT examination and the most effective SPECT tracer. The absolute rCBF values should also be studied. However, it is evident in acute ischemic stroke that Tc-HMPAO SPECT can demonstrate the presence of large arterial occlusions before the appearance of CT hypodensity and the area with presumed reperfusion following rt-PA infusion. It may therefore be useful in the evaluation of patients for thrombolysis and, with a second study, may indicate perfusion outcome of thrombolytic therapy.

Conclusion

We have examined the usefulness of Tc-HMPAO SPECT in 6 cases before and after rt-PA infusion, and evaluated the cerebral blood flow changes in comparison to clinical and angiographical outcomes. SPECT is useful in the diagnosis, especially in early stages of acute ischemic stroke because it provides information about the presence of large arterial occlusions, and may give an indication of reperfusion following thrombolytic therapy.

Acknowledgments. We would like to express great thanks to Tetsuzo Ogasawara, M.D., Division of Neuroradiology, Yoshisuke Saku, M.D., Takanari Kitazono, M.D., Shinichiro Fujishima, M.D., Yuji Fukudome, M.D. and Haruyuki Goda, M.D., Department of Cerebrovascular Disease, St. Mary's Hospital, Kurume, for their generous assistance. This study is much indebted to their hard work.

References

1. Adams RJ, Meador KJ, Sethi KD, Grotta JC, Thomson DS (1987) Graded neurologic scale for use in acute hemispheric stroke treatment protocols. Stroke 18:665–669
2. del Zoppo GJ, Poeck K, Pessin MS, and 16 coauthors of the rt-PA Acute Stroke Study Group (1992) Recombinant tissue plasminogen activator in acute thrombotic and embolic stroke. Ann Neurol 32:78–86
3. Giubilei F, Lenzi GL, Di Pietro V, et al (1990) Predictive value of brain perfusion single-photon emission computed tomography in acute ischemic stroke. Stroke 21:895–900
4. Herderscheê D, Limberg M, van Royen EA, Hijdra A, Büller HR, Koster RA (1991) Thrombolysis with recombinant tissue plasminogen activator in acute ischemic stroke: Evaluation with rCBF-SPECT. Acta Neurol Scand 83:317–322
5. Limburg M, van Royen EA, Hijda A, Verbeeten B (1991) rCBF-SPECT in brain infarction; When does it predict outcome? J Nucl Med 32:382–387
6. Mori E, Yoneda Y, Tabuchi M, et al (1992) Intravenous recombinant tissue plasminogen activator in acute carotid artery territory stroke. Neurology 42:976–982
7. Okada Y, Sadoshima S, Nakane H, Utsunomiya H, Fujishima M (1992) Early computed tomographic findings for thrombolytic therapy in patients with acute brain embolism. Stroke 23:20–23
8. Okada Y, Yamaguchi T, Minematsu K, et al (1989) Hemorrhagic transformation in cerebral embolism. Stroke 20:598–603
9. Reynaud C, Rancurel G, Tzourio N, et al (1989) SPECT analysis of recent cerebral infarction. Stroke 20:735–740

The Relevance of Neurological and Functional Outcome Scales for Acute Stroke Trials

A. Ferbert and K. Willmes

Research in the field of medical treatment is based on the assessment of variables that are aimed at by the therapy under question. Even if it is tempting and easy to choose a single laboratory parameter for measurement, it is the improvement of the patient's general clinical status that is of utmost importance before introducing a new therapy. The assessment of a stroke patient seems to be particularly difficult, as a stroke commonly leads to a variety of more or less independent signs that may or may not be improved by a drug in different ways. Is the treatment of benefit to the patient or not if his or her moderate paresis completely resolves but at the same time Broca's aphasia deteriorates to global aphasia? In the following we will try to analyze how different stroke scales have dealt with this problem. We will focus on scales that attempt to quantify deficit or residual abilities once stroke has occurred. We will not touch on the methodological problems that one has to face in a stroke prevention trial when an ischemic event or death occurs in a previously healthy or at-risk patient.

Requirements for a Clinical Scale

Clinical scales like a stroke scale are based on clinical judgments. Thus, when using a scale we have to take at least three steps:

1. Obtain a certain neurological sign.
2. Transform this sign into a given category of the scale.
3. In many instances, classify the intensity of this sign.

Each of these steps may be subject to bias.

How reliably these steps are taken can be estimated by testing the agreement between different investigators (interrater reliability) and the agreement of two judgements of the same investigator at different points in time (intrarater stability). One of the first papers to look at interrater reliability in neurological examinations [19] found considerable disagreement between two observers even for seemingly unequivocal signs (15% disagreement for "paresis"). Simi-

Department of Neurology, RWTH Aachen, Aachen, Federal Republic of Germany

G. J. del Zoppo, E. Mori, W. Hacke (Eds.)
Thrombolytic Therapy in Acute Ischemic Stroke II

lar results have been obtained from the Stroke Data Bank [18] with kappa values for neurological history-taking even lower than for the neurological examination. The interrater reliability has been investigated for several stroke scales or disability scales [4, 8, 10, 24]. A measure for interobserver agreement is the kappa statistic which ranges between 1 for complete agreement and −1 for complete disagreement. Kappa is corrected for chance agreement [3] and interobserver bias [12].

Less is known about intrarater stability. Here, the problem of the observer being biased by his previous choice may occur. Still less has been discussed about the validity of a stroke scale. At first sight, content validity seems to be obvious for most stroke scales. The issue may, however, be critical for functional scales. Do we want to measure the severity of a syndrome or do we want to quantify how much the patient suffers from a given deficit?

Besides these standard psychometric requirements, a stroke scale should be simple and quick to be completed. A major problem for any stroke scale is the issue of missing data. One sign may prevent the assessment of another. If, for example, the patient has global aphasia, the investigator is commonly unable to assess the patient's orientation even if the latter is undisturbed. If a global test score is calculated, missing scores lead to an incorrect assessment of the patient. The same holds true for patients whose neurological status is not assessable due to the application of sedative drugs.

One Total Score for a Multidimensional Test?

It is very popular to use total scores in stroke scales as well as in other neurological scales that have found widespread application like the Glasgow Coma Scale (GCS). This is because total scores appear to be handled easily and can also be used in group studies. This procedure seems to be justified if just one phenomenon (e.g., disability) is measured. However, the procedure seems to be dubious with multidimensional scales that measure the presence and intensity of several signs. Avoiding total scores would imply that when, for example, comparing a treatment and a placebo group, one would have to deal with a large number of variables. One way of reducing multivariate data is principle component analysis, a method by which the original variables are transformed to a smaller set of new variables (the principle components) which cover most of the variability in the set of original variables. Such an approach has been applied to data from a study using the Glasgow Coma Scale. As a result of this analysis, the authors strongly discourage the use of the GCS sum score [11].

It is not the aim of this paper to cover the problems that arise from statistical analysis of data derived from stroke scales. It should, however, be mentioned that most stroke scales or disability scores are only ordinal, precluding the use of, for example, t or F tests.

Functional Scales

Functional scales are designed to measure the functional status of a patient in terms of activities of daily living or in terms of disability irrespective of the specific neurological deficit causing a given disability. Some of the functional scales are therefore not specifically designed for stroke. It takes some time to assess a patient's activities of daily living. The ability to take a bath independently or control bowel (like in the Barthel index) can not be assessed within a few minutes and, therefore, such scales are not suited for studies that aim at evaluating the neurological status before and after treatment for acute stroke. There are, however, several studies that use both a stroke scale for the acute stage and, in addition, a functional scale in the late phase for comparison of treatment and control groups.

One problem of functional scales lies in the fact that the capabilities of different patients to cope with a given neurological deficit are quite different. A moderate hemiparesis might lead to only mild disability in one patient with excellent compensatory strategies, whereas it may lead to a greater disability in another patient. We will only mention two functional scales that have often been used in previous stroke studies. A more complete account is given elsewhere [23].

Barthel index: The Barthel index [14] is one of the most commonly used scores for testing activities of daily living. It contains the following items: bowel control, bladder control, grooming, toilet use, feeding, transfer, walking, dressing, stairs, and bathing with two or three categories for each item. The score ranges from 0 for complete functional dependence to 100 for independence, with 5-point increments. As this gives a wrong impression of preciseness, one can also use a version with scores ranging from 0 to 20 and 1-point increments. The validity of the Barthel index has been tested [25] by comparing it with other scales and has been found to be sufficient. These authors also reported about a factor analysis leading to three factors, one of which had a high communality for all items. However, some items are not a direct measure of the severity of the stroke but are rather the result of some other deficit: disturbed bowel and bladder control are not a common consequence of a stroke unless the patient suffers from hemiplegia rendering him unable to move. The Barthel index differentiates better between severely disabled patients than between mildly disabled patients. A patient with global aphasia and a mild hemiparesis will get the maximum score similar to another patient whose symptoms and signs have completely recovered, which again points out the multidimensional properties of this index.

Most of the work aimed at testing the psychometric properties has been carried out with patients in the chronic stage, or some days after stroke at the earliest [25]. Therefore, the Barthel index is unlikely to be a valid measure of disability in the first hours after a stroke. In many stroke studies a neurological scale has been used for clinical assessment in the early phase, and the Barthel index has been applied 3 months after the stroke.

Most neurological scales have explicitly or implicitly been designed for strokes in the anterior circulation. This is indeed a crucial point. A pupillary abnormality has a completely different meaning in an anterior versus posterior circulation stroke. Thus, it is not advisable to include patients of either group in one single trial using one neurological scale.

The Rankin scale is a measure of disability. The original version [16] contained 5 grades and was slightly modified later on [22] to 6 different degrees. The latter version ranges from 0 for no symptoms at all to 5 for severe disability, being bedridden, incontinent, and requiring constant nursing care and attention. This scale measures only one facet (disability) which makes it easier to use and for grouping data from many patients, but it is still only ordinal. The interobserver agreement of the Rankin scale has been investigated. In half of the patients, two observers differed by 1 degree and in three patients by 2 degrees [24], which was considered by the authors to be a good yet improvable result in favor of the Rankin scale. The scale has been used in the Dutch TIA Trial [21] as well as in the European Carotid Surgery Trial [6]. A difficulty with this scale as with all disability scales is that a given deficit may be classified completely differently according to the patient's habits. A patient with a mild hemiparesis and Broca's aphasia may feel only mildly disabled if he has retired from work and is under the care of his family. However, a sales manager living on his own will perceive the same deficit as a severe disability.

Neurological Stroke Scales

Neurological stroke scales try to assess neurological signs caused by the stroke irrespective of the particular impact of these signs to the individual. Different scales differ mainly with respect to the comprehensiveness with which signs are recorded. We are used to performing a neurological examination with much scrutiny. However, some of the signs that may be of diagnostic value may not be of use to indicate the efficacy of a new therapy. On the other hand, the more signs we record, the more facets we have to deal with, making comparisons more difficult.

The scales also differ in the way they account for signs that cannot be assessed due to the presence of another deficit (e.g., orientation in a patient with aphasia). Nearly all of them contain an assessment of orientation. This is difficult to understand since disturbed orientation is common in diffuse brain dysfunction but not in focal disease like ischemic infarction. It can, however, be misunderstood as some other neuropsychological sign such as mild Wernicke's aphasia or neglect.

One of the first neurological stroke scales was the *Mathew score* [15]. It was designed for a glycerol study without having undergone any check for validity or reliability, and those studies are still scarce. The interobserver variability is considerable and it has been suggested to avoid items with low interobserver agreement like sensation, hemianopia, etc. [8]. The scale ranges from 100 for the healthy patient to 0 for death. Items include mentation, speech, cranial nerves, motor power, performance or disability, reflexes and sensation. Thus, a functional scale is integrated into the neurological scale. The weighting of these items is unbalanced in that the patient loses only up to 8 points for being in a coma but on the other hand 23 points for severe aphasia. Despite these drawbacks, the scale has been used in a number of studies including those concerned with calcium antagonists [9].

The *Hemispheric Stroke Scale* [1] has incorporated the Glasgow Coma Scale. Apart from that, it has a rather complete list of items of the neurological examination including muscle tone and stereognosis. The maximum score is 100 for the most severely disabled.

The *NIH Stroke Scale* [2] has been developed from three preexisting scales and contains a rather complete list of 15 items that one would expect to be of relevance in stroke. The interobserver reliability has been found to be moderate to substantial in 9 of 13 items and the scale is thought to compare favorably with other scales [10]. The possibility of using an abbreviated form that proved more reliable was discussed [2]. However, it was felt that the lower correlation of the short form with infarct size in CT would indicate lower validity and therefore the short form was dismissed. We think that reliability is of particular importance, and it is not yet clear whether infarct size on CT is an ideal external criterion for assessing the validity of a stroke scale. Therefore, the abbreviated form could still be a valuable option.

The *Scandinavian Stroke Scale* [17] has been developed for a trial of hemodilution in ischemic stroke. Two forms are available: in a short version for the acute stage, the patient can reach a maximum score of 22 with 4 items (consciousness, eye movements, motor power of arm, motor power of leg). The long version comprises 7 items including speech and gait, with a maximum score of 48. The scale represents a first step towards reducing the number of items in the acute stage, even though speech should be included and the weighting of different eye movement abnormalities is not feasible for hemispheric stroke (gaze preponderance to one side occurs prior to a gaze palsy in hemispheric stroke).

The *Canadian Neurological Scale* [4, 5] differs from other stroke scales in that it is shorter and focusses on a few key signs: disturbance of mentation including speech and motor power. These are items that can lead to long- lasting deficit in a hemispheric stroke. The score ranges from 11.5 for the healthy individual to 1.5 for the most severe syndrome. It was the reasoning of the authors to avoid the recording of signs that are of minor relevance for the patient in the long run. In this respect, the Canadian Neurological Scale can be viewed as a link between a neurological scale and a disability scale. Besides other psychometric properties of the scale, its discriminant validity has been investigated and the scale was found to be sensitive to changes in neurological status, more sensitive than the Glasgow Coma Scale [4]. The one thing that is difficult to understand in this scale is the scoring of motor function in the patient with a comprehension deficit: a patient with global aphasia would score 3.5 for undisturbed motor function, whereas a patient without a comprehension deficit would score 6.5 for undisturbed motor function. Therefore, if motor function is normal as seen from observation, it should be scored 6.5 irrespective of the existence of a comprehension deficit.

A number of scales exist for the assessment of single stroke signs like paresis, aphasia, depression, etc. Of these, motor scales seem to be most suited for a treatment trial of acute stroke in that hemiparesis can easily and quickly be assessed. Furthermore, hemiparesis is probably the most common and the most disabling sign in stroke. Several motor assessment scales have been developed [7, 13, 20, 25]. Most of these studies have been used in a rehabilitation setting but it would be worthwhile to investigate their usefulness in an acute stroke study.

Conclusion

The number of available neurological and functional stroke scales indicates that none of them is suited for all kinds of stroke studies. One has to find out the specific demands for a given study, and still an ideal assessment procedure may not be available yet. The psychometric properties of the scales at hand should be investigated more thoroughly. Most important is the question whether all items represent just one homogeneous scale. Otherwise, several independent types of information may be confounded in a single score.

References

1. Adams RJ, Meador KJ, Sethi KD, Grotta JC, Thompson DS (1987) Graded neurological scale for use in acute hemispheric stroke treatment protocols. Stroke 18:665–669
2. Brott T, Adams HP, Olinger CP, et al (1989) Measurements of acute cerebral infarction: A clinical examination scale. Stroke 20:864–870
3. Cohen J (1960) A coefficient of agreement for nominal scales. Educ Psychol Measur 20:34–46
4. Coté R, Battista RN, Wolfson C, Boucher J, Adams J, Hachinski VC (1989) The Canadian Neurological Scale: Validation and reliability assessment. Neurology 39:638–643
5. Cote R, Hachinski VC, Shurtell BL, Norris JW, Wolfson C (1986) The Canadian Neurological Scale: A preliminary study in acute stroke. Stroke 17:731–737
6. European Carotid Surgery Trialist's Collaborative Group (1991) MRC European carotid surgery trial: Interim results for symptomatic patients with severe (70–99%) or with mild (0–29%) carotid stenosis. Lancet 337:1235–1243
7. Fugl-Meyer AR, Jääskö L, Leyman I, Olsson S, Steglind S (1975) I. A method for evaluation of physical performance. Scand J Rehabil Med 7:13–31
8. Gelmers HJ, Gorter K, de Weerdt CJ, Wiezer HJA (1988) Assessment of interobserver variability in a Dutch multicenter study on acute ischemic stroke. Stroke 19:709–711
9. Gelmers HJ, Hennerici M (1990) Effect of nimodipine on acute ischemic stroke pooled results from five randomized trials. Stroke 21(Suppl IV):IV-81–IV-84
10. Goldstein LB, Bertels C, Davis JN (1989) Interrater reliability of the NIH Stroke Scale. Arch Neurol 46:660–662

11. Koziol JA, Hacke W (1990) Multivariate data reduction by principal components, with application to neurological scoring instruments. J Neurol 237:461–464
12. Krauth J (1984) A modification of kappa for intraobserver bias. Biom J 26:435–445
13. Loewen SC, Anderson BA (1988) Reliability of the modified motor assessment scale and the Barthel index. Phys Ther 68:1077–1081
14. Mahoney FJ, Barthel DW (1965) Functional evaluation. The Barthel index. Md Med J 14:61–65
15. Mathew NT, Rivera VM, Meyer JS, Charney JZ, Hartmann A (1972) Double-blind evaluation of glycerol therapy in acute cerebral infarction. Lancet December 23:7791–7793
16. Rankin J (1957) Cerebral vascular accident in patients over the age of 60. II. Prognosis. Scott Med J 2:200–215
17. Scandinavian Stroke Study Group (1985) Multicenter trial of hemodilution in ischemic stroke – background and study protocol. Stroke 16:885–890
18. Shinar D, Gross CR, Mohr JP, et al (1985) Interobserver variability in the assessment of neurologic history and examination in the Stroke Data Bank. Arch Neurol 42:557–565
19. Sisk C, Ziegler DK, Zileli T (1970) Discrepancies in recorded results from duplicate neurological history and examination in patients studied for prognosis in cerebrovascular disease. Stroke 1:14–18
20. Skyhoj-Olsen T (1990) Arm and leg paresis as outcome predictors in stroke rehabilitation. Stroke 21:247–251
21. The Dutch TIA Study Group. (1988) The Dutch TIA Trial: Protective effects of low-dose aspirin and atenolol in patients with transient ischemic attacks or nondisability stroke. Stroke 19:512–517
22. UK TPA Study Group (1988) The UK-TPA aspurin trial. Interim results. Br Med J 296:316–320
23. van Gijn J (1992) Measurement of outcome in stroke prevention trials. Cerebrovasc Dis 2(Suppl 1):23–34
24. van Swieten JC, Koudstaal PJ, Visser MC, Schouten HJA, van Gijn J (1988) Interobserver agreement for the assessment of handicap in stroke patients. Stroke 19:604–607
25. Wade DT, Hewer RL (1987) Functional abilities after stroke: Measurement, natural history and prognosis. J Neurol Neurosurg Psychiatry 50:177–182

Discussion Summary: Diagnosis and Assessment of Outcomes in Acute Cerebral Ischemia

Chaired by S.M. Otis[1] and L. Wechsler[2]

In opening the discussion, Dr. Grotta commented to Dr. Ringelstein: "That was a beautiful presentation. My neurologic fellow lives with our patients for the first 24 h doing serial transcranial Dopplers because of the amount of data that must be obtained. I wonder whether you have noticed a relationship between late recanalization and patients who deteriorate from cerebral edema? In other words, I know you presented your data about improvement in relationship to recanalization, but what about deterioration from edema with patients who have rather late recanalization?" Dr. Ringelstein replied that he could not answer the question because this aspect was not investigated.

Dr. Fieschi then rose: "I have two questions. Both of them concern time. One for Dr. Wolpert and one for Dr. Ringelstein. I think we have to deal with time here at this conference. In fact, it is the only thing we can reliably measure without having to deal with interobserver reliability and without high technology. Now, time is important, even though, as Lou Caplan said once, 'We should not treat time, but patients.' But, time is still very important. So, the first question to Dr. Wolpert. He states that there is a good relationship between early CT signs and both final clinical outcome and final infarct size. But his measurement was done within 24 h. And to me, this is not exactly an early CT scan. Or, at least, I would like to know how many CT scans have you done within 6 h. My question is based on our own findings. In fact, we had positive early CT scans within 5 to 6 h in 44% of patients who eventually had a good outcome clinically. Slightly fewer positive CT scans in the good outcome group than in the bad outcome group were seen, but yet we did not find the correlation that you found within the 24-h CT scans. So, how many studies did you do within 6 h?"

Dr. Wolpert replied: "I think I probably did not make myself clear. The early signs of ischemia were assessed on the initial CT scan obtained in all patients prior to being allowed to get into the study. Early CT signs, i.e., the effacement

[1] Division of Neurology, Scripps Clinic & Research Foundation, La Jolla, CA, USA
[2] Pittsburgh Neurology Group, Inc., Pittsburgh, PA, USA

G.J. del Zoppo, E. Mori, W. Hacke (Eds.)
Thrombolytic Therapy in Acute Ischemic Stroke II

of the sulcus size and the slight hypodensity, were assessed on the first scan (the entry CT scan), all within 8 h. The size of the infarct was assessed on the 24-h scan that every patient had. I did not deal with clinical outcome."

Dr. Fieschi, again: "The second question is for Dr. Ringelstein. I completely agree with your statement that there is a marginally significant relation between spontaneous recanalization and final outcome. But, here again, spontaneous recanalization between the first TCD, and the second TCD – I should not call it early, since early, clinically, is only if the recanalization takes place within the initial 6 to 8 h. You have the second TCD showing recanalization done at 24 h, if I am correct. That is already late for the clinical benefit to the patient. This is perhaps a matter of terminology: what should be called 'early' and what should be called 'late'?" Dr. Ringelstein responded "Yes, the correlations that we calculated between the time of recanalization and the outcomes of infarct size and neurological score were only related to those patients who were subdivided into the groups *very early*, which is up to 4 h, *early*, which is up to 8 h (so we agree in defining 'early'), and *late*, which means later than 8 h. So, the numbers refer to this subdivision. The correlation that we found between the rapidity of recanalization and outcome by infarct size and neurological score was only true for patients with either *very early* recanalization (i.e., within 4 h after stroke onset), or with *early* recanalization (i.e., within 8 h after stroke). An unfavorable outcome was significantly more frequent if recanalization occurred 'late,' i.e., later than 8 h."

Dr. Forsting presented a question to Dr. Furlan regarding any additional future advantages of MRI. He noted that their group had performed work on perfusion MR imaging using an animal stroke model and superparamagnetic contrast agents. They were able to detect the perfusion defects (transforming to the definite complete infarction area later on) within 45 min after occlusion of the MCA.

Dr. Furlan replied that the most useful imaging modality for detecting early ischemia-related changes appears to be diffusion-weighted MR imaging. Experience at the Cleveland Clinic with animal models has demonstrated similar diffusion-weighted changes within an hour of vessel occlusion which are most probably related to early cytotoxic edema and intracellular sodium accumulation. These observations are promising, although one logistical problem which must be overcome is the current requirement for special coils adapted for human imaging studies. Further developments along these lines should make this a very sensitive index of ischemia. Dr. Furlan continued, regarding MR perfusion imaging. "I think potentially this has great promise, because we can now do functional flow correlation. Some of this data is starting to come out analogous to some of the PET work. Again, the beauty of MR is that with this single basic technology, we can manipulate the signal to get not only anatomic, but also vascular and functional imaging. The trick is how to bring this all together in what I call a 'stroke-o-gram.' What kind of information do we need? How fast do we need it? A lot of this will depend on what kind of patient we are looking at, what kind of drug we are looking at, what kind of question we are trying to answer."

Dr. von Kummer presented a comment on Dr. Furlan's presentation. "We observed vascular enhancement with MR in one patient with bilateral carotid occlusion, but without an infarct. So I think this sign indicates the flow disturbance, but not early infarct."

Dr. von Kummer followed with a question to Dr. Ringelstein regarding his slide showing the effect of rt-PA and heparin on recanalization: "Do you think that the minimal difference is due to rt-PA, in general, or due to the dosage used?" Dr. Ringelstein replied, "As we have heard in a previous paper, the rt-PA Acute Stroke Study Group trial had prematurely been stopped, and the intended full rt-PA dosage was never reached. Although some of the patients received rt-PA doses in the range of 0.9 mg/kg (sic) during their 1-h treatment, one may argue that the patients underlying the recanalization curve of the rt-PA group did not reflect a beneficial effect of fibrinolysis since the dose-rates were ineffective. So there are, indeed, two ways to interpret our findings, either to state that there is no detectable difference in the rapidity of MCA recanalization between rt-PA-treated and heparin-treated patients, or, alternatively, that rt-PA applied in the doses used during the study are ineffective and do not accelerate renewal of MCA blood flow. In any case, our findings prove that a favorable effect of rt-PA in terms of recanalization time remains questionable and that the therapeutic time window is extremely narrow, presumably less than 4 h."

Ancillary Therapy for Cerebrovascular Reperfusion

Neuronal Protection and Recanalization Strategies: Is More Better?

J. Grotta

The very title of this section of the symposium, i.e., "*Ancillary* Therapy for Cerebrovascular Reperfusion," underscores the prominent hopes and expectations that the stroke community has invested in thrombolytic therapy. Thrombolysis makes intuitive sense, is effective in other circulatory beds, and may result in dramatic clinical changes. Furthermore, it requires mobilization of emergency personnel which requires neurologists to depart from their traditional passive therapeutic attitude towards stroke.

All of these features are lacking with neuronal protective therapy, hence its relegation in this symposium to the stepchild category of "ancillary" therapy. Neuroprotective therapies are based on manipulating a complex and interacting group of pathways leading to cell destruction which still are poorly understood. Such therapies have not been proven useful in other organ systems, and in experimental animal and human studies to date they have been of only marginal benefit. Finally, as they have been employed in clinical trials, the use of these agents has more or less followed the traditional less aggressive practices of our specialty and, except in a few instances, have not generally incorporated the mobilization of emergency medical resources.

This section will review the current state of knowledge about neuronal protective agents focusing particularly on glutamate antagonists. I will not provide an exhaustive review of the vast number of experimental studies carried out using these agents but will select a few which demonstrate the methods of action and potential potency of these drugs, their side effects, and most importantly how they might be combined with reperfusion therapies. This last question remains largely speculative but deserves careful thought and planning as we analyze the first round of thrombolytic clinical trials in an attempt to augment the effect of thrombolytics, reduce their side effects, and extend the time window of opportunity for safe recanalization.

Department of Neurology, University of Texas Medical School, Houston, TX, USA

G. J. del Zoppo, E. Mori, W. Hacke (Eds.)
Thrombolytic Therapy in Acute Ischemic Stroke II

Biology of Neuronal Protection

Interest in protecting nerve cells against ischemic injury was stimulated by the observation of "delayed neuronal damage" in models of global cerebral ischemia [16]. The recognition that brief periods (i.e., up to 30 min) of near total ischemia did not produce immediate cell death, but rather selective damage in vulnerable cell populations occurring over 72 h led researchers to explore the biochemical pathways responsible for these changes. The "calcium hypothesis" linking an increase in intracellular ionic calcium and consequent activation of proteases, phospholipases, and kinases has been the most studied and has resulted in the most potential pharmacological manipulations. However, much of the early work relating calcium to neuronal death was based on cell culture and hippocampal slice preparations and not on in vivo models more analogous to the human stroke situation. It has only been in the last few years that calcium influx has been causally linked to ischemic injury, and more importantly, it has been recognized that changes in calcium homeostasis and activation of potentially damaging enzyme systems occurs almost instantaneously. Therefore, although the histologic appearance of cell death may be delayed for 72 h, if calcium is the culprit, the damage is done within the first few minutes.

In our laboratory, we have studied calcium–calmodulin (CaM) binding and CaM kinase II activation after both global and focal ischemia in an attempt to determine a time window for potential neuroprotective therapy aimed at preventing calcium-mediated events. After global ischemia, calcium–calmodulin binding was maximal by 24 h after a threshold of 10 min of ischemia [2, 15]. Ischemic intervals below 10 min resulted in little damage and reversal of histologic damage. Ischemic intervals longer than 10 min resulted in progressively more calcium–calmodulin binding which became maximal by 24 h.

In a model of focal middle cerebral artery occlusion in spontaneously hypertensive rats, temporary occlusion as brief as 1 h resulted in infarct volumes that were almost 50% as large as those infarcts that were found when the artery was permanently occluded. In almost an exact correlation, irreversible calcium–calmodulin binding was found in those same regions that became infarcted, and partial binding was found in border zone regions. Within 2 to 4 h of occlusion, maximal calcium–calmodulin binding was seen throughout the entire middle cerebral artery distribution in proportion to the histologic damage found at 24 h (Fig. 1) [5].

Even more rapid changes can be found using an assay of CaM kinase II activity. Ischemic durations of 5, 30, and 60 min resulted in progressively greater inactivation of CaM kinase II in a central core surrounded by progressively less reduction in activity as tissue samples were obtained further away from the site of maximal injury (A. Hanson and J. Grotta, unpublished). Even after only 5 min of temporary middle cerebral artery occlusion, CaM kinase II activity had not recovered to normal by 24 h in the central core.

From these data, it is clear that 10 min of severe global ischemia analogous to cardiac arrest, and 2 to 4 h of reversible focal ischemia analogous to clinical

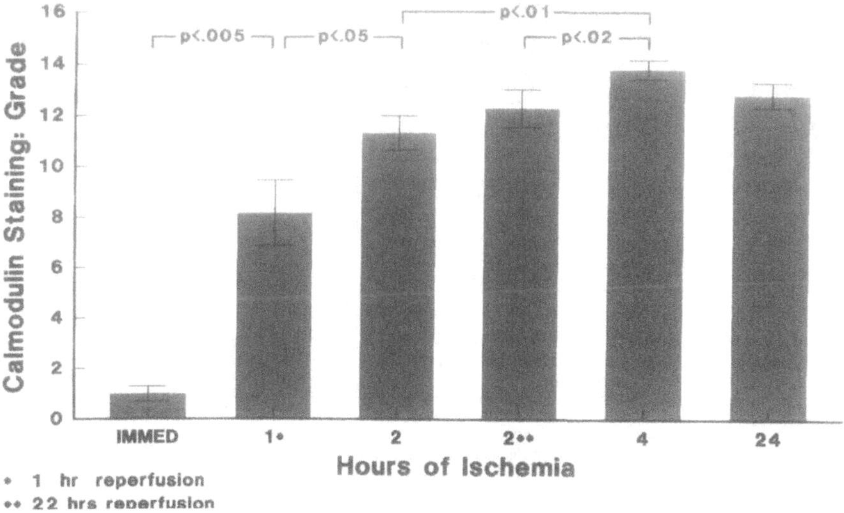

Fig. 1. Grading of calmodulin (*CaM*) staining by an anti-CaM antibody (which recognizes only CaM unbound to calcium ions and target protein) in parietal cortex after middle cerebral artery occlusion. Staining was evaluated immediately after ischemia, after 1 h of occlusion and 1 h of reperfusion, 2 h of occlusion, 2 h of occlusion and 22 h of reperfusion, 4 h of occlusion, and 24 h of occlusion. Staining was graded on a 15-point scale, with 0 being normal and 15 representing total loss of staining due to binding of CaM to calcium and target protein (mean ± SEM)

stroke produces maximal disruption of calcium homeostasis unless reperfusion occurs. Furthermore, calcium disruption occurs instantaneously and is probably maximal by 2 to 4 h.

The clinical relevance of these data is that to be effective, neuronal protective agents aimed at preventing calcium-mediated events must be given and be at work in the brain within 2 to 4 h of the onset of the symptoms to have any effect, and that the earlier the therapy the better. This may sound like a familiar refrain to investigators interested in thrombolytic therapy, but as will be demonstrated, clinical trials of neuroprotective therapies carried out to date have not incorporated in their design anything like this sense of urgency.

Another message from these data is that early (i.e., within 1 to 2 h) reperfusion salvages neurons in proportion to consequent normalization of calcium homeostasis, but reperfusion by itself does not completely reverse calcium–CaM enzyme activation or prevent neuronal damage. Therefore, there is reason to expect that a combination of reperfusion and neuronal protective therapies would be more effective.

Strategies for manipulating the calcium system have focused on the dihydropyridine antagonists of voltage-operated calcium channels and on inhibitors of the receptor-operated channels activated by glutamate. These include the NMDA and quisqualate-operated channels (Fig. 2). Calcium enters cells after membrane depolarization (voltage-operated channels), and after the release of excitatory neurotransmitters such as glutamate (NMDA channel).

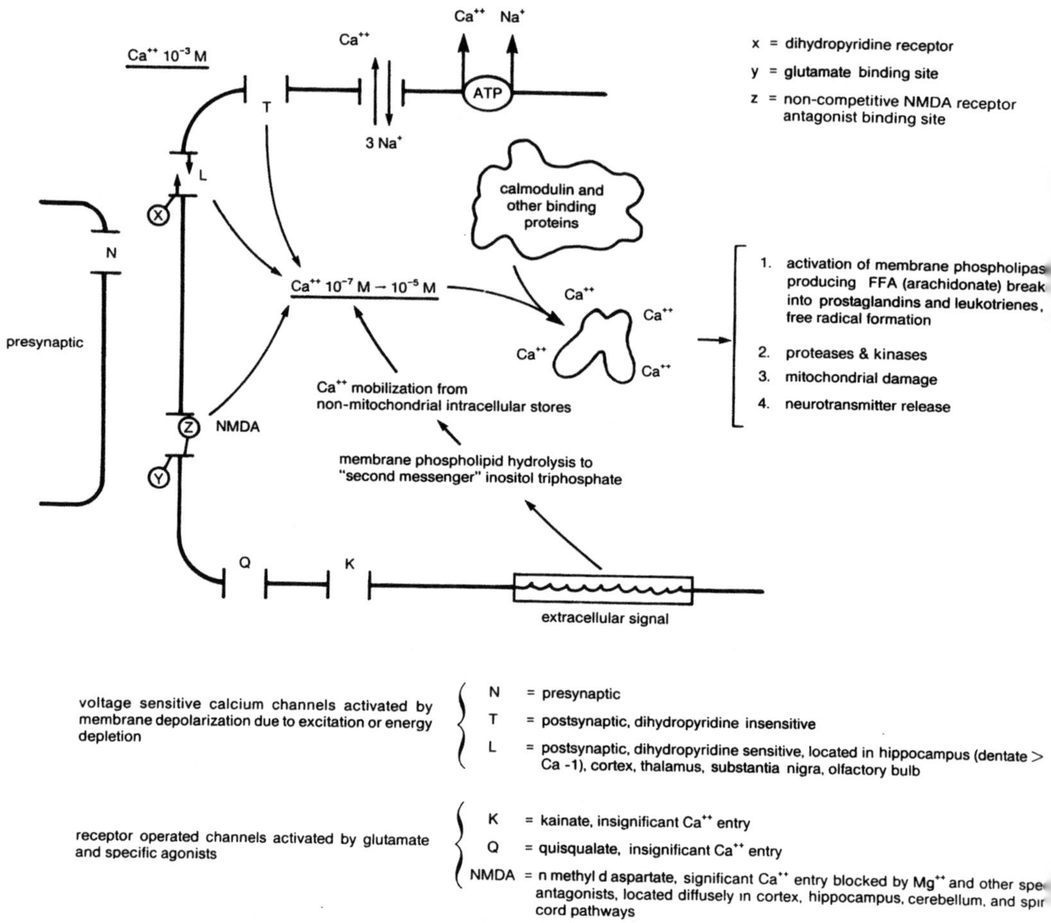

Fig. 2. Calcium entry channels and the fate of calcium ions in the postsynaptic terminal

Glutamate also activates the quisqualate receptor-operated channel which primarily gates sodium movement which has a secondary effect on maintaining activity of the NMDA channel. Consequently, neuronal protective strategies have been aimed at: 1) blocking voltage-operated calcium channels; 2) blocking glutamate release; 3) competitive and noncompetitive blockade of the NMDA channel; and 4) blockade of the quisqualate channel.

Animal Studies

To summarize a huge body of animal experimental data using calcium antagonists, these drugs have been shown to increase cerebral blood flow by producing vasodilation, and have a modest effect on preventing calcium influx in doses which do not produce unacceptable cardiovascular side effects [6, 8]. Modest neuronal protection has been found in some models, particularly after pretreatment of focally ischemic animals [4, 12].

Glutamate antagonists have enjoyed somewhat greater success in animal studies, though interpretation of results has been confused by the propensity of these drugs to cause cerebral hypothermia which by itself has a substantial

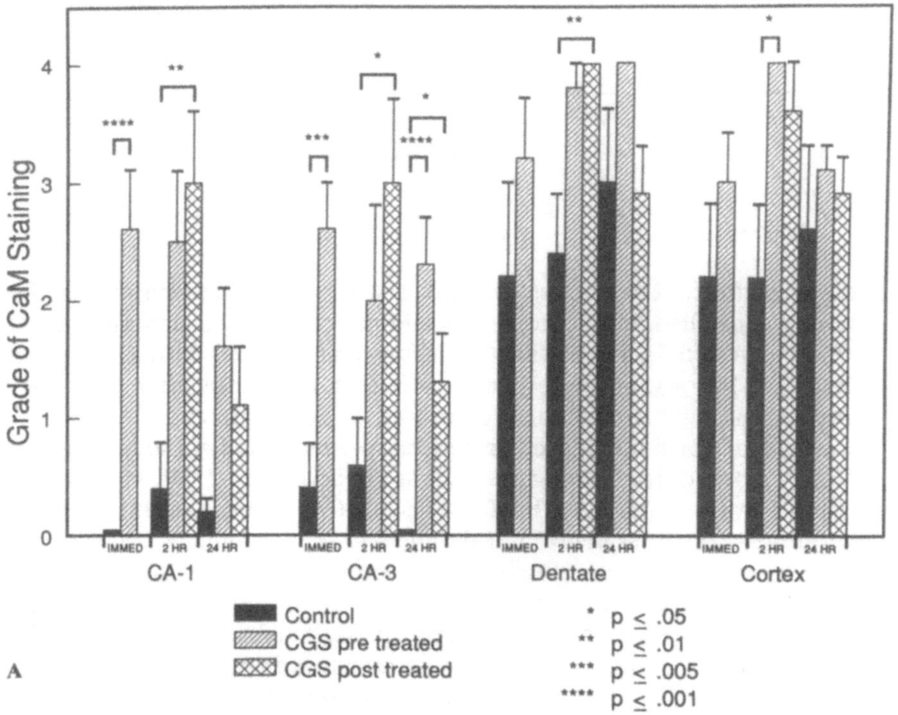

A

Fig. 3. A Grading of calmodulin (CaM) staining by an anti-CaM antibody (which recognizes only CaM unbound to calcium ions and target protein) in CA1, CA3, dentate, and cortex immediately after ischemia, and after 2 and 24 h of reperfusion. Results in ischemic controls and animals treated with CGS 19755 10 mg/kg immediately before ischemia and repeated every 1 to 2 h. Staining was graded on a 4-point scale, with 4 being normal and 0 representing total loss of staining due to binding of CaM to calcium and target protein (mean ± SEM). **B** Grading of histological damage, demonstrated by light microscopy in the cortex and 7 hippocampal regions in ischemic control animals compared to animals given CGS 19755 30 mg/kg immediately prior to ischemia. Damage was graded on a 4-point scale, with 0 being normal and 4 representing 75 to 100% of neurons damaged (mean ± SEM)

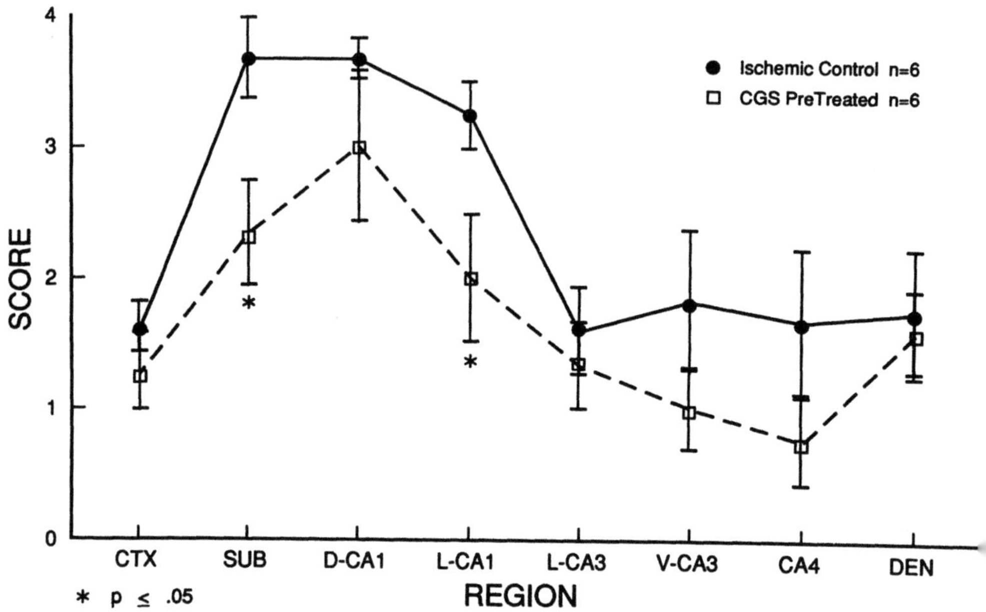

Fig. 3 B

protective effect. Nevertheless, in studies where head temperature has been carefully controlled, both competitive and noncompetitive glutamate antagonists have resulted in less calcium influx and reduced histologic damage (Fig. 3) [9, 14]. Again, more benefit was seen after focal than after global ischemia, and with pretreatment compared to posttreatment.

Because of their binding characteristics, some glutamate antagonists will probably share some of the same effects as phencyclidine (PCP) and other psychoactive drugs which also bind in the NMDA receptor-operated channel. High doses have resulted in sedation in animal models. Furthermore, vacuolization in certain brain regions has been found after dosing in normal animals [13]. Consequently, the potential toxicity of these drugs is a major impediment to their use in humans. Recent studies have shown that some of the damage induced by these drugs may be attenuated by concomitant therapy with haloperidol [18], thereby suggesting a possible mechanism to both counteract the behavioral side effects of the drug and protect against cytotoxicity.

Other strategies to increase the efficacy:toxicity ratio are to focus on inhibitors of glutamate release and on sites having an indirect effect on the NMDA channel. Blockade of glutamate release has been particularly effective in some experiments (S. Graham, unpublished), and other laboratories have reported striking success with NBQX, an inhibitor of the quisqualate channel [19]. However, in our hands, neither intravenous nor intraperitoneal administration of this drug resulted in a beneficial effect on calcium metabolism or infarct size in a focal model of ischemia [3].

Recently, investigators have tried combining glutamate and calcium antagonists. Although we found no benefit combining CGS 19755 and nicardipine [7], combination therapy of MK801 and nimodipine reduced cytosolic-free calcium and histologic damage in a temporary focal model in cats when started within 5 min after ischemia [21]. A combination of MK801 and nicardipine was effective after global ischemia [10]. In both studies, the combination treatment was superior to either drug given alone. Furthermore, these studies demonstrated that reperfusion alone without "neuroprotective therapies" did not result in normalization of disrupted calcium homeostasis.

In summarizing animal experiments with glutamate antagonists, it is fair to say that, as with calcium antagonists, therapy has to be started prior to ischemia to be most effective, with less effect seen after postischemic therapy. Equally important, fear of side effects has substantially tempered enthusiasm for presently available drugs. Nevertheless, manipulation of the glutamate receptor-operated channels remains an area of intensive investigation, and it is possible that second or third generation drugs will be more effective and less toxic. The most effective strategy may be to prevent glutamate release. Alternatively, a drug which acts on the post- synaptic ion channel but in a selective and short-acting fashion might be less toxic.

Clinical Trials

The major group of neuroprotective agents that has undergone the most widespread clinical trials in human stroke patients to date is that of the calcium antagonists. The results of some of those studies have already been reviewed in this Symposium. Since they are the first clinical studies conducted of neuronal protective therapy, they provide important lessons for subsequent work in this field. Studies of dihydropyridine calcium antagonists have mainly focused on nimodipine because of its relative effect on the cerebral vasculature and relative lack of systemic side effects, namely hypotension. Most clinical trials of this drug have used doses that did not produce overt hypotension, i.e., up to 180 mg per day orally. In most cases the drug was started 24 to 48 h after the onset of ischemia [1]. As has already been extensively discussed, such time windows are far beyond the point at which such therapy could possible be effective in preventing neuronal calcium entry. Furthermore, as all of us who are interested in reperfusion therapy know, any effect of calcium antagonists on cerebral blood flow is probably irrelevant beyond the first few hours after infarction. Therefore, it is little surprise that these clinical studies were consistently negative. However, a recent meta-analysis of all nimodipine trials carried out to date included 333 patients treated within 12 h compared to 286 placebo-treated patients. In this subset, there was a highly significant benefit of nimodipine therapy [11]. Furthermore, analyzing dose response data, high doses of intravenous or oral therapy were detrimental because of hypotensive effects.

While a general perception exists that calcium antagonists have been proven ineffective because of these negative studies, a more accurate conclusion is that the drugs have not been adequately tested in a well-designed clinical trial including patients most likely to benefit. We carried out a small pilot study of intravenous nicardipine in an attempt to find a dose that was tolerated without hypotension. While there were no placebo controls in this study, all patients were started on therapy within 12 h of symptom onset, and those started within 6 h did much better than those treated from 6 to 12 h [17]. Based on these results as well as animal studies, the outer limit for onset of treatment after stroke for human studies of neuronal protective therapy should be 6 h.

Clinical trials with glutamate antagonists are just beginning. The FDA has given permission to several pharmaceutical companies to begin small dose escalation studies to determine the maximal tolerated dose in stroke patients. Such a study is underway with CGS 19755, and this study has now entered into a randomized controlled phase in an attempt to make a preliminary determination of efficacy. All patients are started on therapy within 6 h of the onset of symptoms.

A similar study is underway with dextrorphan. Steinberg and colleagues carried out a dose escalation safety study of dextrorphan in neurosurgical patients and administered doses up to 330 mg every 6 h which resulted in blood and brain levels comparable to those resulting in neuroprotection in animal models. High doses resulted in dizziness and ataxia which resolved after discontinuation of therapy [20].

The challenge with glutamate antagonist therapy will be to see if sufficient doses can be given without side effects in stroke patients who already have neurologic impairment which can be magnified by the central actions of these drugs.

Neuroprotection and Reperfusion

Zivin and Mazzarella published a study in which the glutamate antagonist MK801 or the calcium antagonist nimodipine were administered 5 min after the injection of clots into rabbit carotid arteries. Sixty minutes later, t-PA treatment was begun. Animals which had been treated with MK801 had substantially greater benefit from t-PA therapy than those animals treated with either t-PA or MK801 alone or with the combination of nimodipine and t-PA [22]. These data suggest that a safe and easily administered neuroprotective agent might be given in the emergency room setting while evaluating the patient for t-PA or other thrombolytic therapy. Not only might a neuroprotective drug used in this fashion augment the effect of reperfusion therapy, but because of its protective effect on marginally perfused neurons, such therapy may extend the time window during which reperfusion might be efficacious.

Most of us using thrombolytic therapy have observed patients who have improved with reperfusion only to deteriorate several hours later. In our experience using transcranial Doppler and SPECT, reocclusion of cerebral vessels is rare after thrombolytic therapy. Furthermore, in most of these cases, significant edema and hemorrhage is found in the effected region coincident with the late deterioration. Most likely this represents "reperfusion injury." Because such patients have transiently recovered from their neurological deficit, it is likely that neurons have been salvaged by timely reperfusion, but that sufficient endothelial damage has occurred to result in vasogenic edema and hemorrhage as reperfusion progresses. An important objective of neuronal protective therapy in future studies will be to prevent this reperfusion injury. Consequently, future studies of "ancillary" therapy to be coupled with thrombolysis should be based on a better understanding of the pathology of the cerebral vasculature injured by cerebral ischemia. What are the roles of calcium, white blood cells, arachidonic acid metabolites, and free radicals in vascular injury. The concept of "neuronal protective" therapy should be expanded to include protection of the reperfused vascular endothelium which may represent the "Achilles heel" of cerebral thrombolytic therapy.

References

1. American Nimodipine Study Group (1992) Clinical trial of nimodipine in acute stroke. Stroke 23:3–8
2. DeGraba T, Grotta J (1991) Ca^{++} influx an a predictor of neuronal damage after graded global ischemia. Stroke 22:140
3. DeGraba T, Hanson S, Ostrow P, Grotta J (1992) Calcium influx, histologic damage, and motor performance in rats treated with NBQX after focal ischemia. Neurology 42(Suppl III):361
4. Gotoh O, Mohammed A, McCullough J, Graham D, Harper A, Teasdale G (1986) Nimodipine and the hemodynamic and histopathologic consequences of middle cerebral artery occlusion in the rat. J Cereb Blood Flow Metab 6:321–331
5. Grotta J, DeGraba T (1992) How fast must we start neuroprotective therapies after cerebral ischemia? Stroke 23:147
6. Grotta J, Pettigrew L, Reid C, Rosenbaum D, McCandless D, Rhoades H (1988) Studies on the efficacy and mechanism of action of a calcium blocker after global cerebral ischemia. Stroke 19:447–454
7. Grotta J, Picone C, Dedman J, et al (1990) Neuronal protection correlates with prevention of calcium-calmodulin binding. Stroke 21(Suppl III):28–31
8. Grotta J, Picone C, Earls R, Strong R, Yao L, Dedman J (1990) Calcium- calmodulin binding in ischemic rat neurons after calcium channel blocker therapy. Stroke 21:948–952
9. Grotta J, Picone C, Ostrow P, et al (1990) CGS 19755, a competitive NMDA receptor antagonist, reduces calcium-calmodulin binding and improves outcome after global cerebral ischemia. Ann Neurol 27:612–619
10. Hewitt K, Corbett D (1992) Combined treatment with MK-801 and nicardipine reduces global ischemic damage in the gerbil. Stroke 23:82–86
11. International Nimodipine Study Group (1992) Meta-analysis of nimodipine trials in acute ischemic stroke. Stroke 23:148
12. Jacewicz M, Brint S, Tanabe J, Pulsinelli A (1990) Continuous nimodipine treatment attenuates cortical infarction in rats subjected to 24 hours of focal cerebral ischemia. J Cereb Blood Flow Metab 10:89–96
13. Olney J, Labruyere J, Price M (1989) Pathological changes induced in cerebrocortical neurons by phencyclidine and related drugs. Science 244:1360

14. Park C, Nehls D, Graham D (1988) Focal cerebral ischemia in the cat: Treatment with the glutamate antagonist MK-801 after induction of ischemia. J Cereb Blood Flow Metab 8:757
15. Picone C, Grotta J, Earls R, Strong R, Dedman J (1989) Immunohistochemical determination of calcium-calmodulin binding predicts neuronal damage after global ischemia. J Cereb Blood Flow Metab 9:805–811
16. Pulsinelli W, Brierley J, Plum F (1982) Temporal profile of neuronal damage in a model of transient forebrain ischemia. Ann Neurol 11:491–498
17. Rosenbaum D, Zabramski J, Frey J, et al (1991) Early treatment of ischemic stroke with a calcium antagonist. Stroke 22:437–441
18. Sharp F, Jasper P, Butman M (1992) Haloperidol prevents induction of HSP72 heat shock protein in posterior cingulate neurons injured by MK801, ketamine, and PCP: Implications for stroke therapy and psychosis. Neurology 42(Suppl III):360
19. Sheardown M, Nielsen E, Hansen A, Jacobsen P, Honore T (1990) 2, 3-dihydroxy-6-nitro-7-sylfamoyl-benzo (F) quinoxaline: A neuroprotectant for cerebral ischemia. Science 247:571–574
20. Steinberg G, Bell T (1991) Clinical dose-escalation safety study of the NMDA antagonist, dextromethorphan in neurosurgical patients. Stroke 22:141
21. Uematsu D, Araki N, Greenberg JH, Sladky J, Reivich M (1991) Combined therapy with MK-801 and nimodipine for protection of ischemic brain damage. Neurology 41:88–94
22. Zivin J, Mazzarella V (1991) Tissue plasminogen activator plus glutamate antagonist improves outcome after embolic stroke. Arch Neurol 48:1235–1238

Strategies Which Decrease Post-Reperfusion Lipid Peroxidation

E. D. Hall

The rapid treatment of acute thromboembolic stroke with thrombolytic agents to restore perfusion to the ischemic brain tissue is, of course, a rational therapeutic approach. However, the sudden reperfusion of ischemic brain tissue is known to lead to the generation of oxygen-free radicals and the possibility of secondary reperfusion injury. The potential sources of oxygen radicals within the reperfused nervous system include the arachidonic acid cascade (i.e., prostaglandin synthase and 5-lipoxygenase activity), catecholamine oxidation, mitochondrial "leak," and later infiltrating neutrophils. The radical-initiated peroxidation of neuronal, glial, and vascular cell membranes and myelin lipids is catalyzed by free iron released from hemoglobin, transferrin, and ferritin by either ischemia-lowered tissue pH or oxygen radicals. The mechanism of reperfusion injury is believed to mainly involve progressive cell membrane lipid peroxidation [6, 11]. If unchecked, lipid peroxidation is a geometrically progressing process that will spread over the surface of the cell membrane causing impairment to phospholipid-dependent enzymes, disruption of ionic gradients and, if severe enough, membrane lysis.

Thus, efforts have been made to discover pharmacological agents which can effectively inhibit post-reperfusion brain lipid peroxidation that would serve as adjuncts to thrombolytic therapy. Extensive studies with methylprednisolone had indicated that large intravenous doses (30 mg/kg) could ameliorate many of the pathophysiological consequences of traumatic or ischemic injury in the central nervous system (CNS), and promote the functional recovery of experimentally injured animals by inhibiting posttraumatic lipid peroxidation [10]. The definition of this high-dose non-glucocorticoid antioxidant action led to the synthesis of a number of non-glucocorticoid steroid analogues of methylprednisolone (e.g., U-72099E) which also weakly inhibited lipid peroxidation in high concentrations, and at high doses were active in models of experimental CNS trauma [12]. However, synthetic efforts continued that were aimed at preparation of compounds that were even more potent and effective inhibitors of lipid peroxidation, with greater activity in experimental models of CNS trauma and ischemia. This resulted in the discovery of a novel group

Central Nervous System Diseases Research, The Upjohn Company, Kalamazoo, MI, USA

G. J. del Zoppo, E. Mori, W. Hacke (Eds.)
Thrombolytic Therapy in Acute Ischemic Stroke II

of 21-aminosteroids ("lazaroids") which are effective inhibitors of oxygen radical-initiated, iron-catalyzed lipid peroxidation.

From the 21-aminosteroid series, U-74006F (tirilazad mesylate) has been selected for clinical development for the acute treatment of brain and spinal injury, subarachnoid hemorrhage and ischemic stroke. In the present discussion, the focus will be on the known antioxidant mechanisms of U-74006F and the compound's effect in experimental models of focal brain ischemia with reperfusion.

Tirilazad Mesylate-free Radical Scavenging/Antioxidant Mechanisms

The 21-aminosteroids have been shown to be potent inhibitors of lipid peroxidation in vitro. Using rat brain homogenates or purified rat brain synaptosomes as the lipid source, U-74006F potently inhibits iron-dependent lipid peroxidation, with an efficacy greatly surpassing that of the glucocorticoid steroid methylprednisolone, or the earlier non-glucocorticoid steroid U-72099E [8, 14]. U-74006F has further been found to decrease iron-induced damage to cultured cortical neurons [15].

Although U-74006F is a potent inhibitor of iron-dependent lipid peroxidation in intact phospholipid environments, it also inhibits lipid peroxidation in systems that do not contain membranes and are free of iron. By using the free radical generator 2, 2′-azobis(2, 4-dimethyl valeronitrile) to initiate lipid peroxidation in a homogeneous methanol solution of linoleic acid, the 21-aminosteroids have been found to inhibit peroxidation by scavenging lipid peroxyl radicals ($LOO^{\bullet}$) and thus block lipid radical chain reactions in a manner similar to vitamin E [7, 8]. The $LOO^{\bullet}$ scavenging action of U-74006F resides in the amine portion of the molecule, and yields an as yet uncharacterized product. During the inhibition of lipid peroxidation, U-74006F competes for the same reaction as vitamin E and slows its degradation [7]. In vivo studies have demonstrated that U-74006F indeed acts to preserve tissue vitamin E levels in ischemic brain tissue [13].

In addition to scavenging of lipid peroxyl radicals, U-74006F also reacts with hydroxyl radicals generated during in vitro Fenton reactions (i.e., $Fe^{++} + H_2O_2 \rightarrow Fe^{+++}\ OH^- + \cdot OH$). Recently, data has been obtained from rodent models of head trauma and global ischemia suggesting that the compound may also reduce hydroxyl radical concentration in vivo. Administration of salicylate, a hydroxyl radical trap, leads to the posttraumatic or postischemic formation of dihydroxybenzoic acid (DHBA) in brain tissue when it reacts with hydroxyl radical. U-74006F dosing leads to a decrease in DHBA formation, implying either a decreased formation or a scavenging of hydroxyl radicals [1, 2].

U-74006F also has stabilizing effects on cell membranes. The iodoacetate or iron(lipid peroxidation)-induced release of free arachidonic acid from injured cell membranes is blocked by the compound [5]. This effect is not due to glucocorticoid activity (i.e., phospholipase A2 inhibition), but may rather be due to its antioxidant actions. In other studies using cultured bovine brain microvascular endothelial cells, U-74006F has been shown to localize within the hydrophobic core of cell membranes and cause an increase in lipid ordering (i.e., decreased fluidity) of the phospholipid bilayer [3]. This action may help to inhibit the propagation of lipid peroxidation by restricting the movement of lipid peroxyl and alkoxyl radicals within the membrane.

Concerning other possible cerebroprotective mechanisms of action, U-74006F does not produce hypothermic or CNS depressant effects (Hall and coworkers, unpublished results). Moreover, the compound does not directly antagonize excitatory amino acid-induced neurotoxicity in vitro [i.e., they do not interact with NMDA receptors [15]]. Finally, it does not exhibit any significant competition for cholinergic, adrenergic, serotonergic, dopaminergic, opiate, or benzodiazepine receptors with standard ligands (Hall and coworkers, unpublished results). Thus, the only demonstrated cerebroprotective mechanism of U-74006F concerns its ability to block oxygen radical-induced lipid peroxidation.

Effects of Tirilazad Mesylate in Models of Focal Cerebral Ischemia

Protective effects of the 21-aminosteroid U-74006F have been observed in several experimental models of focal cerebral ischemia with reperfusion. First of all, in a model of temporary hemispheric cerebral ischemia produced in the Mongolian gerbil by unilateral occlusion of a carotid artery, U-74006F has been examined for its ability to promote survival and reduce neuronal necrosis [14]. Gerbils were pretreated by intraperitoneal (IP) injection with either vehicle or U-74006F 10 min before and again immediately after a 3-h temporary occlusion of the right carotid artery. U-74006F improved both 24- and 48-h survival compared with vehicle-treated animals. Histological examination of the brains of vehicle-treated animals at 24 h revealed marked neuronal cell loss (as much as 90% below control) in the hippocampus and lateral cerebral cortex. In contrast, the neuronal densities in the ischemic hemisphere of gerbils treated with U-74006F showed a dose-related and statistically significant preservation of neurons in both brain regions.

Mechanistic studies have been undertaken in the same gerbil model to determine the effects of a double-dose 10 mg/kg IP regimen of U-74006F on postischemic lipid peroxidation, measured in terms of brain vitamin E depletion, and on recovery of cerebral cortical extracellular calcium (i.e., reversal of intracellular accumulation) [13]. In both vehicle- and U-74006F-pretreated gerbils, the vitamin E content of the ischemic brain hemisphere was not affected after 3 h of carotid occlusion without reperfusion in relation to sham-occluded animals. However, at 2 h following reperfusion in vehicle- treated gerbils, the vitamin E levels of the previously ischemic hemisphere fell by an average of 60% compared to sham-occluded animals. In U-74006F-treated gerbils, the postischemic decrease in vitamin E was only 27.0% ($p<0.002$ vs vehicle).

Hemispheric ischemia secondary to carotid occlusion (75% reduction in cerebral blood flow) resulted in a drop in extracellular calcium from 1.05 ± 0.03 (SEM) mM before ischemia to 0.11 ± 0.02 mM at 3 h in vehicle-treated gerbils. This decline was unaffected by U-74006F pretreatment. Following 2 h of reperfusion, calcium recovered slightly to 0.22 ± 0.05 mM in vehicle-treated animals, while in the U-74006F-treated animals the 2-h recovery reached 0.56 ± 0.13 mM ($p<0.03$ vs vehicle). Interestingly, the time course of cerebral blood flow was not significantly different between the two groups.

These results provide evidence that the ability of U-74006F to reduce postischemic neuronal degeneration [14] is indeed due to an inhibition of postischemic lipid peroxidation as judged from the significant drug-induced maintenance of endogenous vitamin E. A similar 2-h postischemic preservation of ascorbic acid levels has also been observed with U-74006F [17]. The most likely explanation is that after the ischemic insult, tissue vitamin E and ascorbate are being utilized to quench post-reperfusion membrane lipid peroxidative reactions, while U-74006F spares tissue antioxidant content by assuming this responsibility. Secondary to this membrane protective mechanism, the drug acts to preserve cellular processes responsible for the reversal of the ischemia-triggered intracellular calcium accumulation.

In other work with the gerbil 3-h unilateral carotid occlusion model, U-74006F has been shown to attenuate neutrophil influx into the reperfused hemisphere [16]. Considering the production of oxygen radicals and other toxic products by neutrophils, the lessened postischemic infiltration would also likely contribute to the neuroprotective action. Indeed, these investigators showed a significant correlation between the extent of neutrophil infiltration and neuronal damage over a 24-h period after reperfusion.

U-74006F has also been examined in the cat following a 1-h temporary occlusion of the middle cerebral artery (MCA) [18]. Beginning 15 min after occlusion release, U-74006F was administered as a multiple bolus regimen that was continued for 12 h. At 1 week, using classical histological and quantitative 2-deoxy-glucose autoradiographic techniques, the area of cerebral infarction was assessed. Postischemic treatment with U-74006F significantly reduced the infarction volume compared to that in vehicle-treated cats. However, in another cat study employing a longer period of temporary MCA occlusion (3 h), no effect of the compound was observed [9]. In contrast, Boisvert [4] has recently reported a near complete prevention of 3-h postischemic brain edema in cynomolgous monkeys subjected to 3 h of MCA occlusion but treated with U-74006F intravenously (3 mg/kg IV) 10 min prior to reperfusion.

The compound has further been shown to reduce infarct size in a rat model of temporary MCA occlusion [19]. In Wistar rats pretreated with a 10 mg/kg intravenous dose followed by a 2-h episode of MCA occlusion, there was a 67.3% reduction in the 24-h postischemic infarct volume compared to vehicle-pretreated rats. The same group has shown a 25% reduction in infarct size in a model of 2 h of MCA occlusion plus 24 h of reperfusion in spontaneously hypertensive rats [20].

Most recently, U74006F has been evaluated in a baboon model of 3 h of MCA occlusion plus 2 weeks of postischemic reperfusion (E. Mori and G. del Zoppo, personal communication). U74006F was administered 15 min prior to reperfusion and at 2, 4, 12 and 24 h thereafter. Two-week infarct volume in the cortex and underlying white matter was reduced by 50% compared to vehicle-treated baboons. Although this effect was not statistically significant ($p < 0.163$), analysis of infarct area near the center of the infarct did reveal a significant decrease in the U74006F-treated animals. An early and persistent improvement in neurological score was also associated with U74006F treatment.

Summary

In conclusion, it is apparent that although early reperfusion of ischemic brain is clearly a desirable clinical approach to the acute treatment of stroke, the successful achievement of sudden reperfusion can lead to a burst of oxygen radical formation and the initiation of cell membrane lipid peroxidation. If severe enough, secondary cell damage and necrosis will take place. Lipid peroxidative injury is catalyzed by free iron that is known to be released from storage sites (e.g., hemoglobin, ferritin, transferrin) due to both ischemic lactic acidosis and oxygen-free radicals. Therefore, the administration of an inhibitor of oxygen radical-initiated, iron catalyzed lipid peroxidation such as tirilazad mesylate (U-74006F) either just before or immediately after thrombolytic therapy represents a more rational approach to the therapy of thromboembolic stroke.

References

1. Althaus JS, Williams CW, Andrus PK, VonVoigtlander PF, Hall ED (1991) In vitro and in vivo analysis of tirilazad mesylate (U74006F) as a hydroxyl radical scavenger. Soc Neurosci Abs 17:164
2. Andrus PK, Hall ED, Althaus JS, Williams CW, VonVoigtlander PF (1991) Post- ischemic detection of hydroxyl radicals in gerbil brain: Attenuation by the 21-aminosteroid tirilazad mesylate (U74006F). Soc Neurosci Abs 17:1086
3. Audus KL, Guillot FL, Braughler JM (1991) Evidence for 21-aminosteroid association with the hydrophobic domains of brain microvessel endothelial cells. Free Radic Biol Med 11:361–371
4. Boisvert DP (1991) Effectiveness of postischemic 21-aminosteroid U74006F in preventing reperfusion brain edema. J Cereb Blood Flow Metab 11 (Suppl 2):S135
5. Braughler JM, Chase RL, Neff GL, et al (1988) A new 21-aminosteroid antioxidant lacking glucocorticoid activity stimulates ACTH secretion and blocks arachidonic acid release from mouse pituitary tumor (AtT-20) cells. J Pharmacol Exp Ther 244:423–427

6. Braughler JM, Hall ED (1989) Central nervous system trauma and stroke: I. Biochemical considerations for oxygen radical formation and lipid peroxidation. Free Radic Biol Med 6:289–301
7. Braughler JM, Pregenzer JF (1989) The 21-aminosteroid inhibitors of lipid peroxidation: Reactions with lipid peroxyl and phenoxyl radicals. Free Radic Biol Med 7:125–130
8. Braughler JM, Pregenzer JF, Chase RL, Duncan LA, Jacobsen EJ, McCall LM (1987) Novel 21-aminosteroids as potent inhibitors of iron-dependent lipid peroxidation. J Biol Chem 262:10438–10440
9. Gelb AW, Henderson SM, Zhang C (1990) U-74006F, a 21-aminosteroid, does not ameliorate feline focal cerebral ischemia. J Neurosurg Anesthesiol 2:240
10. Hall ED (1992) The neuroprotective pharmacology of methylprednisolone: A review. J Neurosurg 76:13–22
11. Hall ED, Braughler JM (1989) Central nervous system trauma and stroke. II. Physiological and pharmacological evidence for the involvement of oxygen radicals and lipid peroxidation. Free Radic Biol Med 6:303–313
12. Hall ED, McCall JM, Yonkers PA, Chase RL, Braughler JM (1987) A non-glucocorticoid analog of methylprednisolone duplicates its high dose pharmacology in models of CNS trauma and neuronal membrane damage. J Pharmacol Exp Ther 242:137–142
13. Hall ED, Pazara KE, Braughler JM (1991) Effects of tirilazad mesylate on postischemic brain lipid peroxidatoin and recovery of extracellular calcium in gerbils. Stroke 22:361–366
14. Hall ED, Pazara KW, Braughler JM (1988) 21-aminosteroid lipid peroxidation inhibitor U74006F protects against cerebral ischemia in gerbils. Stroke 19:997–1002
15. Monyer H, Hartley DM, Choi DW (1990) 21-aminosteroids attenuate excitotoxic neuronal injury in cortical cell cultures. Neuron 5:121–126
16. Oostveen JA, Williams LR (1991) Tirilazad mesylate (U74006F) attenuates the accumulation of neutrophilic leukocytes (NLs) in ischemic gerbil brain. Soc Neurosci Abs 17:1092
17. Sato PH, Hall ED (1992) Tirilazad mesylate protects vitamins C and E in brain ischemia-reperfusion injury. J Neurochem (In Press)
18. Silvia RC, Piercey MF, Hoffmann WE, Chase RL, Braughlerr JM, Tang AH (1987) U74006F, an inhibitor of lipid peroxidation protects against lesion development following experimental stroke in the cat: Histological and metabolic analysis. Neurosci Abst 13:1499
19. Xue D, Bruederlin B, Heinecke E, Li H, Buchan AM (1990) U74006F reduces neocortical infarction but does not attenuate selective hippocampal CA1 necrosis. Stroke 21:178
20. Xue D, Slivka A, Buchan A (1992) Tirilazad reduced cortical infarction following transient but not permanent focal cerebral ischemia. Stroke 23:894–899

Anti-PMN Leukocyte Strategies and Their Application to Focal Cerebral Ischemia *

G. W. Schmid-Schönbein [1] and G. J. del Zoppo [2]

In capillaries, the physical properties of individual cells contribute significantly to the rheology of blood and to organ perfusion. In this summary we consider the biophysical properties of circulating cells that determine their motion in the microcirculation and its disturbance in ischemia. The focus is on polymorphonuclear (PMN) leukocytes, their deformability, adhesive properties and cytotoxicity. The intravascular pool of PMN leukocytes will be considered and the mechanism of the non-reflow phenomena in the cerebral microcirculation.

The Kinetics of PMN Leukocytes in the Microcirculation

In the past decade, a body of evidence has accumulated which suggests that despite relatively small numbers in the circulation, PMN leukocytes may be involved in a wide range of cardiovascular complications in addition to classical inflammatory reactions and host defense. The distinction between a beneficial role and an injurious role of granulocytes to the host has become blurred and no organ may escape the potentially cytotoxic effects of these circulating activated cells. Insights have come from a range of approaches. Biophysical and biochemical studies have shown that leukocytes are made up of a relatively stiff viscoelastic actin-containing cytosolic matrix that is difficult to deform by the fluid stresses in the circulation. Furthermore, the cells have the ability to polymerize, which leads to further stiffening of the cell cytoplasm [25]. Granulocytes are larger than other circulating cells, yet they need to pass through capillaries which may be as narrow as almost half their resting dimension. PMN leukocytes can adhere readily to vascular endothelium and other substrates by a mechanism which includes adhesion glycoproteins, such as the in-

* Supported in part by a grant from NS26945 (GJdZ) of the National Institutes of Health. This is publication number 7427-MEM from The Scripps Research Institute, La Jolla, CA, USA.
[1] Institute for Biomedical Engineering, University of California, San Diego, CA, USA
[2] Department of Molecular and Experimental Medicine, The Scripps Research Institute, La Jolla, CA, USA

G. J. del Zoppo, E. Mori, W. Hacke (Eds.)
Thrombolytic Therapy in Acute Ischemic Stroke II

tegrins CD11a,b,c/CD18 and several selectins [1, 13, 20]. The underlying molecular mechanisms may involve different membrane adhesion energies and cell activation of both PMN leukocytes and endothelial cells. These conditions may lead to microvascular entrapment of granulocytes with capillary occlusion and an associated capillary "no-reflow" phenomenon during pathophysiological states, and accumulation of neutrophils in postcapillary venules [23]. Attachment of neutrophils and monocytes to the endothelium causes elevation of endothelial and microvascular permeability [38] by a mechanism which involves the adhesion glycoproteins [3]. Release of oxygen free radical products occurs as a result [30].

Even under normal physiological conditions, the presence of PMN leukocytes in microvessels causes disturbance of microvascular flow. Their entry time into the orifices of capillaries with single file flow is considerably longer than that of the more flexible red cells [37]. The entry deformation depends critically on the pressure drop across the cell and the dimension of the capillary channel [22] (Figs. 1, 2). After entry into capillaries, PMN leukocytes move with a lower velocity than red cells, a condition that leads to a cellular train formation, i.e., a leukocyte with high numbers of erythrocytes accumulated upstream and a cell-depleted region downstream [23]. The significance of the cell transformation lies in the fact that the hemodynamic resistance in such capillary vessels is elevated [33], which in turn manifests itself by a significant eleva-

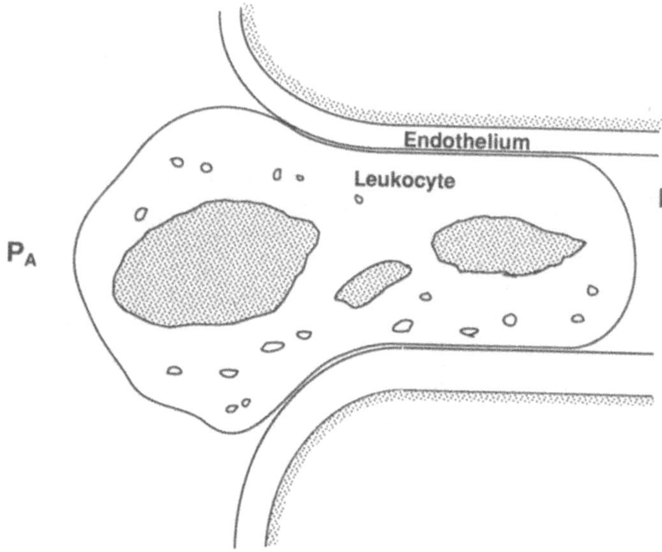

Fig. 1. Schematic of a leukocyte entering a capillary. The pressure drop across the cell, $P_A - P_V$, serves to deform the leukocyte from its undeformed shape into an elongated cylinder, sufficiently narrow to fit into the lumen of the capillary. The time required for this deformation is considerably longer for leukocytes than for the more deformable erythrocytes, associated with temporary plugging of the leukocytes. During the course of entry, the leukocyte membrane comes into close contact with the endothelial cell membrane

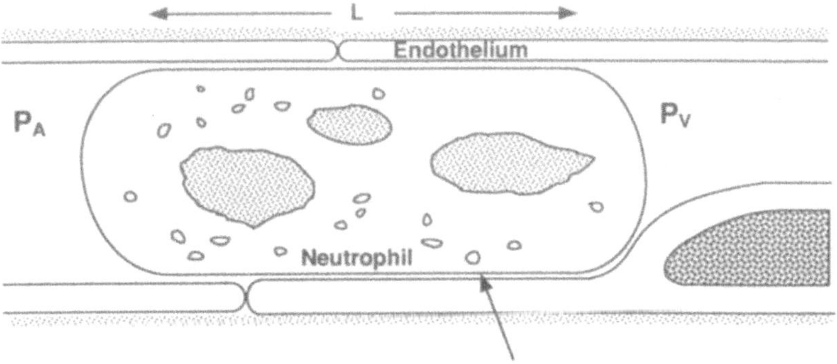

Fig. 2. Schematic of a leukocyte (*L*) trapped in a capillary at a point with endothelial protrusion. Such situations occur frequently in low-flow states, when the capillary distending pressure and lumen dimensions are reduced, while in addition the driving pressure P_A-P_V forcing the leukocyte along the capillary is compromised. Leukocytes may become entrapped in capillaries even without the aid of any membrane adhesion stress, σ. Nonadhering cells can be removed upon restoration of a normal arterial-venous pressure drop, due to the fact that leukocytes have viscoelastic cytoplasmic properties, which permit the cells to deform in the presence of a stress until they can pass through the capillary lumen

tion of whole organ hemodynamic resistance out of proportion to the numbers of granulocytes in the blood [31]. In the brain the elevation of organ resistance by granulocytes is currently unexplored.

Under certain pathophysiological conditions, the motion of PMN leukocytes is impaired. A decrease in perfusion pressure, due to central pressure reduction or to elevation of flow resistance as in atherosclerotic arteries, compromises the driving force for these cells in the microcirculation. Pressure reduction causes relaxation of blood vessels and narrowing of the vascular lumen. Thus, PMN leukocytes must enter narrowed capillaries at a reduced perfusion pressure. Consequently, the cell entry times at capillaries are increased, and complete obstruction may occur. This occurs even in the absence of adhesion to the endothelium. Alternatively, an increase in the membrane adhesion energy to the endothelium may entrap PMN leukocytes in the microcirculation without perfusion pressure reduction [23]. This is most readily seen in situations where leukocyte activators have been administered [6]. In acute ischemia, the attachment of granulocytes is limited to capillaries and postcapillary venules, with less involvement of arteries and arterioles. Any combination of PMN leukocyte activation and pressure reduction greatly increases the risk for microvascular entrapment (Fig. 3).

Restoration of the perfusion pressure, after a low-flow period, may restore flow in some vessels of the microcirculation, but this is inhomogeneous and depends on the details of the events before and during the low-flow state. Some variables that influence the reperfusion pattern include the activation state of the PMN leukocyte before flow reduction [5], the duration of ischemia, its severity, the levels of plasma-derived activators, and endothelial activation. After

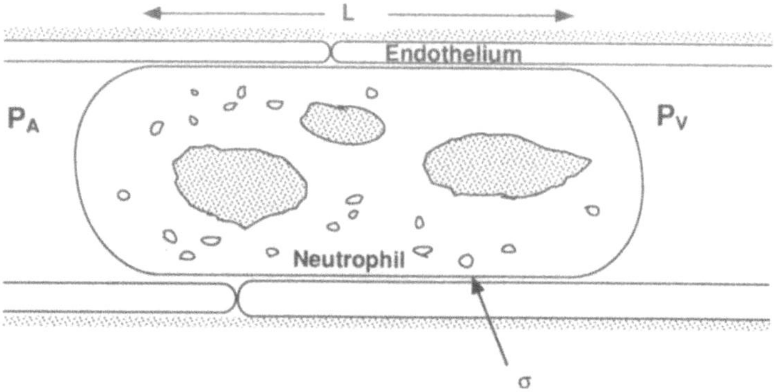

Fig. 3. Schematic showing the adhesion of a leukocyte (L) to capillary endothelium. Such leukocytes completely obstruct the capillary lumen, form a close membrane contact with the endothelium and adhere with an adhesive stress, σ. In equilibrium the magnitude of the membrane adhesive shear stress is determined by the pressure drop across the cell $P_A - P_V$ according to the equilibrium condition

$$\sigma(L\, d\, \pi) = (P_A - P_V)\, \pi\, (d/2)^2$$

between the resultant shear force (left-hand side) and the resultant pressure force (right-hand side). If $(P_A - P_V)\, d/4L$ exceeds the maximum membrane shear stress σ_{MAX} which can be supported by the molecular forces between the two membranes, the leukocyte will be dislodged

acute focal ischemia, the primary vessels showing "no reperfusion" upon restoration of flow are the capillaries. This has been observed in different end organs, including the brain [10]. Under acute conditions larger microvessels, the arterioles and venules, are reperfused almost without exception, although the venules may be lined by adherent leukocytes (Figs. 4, 5). Investigation of the capillaries after ischemia and reperfusion with high resolution light microscopy or electron microscopy demonstrates placement of leukocytes in close contact with the luminal endothelium membrane and virtually complete occlusion of the capillary lumen. This process does not require endothelial swelling or extrinsic compression of capillaries by tissue stresses. Removal of PMN leukocytes by purely hydrodynamic means, such as arterial pressure elevation, is compromised due to the network arrangement of the capillaries since the pressure drop across an obstructing granulocyte cannot be raised above the level of the viscous pressure drop in a neighboring capillary. Obstructed capillaries also contain high numbers of erythrocytes and platelets, but these cells are passively entrapped and rapidly removed if the leukocytes themselves are dislodged [4].

PMN Leukocytes in Cerebral Tissues

Antigranulocyte strategies in noncerebral ischemia/reperfusion (I/R) models have demonstrated a significant improvement in post-I/R function and mor-

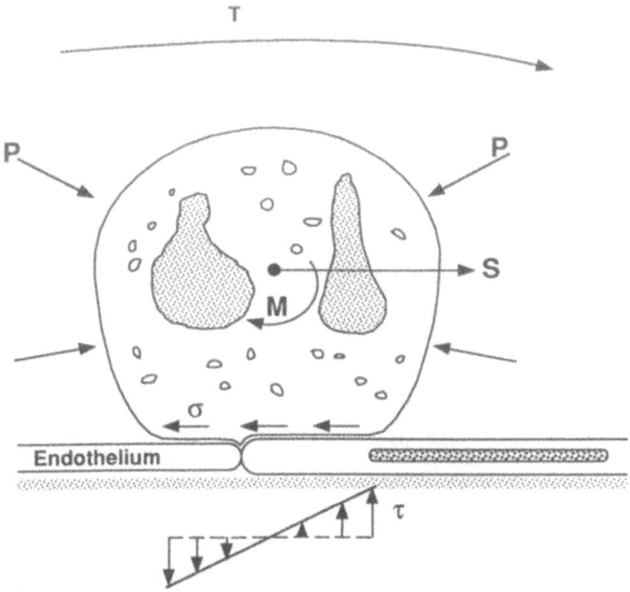

Fig. 4. Schematic drawing of a leukocyte adhering to the endothelium in a postcapillary venule. The portion of the leukocyte sticking into the lumen is subject to a plasma shear stress *T* and pressure *P* by the passing blood stream, with a resultant axial force *S* and moment *M* acting on the leukocyte. In equilibrium, i.e., in a stationary adhering leukocyte or a leukocyte rolling at steady state along the endothelium, the force S and moment M are in equilibrium with the membrane adhesive shear stress σ and the normal stress τ in the region of contact between the leukocyte and endothelium. If the maximum shear force S exerted by the blood stream exceeds the resultant force due to the membrane adhesive shear stress σ (i.e., σ times the contact area), the cell will be sheared away. If the moment M exerted by the blood stream exceeds the maximum resultant moment due to the membrane adhesive normal stress, the cell will roll away. The molecular forces underlying the membrane adhesive stresses σ and τ are due to specific integrins and selectins, as well as nonspecific binding forces due to a charge and dipole distribution in the gap between the cell membranes

tality, suggesting the participation of PMN leukocytes in reperfusion events [8, 28, 35, 36]. Indirect evidence of PMN leukocyte involvement in cerebrovascular reflow has been reported using polyclonal antineutrophil serum or leukopenia strategies [7, 14, 34]. Preischemia depletion of circulating PMN leukocytes by intraperitoneal injection of antineutrophil serum was associated with an increase in local cortical cerebral blood flow (CBF), but not in the ischemic basal ganglia in a rat hypotension/carotid occlusion model of hemispheric ischemia/reperfusion [14]. However, an increased CBF accompanied preischemia infusion of an antineutrophil serum, with a decreased PMN leukocyte count in a rabbit cerebral embolic/hypotension model [7]. Improvement in neuronal functional outcome following vinblastine-induced leukopenia in a rat reversible incomplete forebrain ischemia model was indicated by improvement in EEG and somatosensory evoked potentials [34]. Polyclonal antineutrophil sera and antineoplastic agents, however, have complex effects

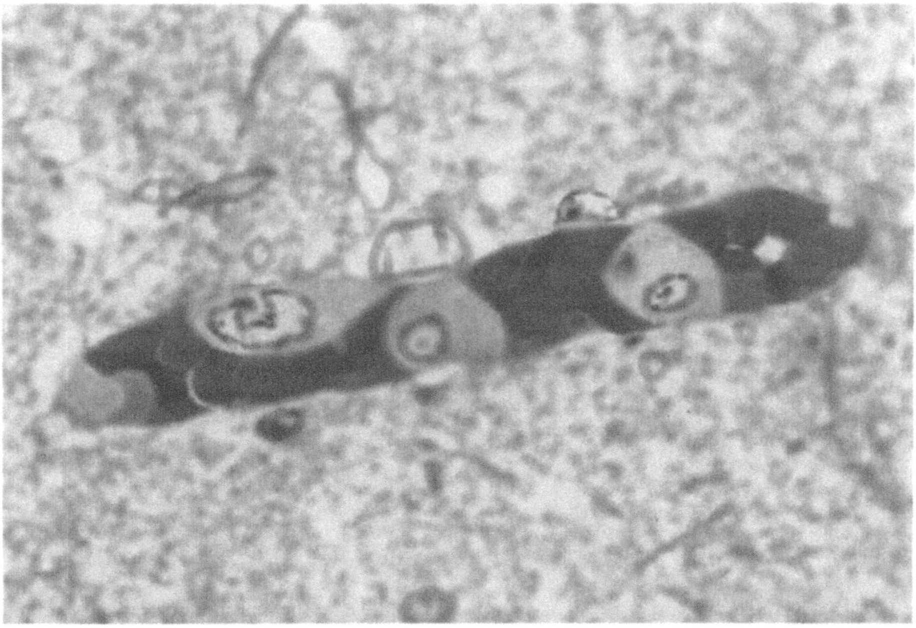

Fig. 5. Postcapillary venule in I/R territory 60 min post- reperfusion demonstrating PMN leukocytes in apposition to the microvascular endothelium

which may also alter platelet count and function. These observations suggest a potential role for the PMN leukocyte in postischemia reperfusion microvascular events.

The finding of microvascular reflow abnormalities by carbon tracer techniques early following MCA occlusion/reperfusion in the nonhuman primate [10] is reminiscent of the "no-reflow" defects seen in rabbits following global cerebral ischemia originally described by Ames and collaborators [2]. A potential role for PMN leukocytes in the development of post-reperfusion defects in focal cerebral ischemia is supported by their presence in capillaries and postcapillary venules of the ischemic territory [9, 10]. Adherence of PMN leukocytes to the endothelium of postcapillary venules of non-cerebral organs is mediated by the leukocyte β_2 integrin CD11b/CD18 (Mac-1, Mo1) [16]. The murine anti-CD18 monoclonal antibody (MoAb) IB4 (60.3) inhibits aggregation, endothelial adherence, and endothelial injury of activated PMN leukocytes in several settings [3, 15, 17–19, 32, 36].

Microvascular Patency Following an Anti-PMN Leukocyte Strategy

To test the concept that adhesion of PMN leukocytes to cerebral microvascular endothelium may contribute to MCA territory microvascular perfusion defects, the effect of prereperfusion blockade of the leukocyte CD11b/CD18 adhesion complex by IB4 (60.3) on microvascular patency was studied. A well-characterized purified endotoxin-free preparation of IB4 which is known to inhibit the sticking of PMN leukocytes [36] and also attenuate reperfusion injury has been employed.

Non-human primates (*Papio anubis/cynocephalus*) fitted with a reversible MCA occlusion device were randomly assigned to receive i) IB4 (2–4 mg/kg) by intravenous infusion 15 min prior to MCA reperfusion following 180 of MCA occlusion, or ii) no intervention. The surgical procedure and anesthesia protocol for preparation of the non-human primate MCA occlusion/reperfusion model has been described in detail elsewhere [10]. Halothane (1.5%–5.0%) was administered, following ketamine HCl analepsis (10 mg/kg), as the sole anesthetic during the 1.5-h procedure. Recovery was prompt. All subjects were allowed a 7-day procedure-free interval prior to experimentation. During this period, the responses of PMN leukocytes to C_{5a} (β-glucuronidase release, O_2^- production, and polarization) and chemotaxis were studied. Normal neurological status (score = 100 [29]) was a requirement for study entry. Each experiment was terminated at 60 min MCA reperfusion by pressure perfusion with isosmotic fluid under antithrombotic conditions, followed by isosmotic fixation (2% paraformaldehyde/0.5% glutaraldehyde) with carbon tracer (Pelikan Fount India, Pelikan AG, Hannover, FRG) at identical perfusion pressures [10, 21].

After randomization to control ($n = 6$) or IB4 infusion ($n = 7$), occlusion of the MCA was performed by inflation of the extrinsic MCA balloon in the awake subject. In the treatment group, IB4 was infused 15 min prior to reperfusion (balloon deflation) (Fig. 6).

Serial 10 µm thick sections were prepared as described [10, 21] and analyzed automatically with a computer-based video-image acquisition system consisting of a Hamamatsu C2400–07 NTSC video camera staged on a light microscope (Kontron and Carl Zeiss, Munich, FRG). Contiguous fields with total surface area of 25 mm^2 were processed on each section at 30 µm intervals until a minimum of 2000 vessels were counted in the nonischemic basal ganglia. "Percent" reflow, the normalized ratio of patent microvessels in an equal number of fields from the I/R versus non-ischemic regions were computed for the biologically relevant vessel classes of i) capillaries (4.0–7.5 µm); ii) post-

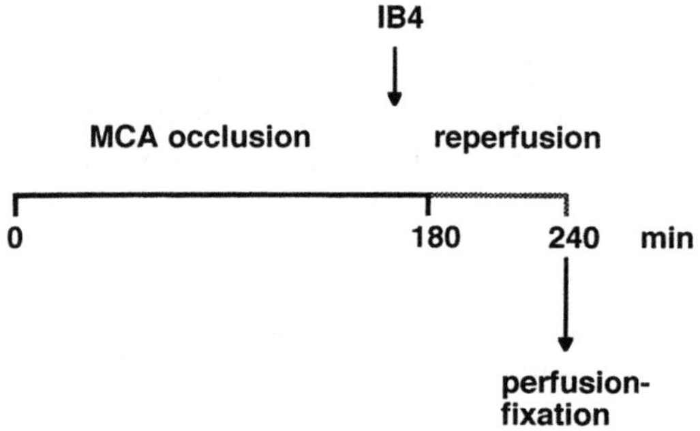

Fig. 6. Experimental protocol. Subjects received either IB4 (*arrow*) or no treatment

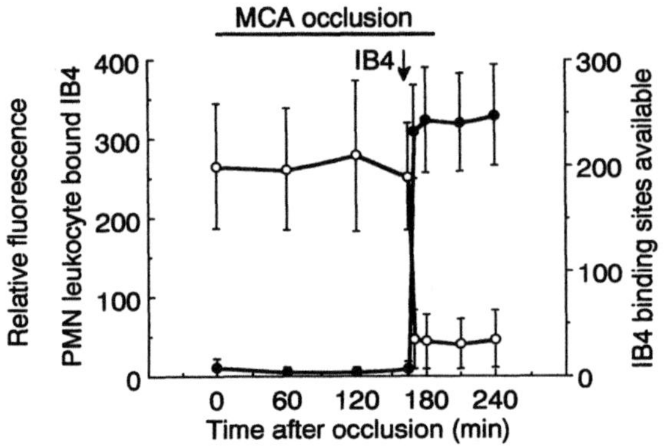

Fig. 7 Binding of FITC-labeled IB4 to baboon PMN leukocytes in vivo by flow cytometry

capillary venules/metarterioles (7.5–30 μm); iii) connecting venules/metarterioles (30–50 μm); and iv) venules/muscular arterioles >50 μm diameter.

Two subjects in the IB4 group were excluded from data analysis because of inhomogeneous tracer perfusion ($n = 1$) and incomplete vascular packing of the carbon elements ($n = 1$). Either condition would cause inappropriate counting by the computer-based acquisition system. Therefore, 5 IB4-treated animals were compared with 6 control animals.

PMN Leukocyte Activation. The surgical procedure for placement of the MCA device did not alter baseline peripheral PMN leukocyte function as determined by PMN leukocyte superoxide production, polarization, or β-glucuronidase release in response to C_{5a}. Chemotaxis to zymogen was depressed at 24 h postsurgery but returned to normal by 7 days and the time of the experiment.

IB4 Binding to PMN Leukocytes. Binding of IB4 to baboon PMN leukocytes in vivo plateaued within 5 min of infusion and remained unchanged throughout the duration of the experiments. An 83.3% reduction of free PMN leukocyte CD18 binding sites was observed by flow cytometry (Fig. 7).

Baseline Cellular Data. Hematocrit, platelet counts, total white cell counts, and neurological scores prior to and following occlusion of the MCA were not significantly different between the groups.

No Reflow (Control Group). In the control group a statistically significant reduction in the number of patent microvessels was observed in the capillary range (4.0–7.5 μm minimum diameter, $p = 0.042$), and the postcapillary venule/ precapillary arteriole range (7.5–30 μm, $p = 0.009$).

Reflow Following IB4 Infusion. Infusion of IB4 immediately prior to MCA reperfusion resulted in a significant increase in the percent reflow in the microvascular classes of 7.5–30 μm diameter ($p = 0.049$) and of 30–50 μm diameter ($p = 0.034$) (Fig. 8).

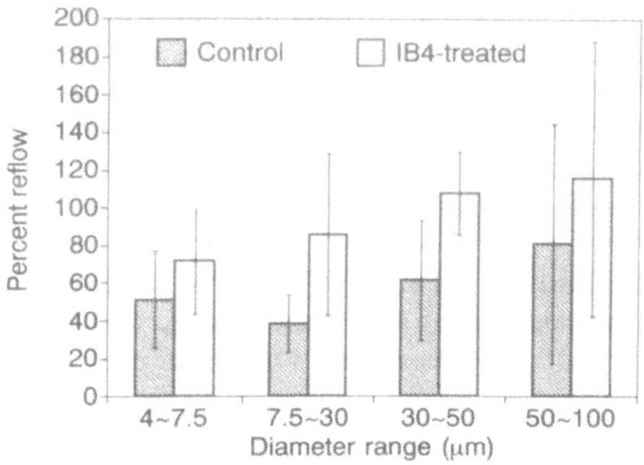

Fig. 8. Comparative microvascular patency (percent of reflow) between IB4-treated and untreated cohorts by microvessel size class (see text)

Vasodilatation. When normalized for vessel number, no significant shift toward larger vessel diameters in the distribution of microvessels undergoing ischemia/reperfusion compared with the nonischemic territory was evident in either the IB4-treated or control distributions.

Neurological Outcome. Following MCA occlusion, a reduction in neurological score was observed in both animal cohorts. However, no improvement of mean score was evident within the 60 min after reperfusion in either the IB4-treated or control groups.

Implications

These data indicate that blockade of the PMN leukocyte adherence complex CD18 increases microvascular reflow following focal cerebral ischemia and reperfusion. Two observations are relevant: i) that exposure of circulating PMN leukocytes to IB4 known to inhibit PMN leukocyte adhesion to postcapillary venules was associated with a significant increase in reflow following MCA occlusion and reperfusion, and ii) the effect on microvascular reflow occurred when IB4 was infused *prior* to reperfusion, but following onset of ischemia. The most significant increase in reflow occurred in 7.5–30 μm diameter (postcapillary venules/precapillary arterioles) and 30–50 μm diameter microvessels. Although computer-assisted imaging techniques do not allow distinction between postcapillary venules and precapillary arterioles, these data are most consistent with reperfusion of postcapillary venules and large microvessels. This is supported by the findings of PMN leukocytes in postcapillary venules following reperfusion in previous experiments [10] (Fig. 5) and the known interaction of activated PMN leukocytes and postcapillary venule endothelium mediated by the CD11/CD18 adherence complex in other organ systems [8, 19, 32].

The "no-reflow" phenomenon is observed during reperfusion following focal cerebral ischemia. This obstruction mirrors the finding of microvascular perfusion defects in other organ systems [24, 26, 27]. As in studies of experimental coronary artery occlusion and reperfusion [11, 12, 26] and resting skeletal muscle [27], granulocytes may obstruct microvessels. Although the MCA microvascular bed has not been described in detail, the perfusion defects may be most readily explained by capillary occlusion, with some contribution by obstruction of postcapillary venules. Of clinical relevance, modulation (improvement) in focal "no-reflow" occurred when IB4 was given just prior to MCA reperfusion. This implies that endothelial adherence by PMN leukocytes leading to microvascular obstruction must occur upon reperfusion. Confirmation of this phenomenon in cerebral ischemia/reperfusion with real-time imaging techniques is necessary.

Acknowledgments. All procedures were approved by the institutional Animal Research Committee and conducted by standards established by the National Institutes of Health, National Research Council, and the USDA in the Animal Welfare Act.

References

1. Albeda SM, Buck CA (1990) Integrains and other cell adhesion molecules. FASEB J 4:2868–2880
2. Ames A, Wright LW, Kowade M, Thurston JM, Majors G (1968) Cerebral ischemia: II. The no-reflow phenomenon. Am J Pathol 52:437–453
3. Arfors K-E, Lundberg C, Lindbom L, Lundberg K, Beatty PG, Harlan JM (1987) A monoclonal antibody to the membrane glycoprotein complex CD18 inhibits polymorphonuclear leukocyte accumulation and plasma leakage in vivo. Blood 69:338–340
4. Bagge U, Amundson B, Lauritzen C (1980) White blood cell deformability and plugging of skeletal muscle capillaries in hemorrhagic shock. Acta Physiol Scand 108:159–163
5. Barroso-Aranda J, Schmid-Schönbein GW (1898) Transformation of neutrophils as indicator of irreversibility in hemorrhagic shock. Am J Physiol 257: H846– H852
6. Barroso-Aranda J, Schmid-Schönbein GW, Zweifach BW, Mathison JC (1991) Polymorphonuclear neutrophil contribution to induced tolerance to bacterial lipopolysaccharide. Circ Res 69:1196–1206
7. Bednar MM, Raymond S, McAuliffe T, Lodge PA, Gross CE (1991) The role of neutrophils and platelets in a rabbit model of thromboembolic stroke. Stroke 22:44–50
8. Carden DL, Smith JK, Korthuis RJ (1990) Neutrophil-mediated microvascular dysfunction in postischemic canine skeletal muscle. Role of granulocyte adherence. Circ Res 66:1436–1444
9. del Zoppo GJ, Copeland BR, Harker LA, et al (1986) Experimental acute thrombotic stroke in baboons. Stroke 17:1254–1265
10. del Zoppo GJ, Schmid-Schönbein GW, Mori E, Copeland BR, Chang C-M (1991) Polymorphonuclear leukocytes occlude capillaries following middle cerebral artery occlusion and reperfusion in baboons. Stroke 22:1276–1283
11. Engler RE, Schmid-Schönbein GW, Pavelec RS (1987) Leukocyte capillary plugging in myocardial ischemia and reperfusion in the dog. Am J Pathol 111:98–111
12. Engler RL, Dahlgren MD, Peterson MA, Dobbs A, Schmid-Schönbein GW (1986) Accumulation of polymorphonuclear leukocytes during experimental myocardial ischemia. Am J Physiol 251:H93–100
13. Entman ML, Michael L, Rossen RD, et al (1991) Inflammation in the course of early myocardial ischemia. FASEB J 5:2529–2537
14. Grogaard B, Schurer L, Gerdin B, Arfors KE (1989) Delayed hypoperfusion after incomplete forebrain ischemia in the rat. The role of polymorphonuclear leukocytes. J Cereb Blood Flow Metab 9:500–505

15. Ham AW, Cormack DH (1979) The circulatory system. In: Histology, 8th edn. JB Lippincott, Philadelphia Toronto, p 581
16. Harlan JM, Killen PD, Senecal FM, et al (1985) The role of neutrophil membrane glycoprotein GMP-140 in neutrophil adherence to endothelium in vitro. Blood 66:167–178
17. Hernandez LA, Grisham MB, Twohig B, Arfors K-E, Harlan JM, Grange DN (1987) Role of neutrophils in ischemia/reperfusion-induced microvascular injury. Am J Physiol 253:H699–703
18. Hossmann KA, Olsson Y (1970) Suppression and recovery of neuronal function in transient cerebral ischemia. Brain Res 22:313–325
19. House SD, Lipowsky HH (1987) Leukocyte-endothelium adhesion: Microhemodynamics in mesentery of the cat. Microvasc Res 34:363–379
20. McEver RP (1991) Selectins: Novel receptors that mediate leukocyte adhesion during inflammation. Thromb Haemost 65:223–228
21. Mori E, del Zoppo GJ, Chambers JD, Copeland BR, Arfors KE (1992) Inhibition of polymorphonuclear leukocyte adherence suppresses no-reflow after focal cerebral ischemia in baboons. Stroke 23:712–718
22. Needham D, Hochmuth RM (1990) The behavior of human neutrophils into a μm pipet and measurement of cytoplasmic viscosity. J Biomech Eng 112:269–276
23. Schmid-Schönbein GW (1987) Leukocyte kinetics in the microcirculation. Biorheology 24:139–151
24. Schmid-Schönbein GW (1987) Capillary plugging by granulocytes and the no-reflow phenomenon in the microcirculation. Fed Proc 46:2397–2401
25. Schmid-Schönbein GW (1990) Leukocyte biophysics. Cell Biophys 17:107–135
26. Schmid-Schönbein GW, Engler RL (1987) Granulocytes as active participants in acute myocardial ischemia and infarction. Am J Cardiovasc Pathol 1:15–30
27. Schmid-Schönbein GW, Skalak TC, Sutton DW (1989) Bioengineering analysis of blood flow in resting skeletal muscle. In: Lee JS, Skalak TC (eds) Microvascular mechanics. Springer-Verlag, Berlin Heidelberg New York, p 65
28. Simpson PJ, Todd RF, Fantone JC, Mickelson JK, Griffin JD, Lucchesi BR (1988) Reduction of experimental canine myocardial reperfusion injury by a monoclonal antibody (anti-Mo1, anti-CD11b) that inhibits leukocyte adhesion. J Clin Invest 81:624–629
29. Spetzler RF, Selman WR, Weinstein P, et al (1980) Chronic reversible cerebral ischemia: Evaluation of a new baboon model. J Neurosurg 7:257–261
30. Suematsu K, Kurose I, Asako H, Miura S, Tsuchiya M (1989) In vivo visualization of oxy-radical-dependent photo emission during endothelium-granulocyte interaction in microvascular beds treated with platelet-activating factor. J Biochem 106:355–360
31. Sutton DW, Schmid-Schönbein GW (1992) Elevation of organ resistance due to leukocyte perfusion. Am J Physiol (In Press)
32. Suzuki M, Inauen W, Kvietys PR, et al (1989) Superoxide mediates reperfusion-induced leukocyte-endothelial cell interactions. Am J Physiol 257: H1740–H1745
33. Thompson TN, LaCelle PL, Cokelet GR (1989) Perturbation of red blood cell flow in small tubes by white blood cells. Pflugers Arch 413:372–377
34. Vasthare US, Heinel LA, Rosenwasser RH, Tuma RF (1990) Leukocyte involvement in cerebral ischemia and reperfusion injury. Surg Neurol 33:261–265
35. Vedder NB, Fouty BW, Winn RK, Harlan JM, Rice CL (1989) Role of neutrophils in generalized reperfusion injury associated with resuscitation from shock. Surgery 106:509–516
36. Vedder NB, Winn RK, Rice CL, Chi EY, Arfors K-E, Harlan JM (1990) Inhibition of leukocyte adherence by anti-CD18 monoclonal antibody attenuates reperfusion injury in the rabbit ear. Proc Natl Acad Sci USA 87:2643–2646
37. Warnke K, Skalak TC (1990) The effects of leukocytes on blood flow in a model skeletal muscle capillary network. Microvasc Res 40:118–136
38. Wedmore CV, Williams TJ (1981) Control of vascular permeability by polymorphonuclear leukocytes in inflammation. Nature 289:646–650

Von Willebrand Factor as a Target for Antithrombotic Intervention

Z.M. Ruggeri

The adhesive protein von Willebrand factor (vWF) is essential for the formation of platelet thrombi under flow conditions characterized by high shear stress. Two distinct platelet receptors, the glycoprotein (GP) complexes Ib-IX-V and IIb-IIIa, are required for these interactions. Interaction with GP Ib-IX-V results in platelet activation, a necessary step for binding to GP IIb-IIIa and stable aggregation. Inhibition of von Willebrand factor binding to GP Ib can be achieved with small recombinant fragments containing the specific functional domain of the von Willebrand factor molecule that interacts with this platelet receptor. Such fragments may provide a new selective approach to antithrombotic therapy.

Background: The Role of von Willebrand Factor in Platelet Function

Considerable progress has been made in understanding the molecular aspects of platelet function in both normal hemostasis and in their contribution to pathological vascular occlusion. Following vessel injury, irreversible contact (adhesion) of the platelet occurs onto a site with a break in endothelial integrity. These interactions are promoted by blood flow conditions of high shear stress. One of the main biological responses is the specific functional requirement for the multimeric, multivalent vWF molecule which may interact with subendothelial components as well as GP Ib–IX–V complex and the GP IIb–IIIa complex of the platelet [15]. Assembly of the complex of the disulfide-linked GP Ib α and β chains with the noncovalently linked GP IX and possibly GP V is required for the normal expression of GP Ib on the surface of platelets and for its signal transducing function. But the vWF-binding site resides exclusively in the amino terminal region of GP Ibα [19]. For this

Roon Research Center for Arteriosclerosis and Thrombosis, Division of Experimental Thrombosis and Hemostasis, Department of Molecular and Experimental Medicine and Committee on Vascular Biology, The Scripps Research Institute, La Jolla, CA, USA

G.J. del Zoppo, E. Mori, W. Hacke (Eds.)
Thrombolytic Therapy in Acute Ischemic Stroke II

reason, vWF binding to the GP Ib-IX-V complex described here will be referred to as the vWF-GP Ib interaction.

The precise mechanisms by which vWF serves its role in hemostasis are still incompletely understood. It is generally assumed that this function is expressed through the interaction with components of the subendothelium, on one side, and platelet membrane receptors on the other. vWF would then act as a "bridging" molecule between platelets and the vessel wall. One significant observation is that the vWF molecule circulating in normal blood does not interact to any major degree with platelet GP Ib, even though the function of this receptor is considered to be independent of activation. As a consequence, the concept has evolved, but has never been proven experimentally, that only vWF in the vessel wall expresses the ability to bind GP Ib, presumably after forming a complex with some subendothelial component that would act as a "modulator" of vWF activity. Another notion is that the binding of vWF to GP Ib can promote events usually associated with the action of agonists like ADP and thrombin, namely GP IIb–IIIa activation and platelet aggregation [5]. In this context, vWF would be more than the "glue" that makes platelets stick to the vessel wall and would, in addition, perform the role of an important inducer and modulator of thrombogenesis.

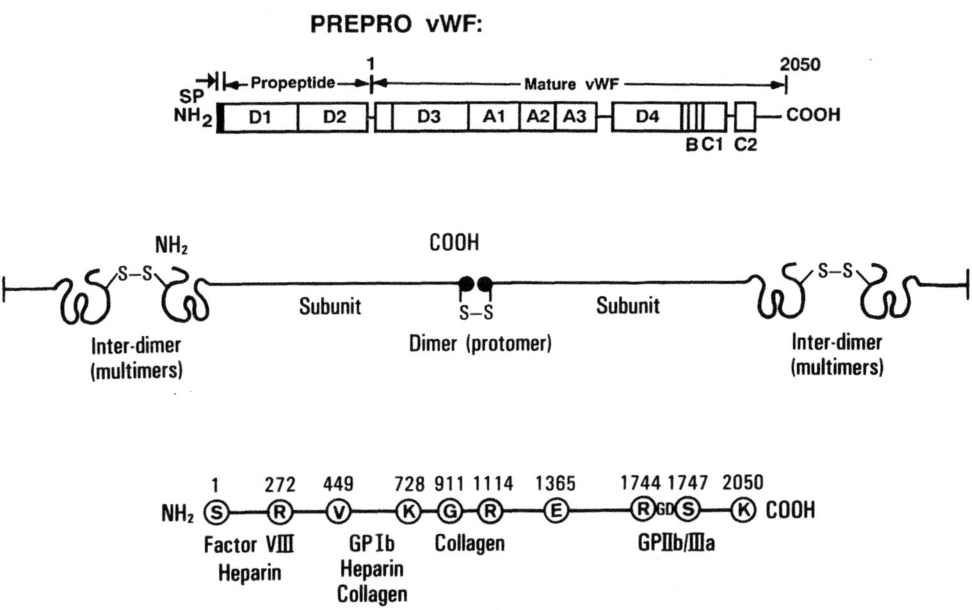

Fig. 1. Schematic representation of the structural organization of vWF. The *top panel* shows the cDNA structure of vWF with the repeats of 4 homologous domains. The *middle panel* represents the assembly of the constituent subunit into dimers by interchain disulfide bonding of C-terminal domains, and the assembly of dimers into multimers by disulfide bonding of N-terminal domains. The *lower panel* represents the topographic location of different functional domains within the constituent subunit

Functionally important specific regions of the vWF subunit have been identified (Fig. 1). One concept that has emerged is that recognition specificities leading to interaction with other molecules reside in distinct domains of the subunit. This implies that because of the larger number of recognition sites there should be a direct correlation between multimer size and affinity of interaction with subendothelial components and platelet receptors. Thus, the larger multimers are more effective in mediating platelet adhesion and aggregation under conditions of high shear stress.

The Domains of vWF Which Interact with Platelet Receptors

The domain of vWF that interacts with GP Ib corresponds to a tryptic fragment containing residues Val^{449}-Lys^{728} (Fig. 2). This fragment inhibits binding of native vWF to GP Ib, whether mediated by ristocetin [9] or botrocetin [6]. One problem with the studies on the interaction between vWF and GP Ib is the still limited understanding of the mechanisms involved in the assays used experimentally and of how they relate to physiologically relevant conditions. For example, the positive electrical charge of ristocetin seems to be essential for its activity, suggesting that this molecule may act by decreasing the negative surface charge of platelets and/or the net negative charge of vWF, thus allowing binding to occur [3]. Botrocetin, on the other hand, forms a bimolecular complex with vWF which then binds to platelets [8]. While this mechanism of

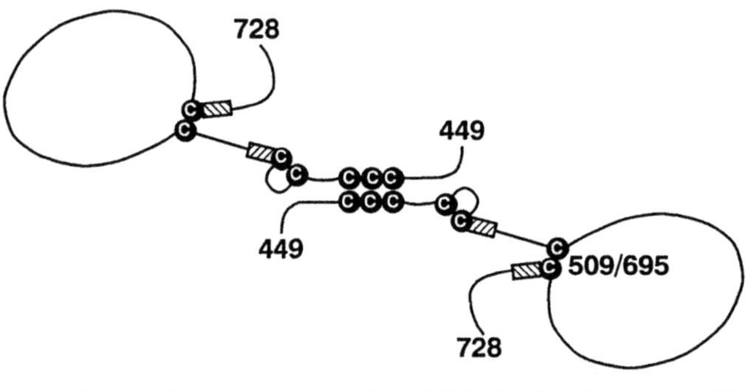

Fig. 2. Schematic representation of the GP Ib-binding domain of vWF between residues 449–728 of the mature subunit. The sequence of residues 449–728 of the mature vWF subunit contains 7 Cys residues (C in one-letter notation): 3 of these (residues 459, 461, 464) form interchain disulfide bonds with the corresponding residues of another subunit, whereas 2 pairs (471–474 and 509–695) form a small and a large intrachain disulfide loop, respectively. The discontinuous elements of sequence thought to be involved in GP Ib binding (residues 474–488 and 694–708) are indicated by the shaded boxes at the two sides of the large loop. In mammalian cells, this fragment of vWF sequence is expressed as a disulfide-linked dimeric species that binds to platelet GP Ib only in the presence of modulators [21]. However, the recombinant fragment expressed in bacteria is used only after reduction and alkylation of cysteine residues and is, therefore, a single chain molecule

action may have interesting analogies with the formation of vWF complexes with molecules in the vessel wall, there is at present no structural knowledge to relate the action of botrocetin to any physiological function of vWF; moreover, it is not known whether the differences in the binding mechanisms elicited by ristocetin and botrocetin reflect variations of pathophysiological relevance in the binding of vWF to GP Ib. Therefore, the correlations between experimental findings and possible in vivo significance, particularly important when evaluating potential inhibitors of function, must be accepted with caution.

The binding of vWF to the other platelet receptor, the GP IIb–IIIa complex, is mediated exclusively by the sequence Arg-Gly-Asp-Ser, located in the carboxyl terminal domain of the vWF subunit (Fig. 1). Monoclonal antipeptide antibodies that bind to epitopes including one or more of the three residues Arg^{1744}, Gly^{1745}, or Asp^{1746} completely inhibit the vWF : GP IIb–IIIa interaction [1]. Of note, these antipeptide antibodies are specific for vWF as they do not cross-react with the other portions of the GP IIb–IIIa complex that contain the identical Arg-Gly-Asp sequence [1].

The functional integration of the two platelet-binding sites in the vWF molecule is demonstrated by the fact that shear-induced platelet aggregation requires vWF interaction with both GP Ib and GP IIb–IIIa [10]. Similarly, platelet thrombus formation under high shear rates requires binding of vWF to both receptors [22]. Recognition of GP Ib is apparently independent of platelet activation, whereas binding to GP IIb–IIIa requires stimulation of platelets. This is in contrast to surface-bound fibrinogen which can interact with GP IIb–IIIa on resting platelets [16]. Therefore, vWF contains in itself structures that, by regulating its binding to platelet GP Ib, can generate a platelet signal which "activates" GP IIb–IIIa independently of any exogenous agonist. This allows a platelet GP IIb–IIIa interaction with either surface-bound vWF (for irreversible adhesion) or circulating vWF (for aggregation). However, it remains to be established whether vWF-mediated platelet adhesion and aggregation require concurrent interaction of vWF with GP Ib and GP IIb–IIIa, or whether the role of GP Ib is mainly that of supporting the initial contact with vWF and generation of an "activation" signal. In the latter case, the subsequent irreversible platelet–surface and platelet–platelet interactions would be mediated exclusively by GP IIb–IIIa.

vWF Domains Which Interact with Components of the Subendothelium

Experiments in purified systems have provided clear evidence that vWF binds to collagen. It is still uncertain, however, whether the collagen is the subendothelial component that modulates vWF function in all instances or whether heparin-like molecules might also be involved. In any case, the important molecular domains involved in these binding activities of vWF have been identified [7, 11, 12, 14]. Proteoglycans containing sequences of sulfated sugars homologous to heparin are present in subendothelial matrices and may represent noncollagenous vWF binding sites in the vessel wall. It has been shown that vWF may bind to endothelial cell-derived extracellular matrices even after enzymatic removal of collagen [20], and that certain monoclonal antibodies may inhibit vWF binding to subendothelium, but not to collagen [4]. It is possible that several vessel wall components may be involved in these interactions.

Strategy: Expression of a vWF Fragment that Inhibits Platelet Function

Recognition of surface-bound vWF by platelets through the GP Ib receptor is the initial role of vWF in thrombogenesis. GP Ib-mediated vWF binding not only promotes the initial platelet contact with the thrombogenic surface but also activates platelets thereby leading them to aggregation [5]. The selective inhibition of vWF binding to GP Ib may be an appropriate early intervention likely to result in a measurable antithrombotic effect in flowing blood [22]. Indeed, the rationale for the use of a recombinant vWF fragment as a novel antiplatelet agent is based on the concept that vWF binding to GP Ib is: 1) essential for initiating the deposition of platelets at sites of vascular injury under conditions of high wall shear rate; 2) involved in the activation of platelets through a complex signaling pathway; and 3) necessary to support platelet aggregation under high shear stress condition. Therefore, blocking the initial interaction between native vWF and platelet GP Ib should prevent any subsequent platelet activation and result in a potent antithrombotic effect.

A peptide containing the GP Ib-binding domain of vWF expressed in *E. coli* has been shown to inhibit the binding of native vWF to GP Ib [18]. To achieve this, the vWF cDNA corresponding to residues 445–733 of the mature vWF subunit was inserted into a vector that contains a promoter selectively recognized by T7 RNA polymerase, and expressed under the control of the lac UV5 promoter [18]. Analysis of samples obtained after expression revealed the presence of a new, quantitatively predominant protein band with an apparent molecular mass of 36 kDa after reduction of disulfide bonds. By 3 h post-induction this fragment constituted more than 25% of total cellular protein. Amino acid sequence analysis and sequence analysis of proteolytic fragments comprising greater than 70% of the 36-kDa peptide provided results in complete agreement with those predicted from the DNA sequence. The recombinant fragment, designated $r\text{vWF}^{445-733}$, was refolded and purified after reduction and alkylation of the seven cysteine residues in the sequence to obtain a single chain polypeptide formulated for in vivo use. Even though reduced and alkylated $r\text{vWF}^{445-733}$ does not represent the native conformation of vWF, its use in animals has not been associated with any unwarranted acute side effects.

$r\text{vWF}^{445-733}$, unlike the native vWF molecule, can bind to GP Ib in the absence of any exogenous modulator. This happens more effectively after reduc-

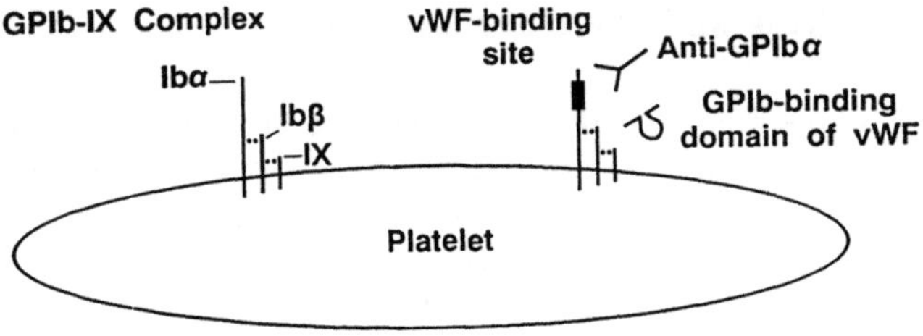

Fig. 3. Schematic representation of the assay used to evaluate the direct binding of $rvWF^{445-733}$ to platelet GP Ib. The recombinant fragment interferes with the binding to GP Ib of a monoclonal antibody directed at the amino terminal domain of this platelet receptor. Since the antibody binds to GP Ib without the need for exogenous modulators, unlike native vWF that binds only when modulators are present, this assay system is suited for demonstrating the direct interaction of the recombinant vWF fragment with the GP Ib-complex

tion and alkylation of all cysteine residues probably because the intrachain disulfide loop between cysteine residues 509 and 695 plays a role in modulating the affinity of vWF for GP Ib [17, 21]. Current in vivo studies with reduced and alkylated $r\mathrm{vWF}^{445-733}$ have demonstrated that it can effectively inhibit the binding of intact multimeric vWF to platelets. For binding induced by ristocetin, the IC_{50} (the concentration necessary to inhibit 50% of binding) was between 66 and 72 nM; for binding induced by botrocetin, the IC_{50} varied between 12 nM and 16 nM. In agreement with the inhibition of vWF binding to GP Ib, $r\mathrm{vWF}^{445-733}$ inhibited in a dose-dependent fashion the agglutination of normal platelets by ristocetin or botrocetin in vitro [18].

The in vitro inhibitory activity of $r\mathrm{vWF}^{445-733}$ can be assessed by testing its ability to interfere with the platelet binding of an anti-GP Ib monoclonal antibody directed at an epitope in the 45 kDa amino terminal region of GP Ib , the same domain of the receptor known to contain the vWF-binding site (Fig. 3). In the presence of the modulators ristocetin or botrocetin, both intact vWF and the recombinant fragment inhibited antibody binding to GP Ib in a dose-dependent manner: the IC_{50} values observed with native vWF were between 6 and 8 nM, and with $r\mathrm{vWF}^{445-733}$ between 30 and 50 nM. Here, the recombinant fragment was approximately 8-fold less effective than native vWF. However, $r\mathrm{vWF}^{445-733}$, but not native vWF, bound to GP Ib in the absence of modulators with an affinity approximately 8-fold to 10-fold lower than in the presence of modulators. The fact that both native vWF and the reduced and alkylated recombinant fragment inhibited platelet binding of the same anti-GP Ib monoclonal antibody in a competitive manner demonstrates that both species bind at the same site on GP Ib. Under no circumstances did the fragment exhibit any interaction with the GP IIb-IIIa complex. This was expected because $r\mathrm{vWF}^{445-733}$ does not contain the GP IIb-IIIa recognition sequence of vWF (Fig. 1).

In short, recombinant technology has allowed the expression of a small 300 amino acid polypeptide fragment of the large subunit which may bind to and block platelet GP Ib functions. Antithrombotic activity in vivo is anticipated from in vitro studies already performed.

Blood Viscosity, Shear Stress and Platelet Function

In recent years it has become increasingly clear that the complex series of events that determine the occurrence of a normal hemostatic response, including chemical reactions that involve cells, the vessel wall and molecules in solution, are influenced by the flow of blood. Rheology is the science that deals with the study of flow and deformation of structures under flow conditions. This subject is described in detail in G.W. Schmid-Schönbein and G.J. del Zoppo (this volume). Blood near the vessel wall moves at a lower speed than at the center of the vessel. This difference in velocity creates a shearing effect between adjacent layers of blood that is greatest near the vessel wall and decreases progressively towards the center of the vessel. Shear *stress* is the force per unit area that can be viewed as the underlying cause of the shearing motion of blood. The *shear* rate, measured in reciprocal seconds (sec^{-1}), is directly proportional to the shear stress and inversely proportional to the viscosity of the fluid.

The role of platelets in hemostasis and thrombosis requires that they become irreversibly attached at a site of injury against the tendency of flow to move adhering platelets with the layer of blood adjacent to the surface. The force opposing a stable adhesion and aggregation is greater with increasing shear rate. The role of vWF in supporting these processes appears to be most significant at high shear rates [2], presumably because of its unique molecular architecture. Thus, it is possible that, under the effect of high shear forces, vWF molecules take the shape of extended filaments, as seen with electron microscopy. The repeating subunit structure in these large multimers offers an array of interaction sites capable of binding in a multivalent manner to receptors on the platelet membrane, thereby increasing the number of contact points and the affinity (strength) of interaction [13]. As a result, the overall force linking platelets to the surface and/or to one another is increased, effectively opposing fluid shear stress. This interpretation of events explains why the role of vWF is less relevant at lower shear rates, since other adhesive molecules may provide sufficient force of interaction to withstand opposing shear forces of lesser magnitude.

These studies, and recent work with shear stress-induced thrombosis, suggest that the definition of crucial amino acid residues involved in vWF interaction with specific substrates should provide information necessary for the rational design and synthesis of peptides and other small organic molecules which specifically interfere with selected pathways of platelet adhesion and aggregation. These may represent a new class of compounds useful for altering the course of thrombotic vascular occlusion in human cerebrovascular disease. Clinical results obtained with the first generation of such compounds may become available in the next few years.

Acknowledgments. Production of the recombinant vWF fragment resulted from a collaboration with the Research and Development group at Rhone-Poulenc Rorer, King of Prussia, Pennsylvania.

References

1. Berliner S, Niiya K, Roberts JR, Houghten RA, Ruggeri ZM (1988) Generation and characterization of peptide-specific antibodies that inhibit von Willebrand factor binding to glycoprotein IIb-IIIa without interacting with other adhesive molecules. J Biol Chem 263:7500–7505
2. Biddison WE, Rao PE, Talle MA, Goldstein G, Shaw S (1982) Possible involvement of the OKT4 molecule in T cell recognition of class II HLA antigens. Evidence from studies of cytotoxic T lymphocytes specific for SB antigens. J Exp Med 156:1065–1076
3. Coller BS, Gralnick HR (1977) Studies on the mechanism of ristocetin- induced platelet agglutination: Effects of structural modification of ristocetin and vancomycin. J Clin Invest 60:302–312
4. de Groot PG, Ottenhof-Rovers M, Van Mourik JA, Sixma JJ (1988) Evidence that the primary binding site of von Willebrand factor that mediates platelet adhesion on subendothelium is not collagen. J Clin Invest 82:65–73
5. De Marco L, Girolami A, Russell S, Ruggeri ZM (1985) Interaction of asialo von Willebrand factor with glycoprotein Ib induces fibrinogen binding to the glycoprotein IIb-IIIa complex and mediates platelet aggregation. J Clin Invest 75:1198–1203
6. Fujimura Y, Holland LZ, Ruggeri ZM, Zimmerman TS (1987) The von Willebrand factor domain mediating botrocetin-induced binding to glycoprotein Ib lies between Val^{449} and Lys^{728}. Blood 70:985–988
7. Fujimura Y, Titani K, Holland LZ, et al (1987) A heparin-binding domain of human von Willebrand factor: Characterization and localization to a tryptic fragment extending from amino acid residue Val-449 to Lys-728. J Biol Chem 262:1734–1739
8. Fujimura Y, Titani K, Usami Y, et al (1991) Isolated and chemical characterization of two structurally and functionally distinct forms of botrocetin, the platelet coagglutinin isolated from the venom of bothrops jararaca. Biochemistry 30:1957–1964
9. Fujimura Y, Titani K, Holland LZ, et al (1986) von Willebrand factor. A reduced and alkylated 52/48 kDa fragment beginning at amino acid residue 449 contains the domain interacting with platelet glycoprotein Ib. J Biol Chem 261:381–385
10. Ikeda Y, Handa M, Kawano K, et al (1991) The role of von Willebrand factor and fibrinogen in platelet aggregation under varying shear stress. J Clin Invest 87:1234–1240
11. Pareti F, Fujimura Y, Dent JA, Holland LZ, Zimmerman TS, Ruggeri ZM (1986) Isolation and characterization of a collagen binding domain in human von Willebrand factor. J Biol Chem 261:15310–15315
12. Pareti FI, Niiya K, NcPherson JM, Ruggeri ZM (1987) Isolation and characterization of two domains of human von Willebrand factor that interact with fibrillar collagen Types I and III. J Biol Chem 262:13835–13841
13. Reichle FA, Rao NS, Chang KHY, Marder V, Algazy K (1977) Thrombolysis of acute or subacute non-embolic arterial thrombosis. J Surg Res 22:202–208
14. Roth GJ, Titani K, Hoyer LW, Hickey MJ (1986) Localization of binding sites within human von Willebrand factor for monomeric Type III collagen. Biochemistry 25:8357–8361
15. Ruggeri ZM, De Marco L, Gatti L, Bader R, Montgomery RR (1983) Platelets have more than one binding site for von Willebrand factor. J Clin Invest 72:1–12
16. Savage B, Ruggeri ZM (1991) Selective recognition of adhesive sites in surface-bound fibrinogen by GPIIb-IIIa on nonactivated platelets. J Biol Chem 266:11227–11233
17. Sugimoto M, Mohri H, McClintock RA, Ruggeri ZM (1991) Identification of discontinuous von Willebrand factor sequences involved in complex formation with botrocetin. A model for the regulation of von Willebrand factor binding to platelet glycoprotein Ib. J Biol Chem 266:18172–18178
18. Sugimoto M, Ricca G, Hrinda ME, et al (1991) Functional modulation of the isolated glycoprotein Ib-binding domain of von Willebrand factor expressed in Escherichia coli. Biochemistry 30:5202–5209
19. Vicente V, Houghten RA, Ruggeri ZM (1990) Identification of a site in the alpha chain of platelet glycoprotein Ib that participates in von Willebrand factor binding. J Biol Chem 265:274–280

20. Wagner DD, Urban-Pickering M, Marder VJ (1984) von Willebrand protein binds to extracellular matrices independently of collagen. Proc Natl Acad Sci USA 81:471–475
21. Ware J, Dent JA, Zauma H, et al (1991) Identification of a point mutation in type IIb von Willebrand disease illustrating the regulation of von Willebrand factor affinity for the platelet GP Ib-IX receptor. Proc Natl Acad Sci USA 88:2946–2950
22. Weiss HJ, Hawiger J, Ruggeri ZM, Turitto VT, Thiagarajan P, Hoffmann T (1989) Fibrinogen-independent platelet adhesion and thrombus formation on subendothelium mediated by glycoprotein IIb–IIIa complex at high shear rate. J Clin Invest 83:288–297

Neuronal Protection: Is There a Role for Gangliosides or Ca^{+2}-Channel Blockers?

G.-L. Lenzi[1], H. Baasch[2], and R. Bruno[3]

Recently developed experimental data, and initial clinical data for ischemic stroke suggest that the sooner therapeutical intervention in ischemic stroke may achieve recanalization, the better the outcome. TIAs are a natural example of this statement, and a model for an effective and safe thrombolytic therapy. The GISSI studies have underlined the validity of this concept for cardiac ischemia [1, 11]. However, for the ischemic brain, reperfusion does not appear to be without side effects [5, 7, 20], which may be not unimportant for a patient's very survival and final clinical outcome.

Thus, a rational approach could be to protect the ischemic neuronal tissue *pari passu* with recanalization from the phenomena involved in the postischemic cascade so that reperfusion will find tissue in its best possible condition. That is, to add to the thrombolytic intervention ancillary therapies aimed at stopping the maturation of ischemic damage, e.g., stop the entrance of calcium ions.

Barbiturate therapy has been applied to clinical conditions of global ischemia so as to decrease neuronal metabolism during the disturbed energy state associated with ischemia. This approach was not found useful, and has not been applied to stroke. In fact, an ancillary therapy must be deprived of serious side effects to be freely utilized in conditions such as the acute stroke. So safety is a primary requirement. Contrarily, the therapy must be applied in an an amount which is clinical relevant. And, we have to underline that a powerful agent cannot be completely deprived of side effects. Therefore, a safe molecule may show only minor positive clinical effects. Considering the significant incidence and prevalence of stroke, even a minor improvement would be expected to result in major social and personal advantage. As recently underlined by Sandercock and Willems [22], "... if a simple, widely practicable treatment such as an oral calcium antagonist ... reduce(s) early mortality by one-sixth from 12% to 10%, this would represent 20 deaths avoided per 1000 patients treated. This reduction would be worthwhile, especially if it were

[1] Department of Neurological Sciences, University of Rome, Rome, Italy
[2] PH-SM, Funzione Medica, Bayer Spa, Milano, Italy
[3] Fidia Spa, Abano Terme, Padova, Italy

G.J. del Zoppo, E. Mori, W. Hacke (Eds.)
Thrombolytic Therapy in Acute Ischemic Stroke II

accomplished by a similar proportional improvement in survival free of disability."

We will here discuss two different ancillary therapies: the gangliosides and the Ca^{+2}-antagonists. Both molecular strategies are aimed at protecting the nervous tissues from ischemic damage. We will review the relevant experimental data and the initial clinical experiences of one compound belonging to each of these two categories: the GM1 ganglioside, and the Ca^{+2}-antagonist nimodipine.

Gangliosides: Monosialoganglioside GM1

We refer the reader for general information and a bibliography to the review of Carolei, Fieschi, and colleagues [6]. GM1 has been shown to be active in the regulation of membrane-mediated neuronal functions – in particular, in the maturation and repair mechanisms. In the experimental setting, GM1 pretreatment may reduce neuronal damage induced in rats by intracerebral injection of NMDA agonists, such as quinolinic and ibotenic acid. In an ischemic–anoxic model, mortality was reduced up to 49% by GM1 posttreatment. Furthermore, in experimental focal cerebral ischemia, GM1 inhibited the edema formation both in the core and in the periphery of the infarction, with a parallel reduction in the functional deficit of the treated animals [4, 14, 17].

In a model of transient middle cerebral artery (MCA) occlusion in cats [26, 29], GM1 attenuated the histologic damage; ICMRG1c was normalized toward control level within 4 h, while it appeared still depressed up to 75% in control animals. Furthermore, protective effects by chronic treatment with a GM1 inner-ester derivative sialoside were observed 21 days after transitory forebrain ischemia on both delayed hippocampal neuronal death and EEG recordings [23]. In conclusion, the experimental data have supported the clinical utilization of GM1 in the treatment of acute ischemic damage, with the rationale of decreasing edema formation and neuronal deaths, and of improving functional outcome.

What are the initial clinical data in trials with this drug? We will review here only the double-blind studies with treatment initiation within the "first hours" after the onset of symptoms (Table 1). In fact, when those studies were planned, the time window for the pharmacological approach was not so clearly defined as it appears today. Also, since the data from the EST study are not yet public, this study cannot be commented on here. The clinical trials have already demonstrated, in general, "positive" results in terms of the neurological scales and indices considered in each study. However, clinical improvement could well be different from a change in a stroke scale index, as significant as that latter might be.

With these limitations and considerations a number of comments may be made. It would be interesting to make an *a posteriori* stratification of outcome on the basis of the time interval between stroke and treatment, and to evaluate

Table 1. Clinical studies of GM1 ganglioside in stroke

Study	Hours From Onset	N	Principal Parameter	Results
Jamieson [13]	72	30	PET scan	Positive
Heiss [12]	48	25	PET scan	Positive
			Stroke Index	$p<0.04$
Angeleri [2]	48	112	Fritz-Werner	$p<0.01$
			Barthel	$p<0.05$
Argentino [3]	12	502	CNS	$p<0.03$
EST	5	805	CNS	?
Papo [21]	coma	137	GSC	$p<0.02$

clinical outcomes accordingly. In addition, the doses used so far might have been too low: pharmacokinetic studies have demonstrated that, following intravenous injection of 30 mg/kg, GM1 reached cerebral concentrations in the nanomolar range [10]. Although man-to-animal dosage comparisons are not always direct, a dose of 30 mg/kg has already been used in animal studies. The cerebral ischemic symptoms must be sufficiently severe to show a clinically relevant effect of GM1. Therefore, a secondary analysis of patients divided into "severe" and "mild" clinical status would be quite relevant.

If GM1 is efficacious in acute ischemic stroke, can further benefit be obtained in combination with thrombolytic therapy? This is, to our knowledge, unexplored. In conditions different from acute stroke, but similar in terms of potential final ischemic damage, such as subarachnoid hemorrhage, GM1 contributes positively to the recovery of the level of consciousness when compared to placebo, as measured by the Glasgow Coma Scale. This improvement was most evident 1 and 2 weeks after the end of treatment, compared to early assessment [21].

Finally, the efficacy of a therapy must be considered also in the light of its costs. We have calculated that the actual cost of a complete treatment with GM1 in acute stroke – that is, 200 mg/day for 20 days – is approximately $2,000 US.

Calcium Antagonists: Nimodipine

The rationale for Ca^{+2}-antagonist therapy is based on the action of glutamate, an excitatory neurotransmitter. Ischemic conditions produce an increased presynaptic release and a decreased reuptake of this molecule, producing an extracellular excess in concentration. With mechanisms yet to be fully elucidated; this results in damage to the tissue. NMDA receptors are involved in this process, and NMDA antagonists (such as MK801) are able to reduce the ischemic damage in animal models. Therefore, it was assumed that calcium channel blockers with a preferential cerebrovascular action [15] could be beneficial, not only through an increase in cerebral blood flow, but also by the postischemic overload of the ischemic tissue with Ca^{+2}. In fact, the ischemic depletion of tissue stores of ATP reduces the effectiveness of Na-K- ATPase as an ion pump and contributes to the self-regenerating introduction of substantial amounts of Ca^{+2} into the cell. An increase in the cytosolic concentration of Ca^{+2} triggers a cascade of reactions, fully described in Siesjo and Wieloch [24], that ultimately lead to cytoclasis.

Experiments with nimodipine have been promising. In 1983, Steen and colleagues [25] reported that pretreatment with nimodipine improved both postischemic blood flow and neurologic recovery in dogs submitted to 10 min of complete ischemia. This positive result was attributed to minor postischemic delayed hypoperfusion. Kazda and Towart have reported that pretreatment with nimodipine reduces acute cerebrovascular damage in cats, and that chronic treatment decreases the lesions caused by dietary salt load in the SHR-SP rats, thereby increasing survival as well [15]. Mabe and coworkers have shown that in pretreated rats submitted to complete occlusion of the cerebral vessels, recovery of ATP was better in the treated group than the untreated group [16]. Mohamed and colleagues [18] have demonstrated a reduction in the size of the ischemic lesion due to MCA occlusion, when animals were pretreated with nimodipine. This effect was due to a decrease in the volume and extent of cellular damage in the periphery (but not in the core) of the lesion. The authors hypothesized that better oxygen delivery, through the increased blood flow, contributed to the final beneficial effect. Combined therapy with MK801 and nimodipine was reported to be beneficial in a temporary MCA occlusion model by Uematsu and coinvestigators [28], reducing histologic damage and enhancing recovery of the EEG abnormalities. In contrast, recent experimental data on the benefits of adding nimodipine to t-PA was negative [30]. However, the animal model utilized was "probably an exceptionally rigorous test."

So far, clinical experience has been controversial. In 1984 and 1988, Gelmers and colleagues published reports on patients affected by stroke and treated with nimodipine within 24 h of the onset of their symptoms [8, 9]. In the larger, controlled trial, 186 patients were randomized. The authors claimed that "... mortality from all causes was significantly reduced with nimodipine as compared with placebo..." In addition, "... a significantly better neurologic outcome, as assessed by the Matthew Scale of neurologic deficit, was also observed in the nimodipine group..."

Several criticisms have been raised against this study: in particular, the number of patients recruited seemed quite low, considering that out of the initial 186 cases, 22 patients were excluded because of protocol violations and other causes, and the further subdivision into subgroups reduced the power of the study. The reduction of mortality, 20.4% in the placebo group and 8.6% in the treated group, must be referred to the figures of early deaths in other studies: 10% after 30 days in the Oxfordshire Community Stroke Project, and 12% after 3 weeks in untreated controls in the TRUST Study [27]. That is, the mortality in the placebo group was unaccountably high.

The results of the TRUST Study, a large trial, were negative [27]. However, in this study, very few cases (13%), were recruited within the first 12 h, a treatment "window" which could well be considered excessive. A similar problem – that is, a large (48-h) entry window – was present in the study coordinated by Mohr [19]. Furthermore, as in similar studies performed with the aim to be "simple and pragmatic," the utilization of CT scan in the TRUST Study was optional: only a small proportion of the patients had a CT scan performed to confirm the diagnosis, and as an entry criterion.

Commenting on those trials, Sandercock and Willems [22] have emphasized that: "... no single trial has been large enough on its own to provide clear evidence of a reduction in mortality. A nonstandard overview of older trials suggested there might be modest benefits (Gelmers and Hennerici, Stroke, 1990), but an up-to-date overview with standard methods, incorporating the much larger recent trials, is clearly needed to determine whether treatment is beneficial or whether further trials are needed..."

Conclusions

The potential benefits of thrombolytic therapy in acute stroke are hampered by the fact that this therapy has to be given within a very narrow window and cannot be given without a minimum of neuroradiological or instrumental workup of the patient. It is necessary, therefore, to study other ways to protect the cerebral tissue at the same time, if not from the principal infarct, then from the secondary, peripheral, maturing postischemic phenomena. Herein lies the rationale for the co-utilization of ancillary therapies with thrombolytic therapy. Both ganglioside GM1 and nimodipine have, on experimental bases, found support for their utilization in ischemic stroke. Clinical results have so far been less supportive than expected, and not infrequently controversial. Problems with the time interval for recruitment and in the dosages utilized may well be major causes for this uncertainty.

References

1. Gruppo Italiano Per Lo Studio Della Streptochinasi Nell'Infarto Miocardico (GISSI) (1990) GISSI-2: A factorial randomized trial of alteplase versus streptokinase and heparin versus no heparin among 12, 490 patients with acute myocardial infarction. Lancet 336:65–71
2. Angeleri F, Scarpino O, Martinazzo C, et al (1992) GM1 ganglioside therapy in acute ischemic stroke. Cerebrovasc Dis (In Press)
3. Argentino C, Sacchetti ML, Toni D, et al (1989) GM1 ganglioside therapy in acute ischemic stroke. Stroke 20:1143–1149
4. Bharucha VA, Wakade GC, Mahadik SP, Karpiak SE (1991) GM1 ganglioside treatment reduces functional deficits associated with cortical focal ischemia. Exp Neurol 114:136–140
5. Brott T (1991) Thrombolytic therapy for stroke. Cerebrovasc Brain Metab Rev 3:91–113
6. Carolei A, Fieschi C, Bruno R, Toffano G (1991) Monosialoganglioside GM1 in cerebral ischemia. Cerebrovasc Brain Metab Rev 3:134–157

7. del Zoppo GJ, Ferbert A, Otis S, et al (1988) Local intra-arterial therapy in acute carotid territory stroke: A pilot study. Stroke 19:307–313
8. Gelmers HJ (1984) The effects of nimodipine on the clinical course of patients with acute ischemic stroke. Acta Neurol Scand 69:232–239
9. Gelmers HJ, Gorter K, De Weerdt C, Wiezer HJA (1988) A controlled trial of nimodipine in acute ischemic stroke. N Engl J Med 318:203–207
10. Ghidoni R, Firoilli A, Trinchera M, Venerando B, Ghigorno V, Tettamanti G (1989) Uptake, cell penetration and metabolic processing of exogenously administered GM1 ganglioside in rat brain. Neurochem Int 15:455–465
11. GISSI (1986) Effectiveness of intravenous thrombolytic treatment in acute myocardial infarction. Lancet i:397–402
12. Heiss WD, Naserke K, Braune S (1988) Effects of gangliosides upon rehabilitation of patients following stroke. In: Krieglstein J, Oberpichler H (eds) Pharmacology of cerebral ischemia. Wissenschaftliche Verlag GmbH, Stuttgart, p 433
13. Jamieson DG, Reivich M, Alves W, et al (1989) The effect of ganglioside GM1 treatment in acute ischemic infarction: A positron emission tomography study. J Cereb Blood Flow Metab 9(Suppl 1):S602
14. Karpiak SE, Wakade CG, Tagliavia A, Mahadik SP (1991) Temporal changes in edema Na^+, K^+ and Ca^{+2} in focal cortical stroke: GM1 ganglioside reduces ischemic injury. J Neurosci Res 30:512–520
15. Kazda S, Towart R (1982) Nimodipine: A new calcium antagonistic drug with a preferential cerebrovascular action. Acta Neurochir 63:1–4
16. Mabe H, Nagai H, Takagi T, Umemura S, Ohno M (1986) Effect of nimodipine on cerebral functional and metabolic recovery following ischemia in the rat brain. Stroke 17:501–505
17. Mahadik SP, Hawver DB, Hungund BL, Li JS, Karpiak SE (1989) GM1 ganglioside treatment after global ischemia protects changes in membrane fatty acids and properties of NA^+ ,K^+, ATPase and Mg^{2+} ATPase. J Neurosci Res 24:402–412
18. Mohammed AA, Gotoh O, Graham DI, et al (1985) Effect of pretreatment with the calcium antagonist nimodipine on local cerebral blood flow and histopathology after middle cerebral artery occlusion. Ann Neurol 18:705–711
19. Mohr JP (1992) Personal communication.
20. Mori E, Tabuchi M, Yoshida T, Yamadori A (1988) Intracarotid urokinase with thromboembolic occlusion of the middle cerebral artery. Stroke 19:802– 812
21. Papo I, Benedetti A, Carteri A, Merli GA, Mingrino S, Bruno R (1991) Monosialoganglioside in subarachnoid hemorrhage. Stroke 22:22–26
22. Sandercock P, Willems H (1992) Medical treatment of acute ischaemic stroke. Lancet 339:537–539
23. Seren MS, Rubini R, Lazzaro A, Zanoni R, Fiori MG, Leon A (1990) Protective effects of the inner ester derivative of monosialoganglioside following transitory forebrain ischemia in rats. Stroke 21:1607–1612
24. Siesjo BK, Wieloch T (1985) Cerebral metabolism in ischemia: Neurochemical basis for therapy. Br J Anaesth 57:47–62
25. Steen PA, Newberg LA, Milde JH, Michenfelder JD (1984) Cerebral blood flow and neurologic outcome when nimodipine is given after complete cerebral ischemia in the dog. J Cereb Blood Flow Metab 4:82–87
26. Tanaka K, Dora E, Urbanics R, Greenberg JH, Toffano G, Reivich M (1986) Effect of the ganglioside GM1 on the cerebral metabolism, microciruclation, recovery period following focal ischemia in cats. Stroke 17:1170–1178
27. Trust Study Group (1990) Randomized, double-blind, placebo-controlled trial of nimodipine in acute stroke. Lancet 336:1205–1209
28. Uematsu D, Araki N, Greenberg JH, Sladky J, Reivich M (1991) Combined therapy with MK-801 and nimodipine for protection of ischemic brain damage. Neurology 41:88–94
29. Urbanics R, Greenberg JH, Toffano G, Reivich M (1989) Effect of GM1 ganglioside on cerebrocortical microflow, NAD/NADH fluorescence, (K+e) and glucose utilization in focal cerebral ischemia in halothane anesthetized cats. Stroke 20:795–802
30. Zivin JA, Mazzarella V (1991) Tissue plasminogen activator plus glutamate antagonist improves outcome after embolic stroke. Arch Neurol 48:1235–1238

Discussion Summary: Ancillary Therapy for Cerebrovascular Reperfusion

Chaired by M. Hennerici[1] and P. Lyden[2]

The discussion was opened by a physician from the audience who criticized all of the animal data that had been presented which were based on models that avoided the use of embolism. The questioner stated that as most human stroke is embolic, an animal model utilizing an embolic approach would be most appropriate.

Dr. Caplan questioned Dr. Ruggeri regarding where in the carotid artery one might find the shear rates necessary for the formation of platelet and fibrin aggregates. Dr. Ruggeri explained that areas of high shear force may occur in a variety of locations, and one could not predict based on, for example, anatomic criteria where such turbulent flow might occur. The comment was also made that blood is a very difficult fluid to model under ideal circumstances and that research in this area is in its infancy. Another questioner asked whether the ex vivo flow experiment that Dr. Ruggeri had presented had been altered so as to use pulsatile flow rather than laminar flow to move the blood through the test device. Dr. Ruggeri indicated that this was a planned future experiment, but also reemphasized that a stimulus to platelet aggregation could occur in a local microenvironment where conditions are significantly different than mean shear force, or mean blood flow. He emphasized the need for further laboratory testing to explore the local microconditions under which aggregation could be optimized.

Another physician asked Dr. Ruggeri where von Willebrand factor is found in the vasculature and what duration of occlusion is necessary to stimulate its expression. Dr. Ruggeri answered that the protein is endogenously present in the subendothelium. It is synthesized by endothelial cells and constitutively secreted. In short, the protein is everywhere in blood and found wherever cell adhesion might occur. It should be noted that the protein is released in high concentration from endothelial cells when they are stimulated. The protein is also found inside platelets in very high concentration, and it is released locally whenever platelets are activated.

[1] Neurologische Klinik, Klinikum Mannheim (Universität Heidelberg), Mannheim, Federal Republic of Germany
[2] Department of Neurology, University of California at San Diego, San Diego, CA, USA

G. J. del Zoppo, E. Mori, W. Hacke (Eds.)
Thrombolytic Therapy in Acute Ischemic Stroke II

The discussion then turned to the nature of focal cerebral ischemia. A physician in the audience indicated to Dr. Grotta that in the Emergency Department patients typically present with "incomplete" ischemia. It was alleged that animal models of complete ischemia may not be relevant. The situation facing this physician in the Emergency Department is that of a patient who requires hemodynamic management. In particular, acute stroke patients tend to be volume depleted and, therefore, may require therapy which amounts to hemodynamic intervention. Is there a role for active hemodynamic intervention? Dr. Grotta agreed that this is a very common situation in stroke patients and in consecutive studies of patients using a Swan-Ganz catheter, that hemoconcentration and volume depletion is found in about one-third of patients. However, clinical trials of hemodilution therapy have not been uniformly successful in treating patients with stroke. Dr. Grotta pointed out that a principal criticism of those previous studies was that they enrolled patients up to 12 h after acute stroke onset. This delay may have provoked serious complications in those patients that may have limited the effectiveness of the therapy. Using a similar logic, Dr. Grotta noted that in studies of high dose nimodipine, serious adverse effects could be attributed to hypotension induced by the drug. This complication again may have obscured any potential benefit.

A question was raised about antileukocyte strategies, as to whether or not a single treatment was necessary or multiple treatments. Dr. Schmid-Schönbein replied that the effect of the antibody on the PMN leukocyte currently in use only lasts 20 to 40 min and then after that alternative mechanisms of cell adhesion begin to take over.

Several questioners addressed the issue of the use of animal experimentation prior to human clinical trials. A consensus was achieved that important insights into the mechanism of ischemia and infarction could be gained from some animal models. However, all agreed that the extrapolation of animal results to the human setting required the utmost caution. In particular, trials of therapeutic agents done in animals require very careful interpretation prior to embarking on a human trial.

Open Communications

A Meta-Analysis of All Published Data on the Use of Thrombolytic Therapy to Treat Acute Ischemic Stroke

J.M. Wardlaw[1] and C.P. Warlow[2]

Acute ischemic stroke is the third most common cause of death in the developed world and leaves many more patients disabled [2]. Despite this, however, there is as yet no treatment of proven benefit. Thrombolysis has been extensively tested in acute myocardial infarction (a vascular disease with some similarities to acute ischemic stroke) for which it is now an established treatment [4], having been shown to reduce the incidence of vascular death by about 25%. Thrombolysis might also improve outcome after acute ischemic stroke by speeding recanalization of occluded cerebral arteries, and reducing the amount of permanent neuronal damage.

Thrombolysis has not been extensively tested in acute ischemic stroke, although the first attempts to use it were in the late 1950's [10]. Early studies were hampered by the inability to distinguish between intracerebral hemorrhage and infarction as the cause of acute stroke symptoms, until the development of CT scanning in the early 1970's. The natural history of acute ischemic stroke is complex and the assessment of any treatment must be by randomized controlled trial, especially with thrombolysis where the likely adverse effects (cerebral hemorrhage and possible severe infarct edema) mimic the natural history of the disease. There have been more than 60 reports of the use of thrombolysis in acute ischemic stroke in the world literature so far, but we have concentrated on the published randomized controlled trials to see whether analysis using the overview technique [3] would show evidence of a beneficial or detrimental treatment effect on stroke outcome.

Subjects and Methods

We have tried to identify all published work on the use of thrombolytic drugs to treat acute ischemic stroke by a thorough literature search using Index

[1] Department of Clinical Neuroradiology, Southern General Hospital, Govan Road, Glasgow, UK
[2] Department of Clinical Neurosciences, Western General Hospital, Crewe Road, Edinburgh, UK

G.J. del Zoppo, E. Mori, W. Hacke (Eds.)
Thrombolytic Therapy in Acute Ischemic Stroke II

Medicus, by tracing references cited in thrombolysis papers, and by discussion with other researchers interested in thrombolysis. We were able to identify 5 published trials which were truly randomized and had a control group. We have not included trials with retrospective control and prospective treated groups, nor trials where it was unclear how the control patients were selected. The overview technique was used to analyze the effect of thrombolysis on death, and on death or deterioration after acute ischemic stroke without and with the benefit of CT scanning.

Results

Five truly randomized controlled trials of thrombolysis in acute "ischemic" stroke were identified. These comprise two trials by Meyer and colleagues in 1963 [6] and 1964 [7], Abe and coworkers in 1981 [1], Ohtomo and colleagues in 1985 [9] and Mori and investigators in 1992 [8]. The two by Meyer were done prior to the development of CT scanning and may inadvertently have included patients with cerebral hemorrhage or hemorrhagic infarction as the cause of stroke rather than true ischemic strokes. Those by Abe, Ohtomo, and Mori and their respective coworkers were all done with the benefit of CT scanning.

The trials added together included a total of 601 patients. Although different drugs, dose of drug, time to treatment, type of ischemic stroke, and endpoint were used in the 5 trials, the overview (or meta-analysis) allows comparison of different trials to look for an overall treatment effect. In the case of the trials by Meyer, Abe, and Ohtomo, the published information was used, but additional information on deterioration was supplied by Professor Mori.

Analysis of all 5 trials shows that the risk of death is increased by 32% with thrombolysis (95% CI: 30% reduction to 150% excess), and the risk of death or deterioration is reduced by 26% (95% CI: 57% reduction to 27% excess). Analysis of the trials by Abe, Ohtomo, and Mori conducted with the benefit of CT scanning (and therefore truly ischemic stroke) shows a reduction in the risk of death of 40% (95% CI: 79% reduction to 70% excess) with thrombolytic treatment, and in the risk of death or deterioration a reduction of 63% (95% CI: 22% – 82% reduction). The reduction in the risk of death or deterioration with thrombolysis in the CT-guided trials is significant ($2p = 0.012$) and provides some evidence that thrombolysis is likely to be beneficial in acute ischemic stroke, and certainly needs to be properly evaluated.

Discussion

Although there is now increasing information on the use of thrombolysis in acute ischemic stroke from uncontrolled "dose escalation" studies, the data from these studies cannot be used to assess treatment, as the major adverse effects of thrombolysis – cerebral hemorrhage and severe infarct edema – were not controlled for (and in this case they mimic the natural history of ischemic stroke).

Information from recent larger randomized controlled trials of thrombolysis in acute ischemic stroke will be available in the near future. Professor Yamaguchi has presented results of the Japanese multicenter randomized controlled trial at this Symposium. Several randomized controlled trials of thrombolysis in acute ischemic stroke are planned or in progress in Europe and the USA.

However, the overview analysis of the scant information from the 5 randomized controlled trials of thrombolysis so far available provides some evidence that thrombolysis may be beneficial, certainly enough to encourage much larger randomized trials. Very large trials, on the scale of the thrombolysis in myocardial infarction studies [5] including many thousands of patients, will be needed to establish the true beneficial and adverse effects of thrombolytic treatment. Trials should allow patient entry up to at least 12 h (and possibly 24) after symptom onset because in many parts of the world stroke patients go to the hospital, if at all, in a "slow ambulance" and it is unrealistic to expect that to change overnight. Studies should include elderly patients and as wide a spectrum of ischemic stroke as possible so that the risk/benefit ratio can be identified for all age groups and types of ischemic stroke. The overview analysis has shown that thrombolysis is a promising treatment for acute ischemic stroke and provides sufficient justification for the testing of thrombolysis in large randomized controlled trials.

References

1. Abe T, Kazama M, Naito I, et al (1981) Clinical evaluation for efficacy of tissue culture urokinase (TCUK) on cerebral thrombosis by means of multicenter double-blind study. Blood Vessels 12:321–341
2. Bonita R (1992) Epidemiology of stroke. Lancet 339:342–347
3. Collins R, Gray R, Godwin J, Peto R (1987) Avoidance of large biases and large random errors in the assessment of moderate treatment effects: The need for systemic overviews. Stat Med 6:245–250
4. Collins R, Julian D (1991) British Heart Foundation Surveys (1987 and 1989) of United Kingdom treatment policies for acute myocardial infarction. Br Heart J 66:250–255
5. ISIS-3 Collaborative Group (1992) Randomized trial of intravenous streptokinase, tissue plasminogen activator or anistreplase among 46, 000 cases of acute myocardial infarction. Lancet 339:753–770
6. Meyer JS, Gilroy J, Barnhart MI, Johnson JF (1963) Therapeutic thrombolysis in cerebral thromboembolism. Neurology 13:927–937
7. Meyer JS, Gilroy J, Barnhart MI, Johnson JF (1964) Anticoagulants plus streptokinase therapy in progressive stroke. JAMA 189:373
8. Mori E, Yoneda Y, Tabuchi M, et al (1992) Intravenous recombinant tissue plasminogen activator in acute carotid artery territory stroke. Neurology 42:976–982
9. Ohtomo E, Araki G, Itoh E, Tougi H, Matuda T, Atarashi J (1985) Clinical efficacy of urokinase in the treatment of cerebral thrombosis. Clinical Evaluation 13:711–751
10. Sussman BJ, Fitch TSP (1958) Thrombolysis with fibrinolysin in cerebral arterial occlusion. J Am Med Assoc 167:1705–1709

Causes of Delayed Treatment of Stroke Patients Enrolled in t-PA Protocols

M. J. Alberts and A. Perry

For thrombolytic therapy of acute stroke patients to be administered in a safe and efficacious manner, it would appear that such therapy has to be initiated very soon after stroke onset. Past studies of fibrinolytic agents in stroke have shown a high mortality and no efficacy when thrombolytic therapy was initiated more than 12 h after stroke onset [6, 8]. More recent studies have reported a reduced complication rate when thrombolytic therapy was begun within 1.5 to 8 h after stroke onset [4, 5]. One major factor in treating stroke patients rapidly is the undue delay between symptom onset and patient presentation. In the course of participating in two trials of recombinant tissue plasminogen activator (rt-PA) in acute stroke patients, we became aware of another source of delay in beginning therapy, namely, in-hospital delays. We have studied various post-stroke time epochs prior to the administration of rt-PA to determine the factors that delayed initiation of therapy.

Subjects and Methods

We have participated in two trials of rt-PA in acute stroke. One trial was undertaken with the rt-PA/Acute Stroke Study Group (employing duteplase), and the other trial was the t-PA Trial in Acute Thrombotic/Thromboembolic Stroke trial (employing alteplase) (in progress at this writing). Both trials have required that patients undergo a neurologic examination, blood tests, and a head CT scan prior to enrollment. All patients had to undergo a cerebral angiogram to document a complete arterial occlusion likely to be responsible for their symptoms. In both cases, rt-PA was given intravenously, and the infusion had to begin within 8 h (for duteplase) or 6 h (for alteplase) of symptom onset.

Three time epochs were studied in detail. The first was the time period from symptom onset to hospital presentation. The second was the period from hospital presentation to the beginning of cerebral angiography. The third was the

Division of Neurology, Department of Medicine, and the Stroke Acute Care Unit, Duke University Medical Center, Durham, NC, USA

G. J. del Zoppo, E. Mori, W. Hacke (Eds.)
Thrombolytic Therapy in Acute Ischemic Stroke II

time period from the beginning of angiography to the initiation of the intravenous rt-PA infusion. Time data on symptom onset was collected from the patient and family. Time of onset was defined as the first time that symptoms of a focal neurological deficit defined as stroke (leading to this admission) were noted by the patient or a family member. Vague or nonspecific symptoms such as headache and dizziness were not used to calculate onset time. Patients whose symptoms were first noted upon awakening were generally excluded. Time data for hospital presentation was collected from the emergency room triage sheet or admission record. Some patients had a stroke while in the hospital, in which case the delay in hospital presentation was considered to be 0. The time of angiography was when the angiogram was started. The exact time when the rt-PA infusion was begun was carefully noted in the study records. For those patients who did not receive rt-PA (due to an angiographic exclusion), the time of the end of the angiogram was used to calculate the expected rt-PA start time. Since this time data was critical to patient enrollment, very accurate records of these times were kept in the patients' study book and the hospital records.

Results

As of January, 1992, we have enrolled a total of 22 patients in the two rt- PA-based protocols cited above. Two patients had a stroke while in the hospital, and 2 patients did not receive rt-PA due to various angiographic exclusion criteria. The mean time delay from symptom onset to hospital presentation was 180 min (range of 0–390 min). Excluding the 2 patients who had a stroke while in-hospital, only 3 patients presented within 90 min of symptom onset, while 12 presented 180 min or longer after symptom onset.

The mean time from hospital presentation to the beginning of cerebral angiography was 184 min, with a range of 0 to 323 min. The patient with no delay was transferred from an outside hospital and was taken directly to the angiography suite. In this one case most of the required studies (head CT and blood tests) were performed at the outside hospital. Excluding that patient, only 4 patients underwent angiography within 90 min of hospital presentation.

Table 1. Mean time delays and ranges

	Onset → Hospital	Hospital → Angio*	Angio → t-PA*
Time Delay:	180 (0–390)	184 (0–323)	33 (5–97)
Mean Total Delay = 397 minutes (6.6 hours)			
% of Delay:	45%	46%	8%

* Angio = cerebral angiogram; t-PA = tissue plasminogen activator

The mean delay from cerebral angiography to initiation of the rt-PA infusion was 33 min (range of 5 to 97 min) (see Table 1).

The total mean delay from symptom onset to the beginning of the rt-PA infusion was 397 min. When the contribution of each time epoch to the total delay was calculated, the results are as follows: the period of symptom onset to hospital presentation was responsible for 45% of the total time; the epoch from hospital presentation to cerebral angiography was responsible for 46% of the total delay; and the period from angiography to rt-PA infusion was responsible for only 8% of the total delay (see Table 1).

Discussion

This study unexpectedly found that the time required to perform a cerebral angiogram once a stroke patient presented to the emergency room was essentially equal to the time delay from symptom onset to hospital presentation. The mean delay of 3 h from symptom onset to hospital presentation is not indicative of the delay seen in all stroke patients. The 22 patients in this study are a highly select group, since they represent only those patients who were enrolled in one of the rt-PA protocols. Several recent studies have noted average delays from symptom onset to hospital presentation ranging from 12 to 24 h [1, 7]. While public and professional education may help to shorten some of these delays [2], additional efforts clearly need to be targeted in this area.

The mean 3-h time lag between hospital presentation and cerebral angiography can be explained by several factors. At times, the Emergency Department (ED) staff may not triage and evaluate stroke patients as rapidly as necessary. This is supported in a study by Saunders [9], who found a correlation between perceived patient stroke acuity and the pace of evaluation. Since many health care providers do not consider stroke a true emergency, delayed triage is not unexpected.

Other explanations for the delayed ED evaluation may include the time needed to do a complete physical examination and neurologic assessment, obtain informed consent from the patient or family, complete blood tests, and obtain a head CT scan. Timerding and colleagues [10] studied several factors that might delay the evaluation and treatment of stroke patients in the Emergency Department. Delays in performing various blood tests and a head CT scan were found to significantly prolong evaluation time. These procedures need not cause extensive delays, since several patients at our center did undergo angiography within 90 min of hospital presentation. Also, the experience reported in an NIH-sponsored trial of rt-PA (alteplase) for stroke [4], which had a 90-min enrollment window and required a similar assessment (excluding a cerebral angiogram), shows that such evaluations can be performed rapidly.

In our experience, much of the 3-h in-hospital time period was spent awaiting preparation of the angiography suite. At times, the suite had to be cleaned following a prior study, while at other times the neuroradiologist and technical staff had to be called in to the hospital during off hours. While these factors may be amenable to modifications, they would require an angiography suite staffed 24 h a day, similar to what is done in many medical centers doing cardiac catheterization. Such an arrangement might be feasible if invasive studies or invasive treatments were performed on a large percentage of acute stroke patients.

While this group of patients was a highly select population (since they were all enrolled in one of the rt-PA protocols), they are indicative of what was seen in larger studies. The time data for other patients enrolled in the complete rt-PA Acute Stroke Study Group trial showed time patterns very similar to what was observed in our cohort of patients [5]. It seems apparent that newer treatments for acute stroke will require improved out- of-hospital recognition of stroke symptoms and more rapid in-hospital triage and evaluation. Several strategies have been described to improve the rapid identification and triage of stroke patients [3]. Our cardiology colleagues have been very successful in a similar endeavor, providing some hope that the identification, evaluation and treatment of stroke patients can be accelerated in the future.

Acknowledgements. We wish to thank Tina Brantley for typing and preparation of this manuscript. We also wish to thank the Burroughs Wellcome Company (Dr. Rose Snipes and Jackie Zinn) and Genentech, Inc. (Dr. Steve Peroutka and Judy Breed) for their assistance in performing the rt-PA studies.

References

1. Alberts MJ, Bertels C, Dawson DV (1990) An analysis of time of presentation after stroke. JAMA 263:65–68
2. Alberts MJ, Perry A, Dawson DV, Bertels C (1992) Effects of public and professional education on reducing the delay in presentation and referral of stroke patients. Stroke 23:352–356
3. Brott T, Haley EC, Levy D, Barsan W, Broderick J, Marler JR (1991) Strategies for early treatment of acute cerebral infarction. In: Hacke W, del Zoppo GJ, Hirschberg M (eds) Thrombolytic therapy in acute ischemic stroke. Springer-Verlag, Berlin Heidelberg New York, pp 196–203
4. Brott TG, Haley EC, Levy D, et al (1990) Safety and potential efficacy of tissue plasminogen activator (t-PA) for stroke. Stroke 21:181 (Abstract)
5. del Zoppo GJ, Poeck K, Pessin MS, and 16 coauthors from the rt-PA Acute Stroke Study Group (1992) Recombinant tissue plasminogen activator in acute thrombotic and embolic stroke. Ann Neurol 32:78–86
6. Fletcher AP, Alkjaersig N, Lewis M, et al (1976) A pilot study of urokinase therapy in cerebral infarction. Stroke 7:135–142
7. Foulkes MA, Wolf PA, Price TR, Mohr JP, Hier DB (1988) The stroke data bank: Design, methods, and baseline characteristics. Stroke 19:547–554
8. Meyer JS, Gilroy J, Barnhart ME, Johnson JF (1965) Therapeutic thrombolysis in cerebral thromboembolism: Randomized evaluation of intravenous streptokinase. In: Millikan CH, Siekert RG, Whisnant JP (eds) Cerebral vascular diseases. Fourth Princeton Conference. Grune and Stratton, New York, p 200
9. Saunders CE (1987) Time study of patient movement through the emergency department: Sources of delay in relation to patient acuity. Ann Emerg Med 16:1244–1248
10. Timerding BL, Barsan WG, Hedges JR, et al (1989) Stroke patient evaluation in the emergency department before pharmacologic therapy. Am J Emerg Med 7:11–15

A Demming Approach to Recruiting: The National Institute of Neurological Diseases and Stroke (NINDS) t-PA Stroke Trial Experience

B. C. Tilley for The NINDS t-PA Stroke Trial Investigators [1,2]

The NINDS t-PA Stroke Trials are two Phase IIB, randomized, double-blind trials comparing recombinant tissue plasminogen activator (t-PA) to placebo. The trials are being carried out by 8 clinical centers and 40 participating hospitals. The primary alternative hypotheses for each trial are that:

1. There is a difference between the t-PA and placebo groups enrolled within 90 min of onset in the proportion showing significant early improvement; and
2. There is a difference between the t-PA and placebo groups enrolled between 91 and 180 min of stroke onset in the proportion showing significant early improvement.

Significant early improvement is defined as a 4-point decrease from baseline on the NIH Stroke Scale or complete resolution of symptoms at 24 h from stroke onset.

Prior to treatment, the investigator must know the results of:

- CBC and platelet count
- Blood glucose
- CT scan (noncontrast) to rule out hemorrhage

Prior to treatment, blood must also be drawn for:

- Serum electrolytes and creatinine
- Prothrombin time (PT)
- Partial thromboplastin time (aPTT)

If the patient has a history of oral anticoagulant (OA) therapy in the 7 days before treatment, prothrombin time results must be known prior to randomization. Patients currently on OA therapy are excluded. Additionally, if the patient received heparin within the previous 48 h, aPTT results must be known. (There are numerous other eligibility and exclusion criteria.)

The underlying philosophy of recruitment for the trial is summarized as follows:

Division of Biostatistics and Research Epidemiology, Henry Ford Health Sciences Center, Southfield, OH, USA for The NINDS t-PA Stroke Trial Investigators. Please see Appendix.
Presented by K. M. A. Welch, William T. Gossett, Chair, Department of Neurology, Henry Ford Health Sciences Center, Detroit, MI, USA

G. J. del Zoppo, E. Mori, W. Hacke (Eds.)
Thrombolytic Therapy in Acute Ischemic Stroke II

- Problems will come from the process, *not* the people carrying out the process.
- Those involved in carrying out the process must help us understand and improve the process.
- The time to identify process problems is before the trial begins.

A Recruitment Coordinator was identified at each Clinical Center. There was a recruitment training program given at the Coordinating Center where recruiters could share experiences, could share documents used for health care professional or public education, and could be trained in health education methods specific to stroke.

Prior to the start of the trial and throughout the local trial, presentations are given to trial physicians, Recruitment Coordinators, and Clinical Coordinators. The audiences include Emergency Medical System (EMS) Units, nurses and physicians at the participating hospitals, the community, and the media.

The recruitment process from arrival at the Emergency Department (ED) to randomization or determination that the patient was ineligible was flow charted for *each* hospital. As a first step in flow charting, a quality improvement (QIP) team was identified at each site. The QIP team included those who carry out the process (i.e., the Stroke Team PI and Clinical Coordinator, the ED physician and nurse, ED phlebotomist (at some sites), supervisor *and* a laboratory technician, a supervisor *and* CT technician, and a pharmacist. The Stroke Team prepared a first draft of the flow chart (sometimes without the help of QIP team members). The Stroke Team then clarified their knowledge of the process at each QIP site by meeting with each team member as the Stroke Team actually walked through the flow chart.

During the walk-through the purpose and importance of the trial was emphasized to each person contacted. Also, during the walk-through potential deviations from the initial flow chart were identified along with potential problems. Those carrying out the process were asked for ideas on how to solve the problems as these were identified. As an example, at one hospital the elevator to the CT area was exceptionally old and slow. The ED nurse showed the Stroke Team a route through the parking garage to a faster newer elevator, saving up to 10 min in time. In another hospital blood samples were sent to one location, but some of the tests were done three buildings away. The laboratory receiving the blood had to wait for a runner to appear and take the blood to the other building. The Stroke Team arranged to have a runner take the blood directly from the ED to the different laboratories. Many small problems similar to these were discovered. Each represented a cost of valuable time.

Currently the t-PA Stroke Trial is 30% ahead of its 14-month recruitment goal. We cannot separate the benefits of each of the three components to recruitment (training, publicity, flow charting). We cannot know what would have happened to our recruitment without any or all of the components. However, we can conclude that:

- Recruitment is ahead of goal in a trial with very restrictive entry criteria.
- Flow charting helped to resolve process issues.

- Should t-PA prove effective, flow charting would be helpful in solving process problems relevant to implementing emergent stroke therapy in the ED setting.
- Flow charting may be helpful for other clinical trials.

Appendix

This paper was presented by K.M.A. Welch, M.D. (Henry Ford Health Sciences Center).

Coordinating Center:
Henry Ford Health Sciences Center
Barbara C. Tilley, Ph.D., P.I.
K.M.A, Welch, M.D., Co-P.I.
Susan Fagan, Pharm.D., Academic Pharm.
Joel Verter, Ph.D., Senior Biostatistician
Edward Mascha, M.S., Biostatistician
Laura Gordon, Data Coordinator
Edward Meehan, Ph.D., Health Educator
Patricia Isaac, Ph.D., Health Educator

Clinical Centers:
Emory University
Bruce Mackay, M.D., P.I.
Barbara Faherty, Clinical Coordinator
Julie MacDonald, Patient Coordinator
Carol Barch, Patient Coordinator

Henry Ford Hospital
Steven Levine, M.D., P.I.
Richard Nowak, M.D., Co-P.I.
Christopher Lewandowski, M.D., Co-P.I.
Nabih Ramadan, M.D., Co-P.I.
Kara Sawaya, Clinical Coordinator
Sheila Daley, Patient Coordinator

Long Island Jewish Medical Center
Steven Horowitz, M.D., P.I.
Thomas Kwiatkowski, M.D., P.I.
Rose Donnarumma, Clinical Coordinator
Mary Okola, Patient Coordinator

University of California, San Diego
Patrick Lyden, M.D., P.I.
Traci Babcock, Clinical Coordinator

University of Cincinnati
Thomas Brott, M.D., P.I.
Bill Barson, M.D., Co-P.I.
Joe Broderick, M.D., Co-P.I.
Judith Spilker, Clinical Coordinator

University of Tennessee
Kenneth Gaines, M.D., P.I.
Maggie Wilson, Clinical Coordinator

University of Texas
James Grotta, M.D., P.I.
Patti Bratina, Clinical Coordinator
Linda Greenberg, Patient Coordinator

University of Virginia
E. Clarke Haley, M.D., P.I.
Gail Kongable, Clinical Coordinator
Karen Parks, Patient Coordinator

NINDS:
John Marler, M.D., Project Officer

Data and Safety Monitoring Committee:
Michael D. Walker, M.D., Chairman
J. Donald Easton, M.D.
John M. Hallenbeck, M.D.
Gordon Lan, Ph.D.
James D. Marsh, M.D.

Local Intra-arterial Fibrinolytic Therapy Within the Cerebral Arteries: Effectiveness of rt-PA Concerning Recanalization Rate and Time*

H. Zeumer[1], H.-J. Freitag[1], F. Zanella[1], A. Thie[2], and C. Arning[3]

At the University Hospital Eppendorf, we have performed local intra- arterial fibrinolytic (LIF) therapy in acute stroke patients with a superselective technique since 1987 [4, 7]. With urokinase a high recanalization rate was achieved, but complete recanalization did not usually occur before 120 min of infusion. Recombinant tissue plasminogen activator (rt-PA) not only has a higher fibrin specificity and less fibrinogen affinity, but it has a much shorter half-life in plasma than urokinase. Even a relatively high dose of rt-PA (20 mg alteplase) in comparison to urokinase (750000/IU) would have less of an influence on systemic hemostasis, but eventually perhaps a better impact on clot lysis. Thus, we have compared the efficacy of rt-PA with urokinase regarding the time to achieve clot resolution in vivo.

Subjects and Methods

A total of 61 consecutive patients have been entered into the study by now. Twenty-one patients have been treated with a local dose of 750000/IU urokinase and 40 patients with 20 mg rt-PA over 2 h. The fibrinolytic effectiveness of 1 mg rt-PA (alteplase) approximately equals 100 000/IU of urokinase. Inclusion and exclusion criteria as well as the technical approach are described elsewhere [5].

Results

Table 1 demonstrates that rt-PA was not superior to urokinase with respect to the rate of recanalization or completeness of recanalization. Recanalization

* Research on methods in interventional neuroradiology is supported by the Deutsche Forschungsgemeinschaft, Grant Nr. Ze 153/4–1-1035/91.
Department of [1]Neuroradiology and [2]Neurology, University Hospital Eppendorf, and [3]Department of Neurology, Allgemeines Krankenhaus Barmbek, Hamburg, Federal Republic of Germany

G. J. del Zoppo, E. Mori, W. Hacke (Eds.)
Thrombolytic Therapy in Acute Ischemic Stroke II

Table 1. Recanilizing capabilities of urokinase *versus* rt-PA

Type of Occlusion	Urokinase (N = 21)		rt-PA (N = 40)	
	Thrombotic	Embolic	Thrombotic	Embolic
Basilar Territory				
Incomplete Recanalization	1	0	6	0
Complete Recanalization	1	6	6	8
Time, Median (minutes)		120	120	120
Time, Average	120	60	115	85
Carotid Territory				
No Recanalization		0		2
Incomplete Recanalization		5		13
Complete Recanalization		8		5
Time, Median (minutes)		60		120
Time, Average		55		80

time in both vertebrobasilar territory groups were similar. The median and average recanalization time, however, in the carotid territory group treated by rt-PA was almost twice as long as in the urokinase group. This result may be biased due to the high frequency of "M-type" occlusions which all occurred in the rt-PA group. In the urokinase group, there were some more small embolic occlusions of the MCA.

The clinical results will be published elsewhere [6].

Discussion

The results reported above do not support the hypothesis that a higher dose of a more fibrin-specific activator might reduce the recanalization time. Lack of response to a fibrinolytic agent is especially possible with pure platelet emboli [3], which do not generally occur. It does not seem plausible that a plasminogen activator inhibitor [1] is the major cause for the lack of response, particularly considering the very high local rt-PA concentration. If, however, an increase of the activating substance is not effective, we have to question if there is a deficit in the amount of plasminogen to be activated into plasmin, or if there is less reactivity in aged thrombi by rt-PA. In fact, there are two aspects supporting this hypothesis:

1. It is known that aged thrombi lose their intrinsically bound plasminogen and that retraction of the thrombus leads to chemical changes of the fibrin molecule making it less reactive to proteolysis [2]. Emboli are dislodged thrombi which may often represent aged thrombotic material.
2. Occlusion of an artery, e.g., the middle cerebral artery, leads to a proximal dead end, or stump. In this stump, only minor turbulent flow exists with little participation by the normal blood circulation. Even if a microcatheter

can be advanced into this stump, the delivery of rt-PA might not find enough plasminogen inside the embolus, or may rapidly consume the small amount in the stagnant blood column within the vessel stump.

The situation with regard to hemostasis and thrombus formation in *embolic stroke patients* seems to be different from the situation with acute coronary artery *thrombotic occlusion*. This may explain why local arterial infusion or intravenous administration of rt-PA may have a significantly lower and delayed recanalization effect in the intracranial vessels than in the coronary arteries or even the peripheral vessels.

From our experience with LIF we are convinced that further improvements in fibrinolytic stroke therapy are closely related to the reduction of the recanalization time. Thus, our experimental and clinical work is focussed on this problem. In our experience, it cannot obviously be solved by using higher doses of plasminogen activator alone.

References

1. Brockmann MJ, Schwendemann G, Stief TW, Heimburger N (1989) Plasminogen aktivator inhibitor bei akuten zerebralen Infarkten. Verh. deut. Ges. f. Neurologie 5:1086–1089
2. Gottlob R (1970) Die Grundlage für die Lyse alter Thromben. In: Pezold FA, Schattauer FK (eds) Fibrinolyse-Therapie Heute. Thieme, Stuttgart New York, p 43
3. Jang IK, Gold HK, Ziskind AA, et al (1988) Resistance to rt-PA is produced by an increased platelet concentration in occluding thrombi. Circulation 78(Suppl II):211
4. Siepmann G, Müller-Jensen M, Goossens H, Lachenmayer L, Zeumer H (1991) Local intra-arterial fibrinolysis in acute middle cerebral artery occlusion. In: du Boulay G, Molyneux A, Moseley I (eds) Proceedings XIV Symposium Neuroradiogicum. Springer-Verlag, Berlin Heidelberg New York, p 69
5. Zeumer H (1992) Fibrinolysis in cerebrovascular diseases of the central nervous system. In: Vineuela F (ed) Interventional neuroradiology: Endovascular therapy of the central nervous system. Raven Press, New York
6. Zeumer H, Freitag HJ, Zanella F, Thie A, Arning C (1992) Local intra-arterial fibrinolytic therapy in stroke patients: Urokinase versus rtPA. Neuroradiology (In Press)
7. Zeumer H, Frietag H-J, Grzyska M, Neunzig H-P (1989) Local intraarterial fibrinolysis in acute vertebrobasilar occlusion. Neuroradiology 31:336–340

Relation of Thrombolytic Reperfusion and of Collateral Circulation to Outcome in Patients Suffering Cerebral Main Artery Occlusion

A. B. Brucker, H. Potuschak, E. Laich, J. Trenkler, H. Böhm-Jurkovic, and E. Deisenhammer

The aim of this study was to investigate the impact of thrombolytic treatment on the clinical course of patients with thromboembolic or atherothrombotic cerebral artery occlusion. Such patients suffered from occlusion of the basilar artery, carotid artery, or the main stem middle cerebral artery. Another aim was to investigate whether the extent of reperfusion and of collateral circulation was of any predictive value for the outcome of patients treated with fibrinolysis. In addition, we wished to look at further prognostic parameters concerning risk and benefit of thrombolytic treatment.

Subjects and Methods

For inclusion into the study, patients must have suffered a very severe and/or rapidly progressive neurological deficit. Occlusion of one of the main arteries mentioned above must be proven by angiography. Hemorrhage and a territorial hypodensity (as a sign of the recent infarction) must be excluded by CT scan. In cases of ischemia in the carotid territory, thrombolytic treatment must start within 6 h after onset of symptoms. Different from similar studies, thrombolysis was adjusted individually in every case according to the estimated chance of reperfusion and to the estimated risk in every patient. The treatment required a maximum of 100 mg rt-PA (alteplase) injected intravenously and/or intra-arterially over a period of 90 to 120 min. In certain cases urokinase (maximum dose 800000 IU) was given intra-arterially only. Heparin was given concomitantly and continued in case of recanalization. Complete cerebral angiography was performed before and immediately after treatment. The extent of reperfusion as well as the quality of collateral circulation was evaluated on the basis of all taken angiograms using two 6-degree rating scales (grade 0–5), as shown in Table 1. Furthermore, brain edema (Table 2) was evaluated with special focus on its mass effects as well as potential cerebral hemorrhagic events (Table 3) after thrombolytic treatment. The ratings were performed by a neurologist and a radiologist and agreement was reached in all cases. Out-

Department of Neurology, Wagner-Jauregg Krankenhaus, Linz, Austria

G. J. del Zoppo, E. Mori, W. Hacke (Eds.)
Thrombolytic Therapy in Acute Ischemic Stroke II

Table 1

	Collateral circulation		Reperfusion
0	No collateral flow visible	0	Unchanged
1	Minimal flow into the ischemic territory, retrograde via sporadic leptomeningeal arteries	1	Minimal improvement of the collateral circulation
2	Retrograde flow into 1/2 of the territory	2	Marked improvement of the collateral circulation, or distal-propagation of the occluding thrombus with reopening of one main branch-artery
3	Retrograde flow via leptomeningeals approximately into 3/4 of the ischemic territory	3	Recanalization of the main artery but persistent occlusion of some arterial branches
4	Leptomeningeal flow into the entire territory	4	Nearly complete recanalization, still occlusion of few terminal-branches
5	Complete filling of the territory, visualization of all leptomeningeal arteries, retrograde flow reaching the occluding thrombus in the main artery	5	Complete reopening of the whole arterial tree

Table 2. Brain edema

	Comparison of the volume of edema to the volume of the definitely infarcted tissue, especially regarding space- occupying effects (mass-shift), by visual evaluation of all CT scans
0	No mass effects visible, early hypodensities equal to later infarcted tissue
1	Mild space-occupying effects, minimal narrowing of ventricular size, no tissue shift between cranial compartments
2	More space-occupying effects, further ventricular compression, but still no tissue shift between compartments
3	Significant space-occupying effects, complete comparison of ventricles, mass shift between cranial compartments (transtentorial, transfalxial herniation of brain tissue)

Table 3. Cerebral hemorrhagic events [6]

Hemorrhagic Transformation	
HT 1	Small petechiae along the margins of the infarct
HT 2	More confluent petechiae along the margins and in the core of the infarct
Parenchymatous Hemorrhage	
PH 1	Small or medium-sized blood clot located in the center of the infarct not exceeding 30% of the infarcted volume, mild space-occupying effect
PH 2	Large, confluent dense blood clot exceeding 30% of the infarcted volume, significant space-occupying effect

Table 4. Karnofsky's Performance Status

	%	
Able to carry on normal activity and to work; no special care is needed	100	Normal; no complaints; no evidence of disease
	90	Able to carry on normal activity; minor signs or symptoms of disease
	80	Normal activity with effort; some signs or symptoms of disease
Unable to work; able to live at home, care for most personal needs; a varying amount of assistance is needed	70	Cares for self; unable to carry on normal activity or to do active work
	60	Requires occasional assistance but is able to care for most of his needs
	50	Requires considerable assistance and frequent medical care
Unable to care for self; requires equivalent of institutional or hospital care; disease may be progressing rapidly	40	Disabled; requires special care and assistance
	30	severely disabled; hospitalization is indicated, although death not imminent
	20	Very sick; hospitalization necessary; active supportive treatment is necessary
	10	Moribund; fatal processes progressing rapidly
	0	Dead

come was rated 4 weeks after treatment using the Karnofsky's Performance Status, also well known as the "Karnofsky Score" (Table 4).

Data analysis included descriptive statistics, rank measures of association, and multiple correlations. For calculation with ordinal variables, nonparametric tests were used such as Goodman-Kruskal's [2–5] tau or gamma (= G = rank measure of association) to estimate the relationship of variables and its asymptomatic property as proposed by Burr [1] and Kendall [7].

Results and Discussion

From March, 1989 to September, 1991 thrombolytic treatment was performed in 28 patients (15 males and 13 females), with a combined age range from 37 to 71 years. Patient characteristics, treatment results, and outcome measures are summarized in Table 5. There were 9 occlusions of the basilar artery, 9 occlusions of the carotid artery, and 11 occlusions of the main stem of the middle cerebral artery. Nine patients died; 5 of them suffered from basilar occlusion and had already been comatose for several hours prior to the treatment procedure. We observed gross hemorrhages in 2 cases (fatal in 1 case), both deriving from the lenticulostriate arteries in cases of recanalized MCA occlusions.

Table 5. Patients-list

Occluded artery	Basilar artery								
Chronolog. case no.	1	9	10	13	16	17	19	22	23
Age	61	53	62	62	69	39	53	46	63
Sex	f	m	m	m	m	m	m	f	m
Embolic occlusion	x		x	x		?	x	x	x
Athero-thrombot. occl.		x			x	?			
Delay of treatment: hrs	12	10	5	6	9	40	7	14	4
Thrombolytic method	Uk i.a.	rt-PA i.a.	Uk i.a.	Uk i.a.	Uk i.a.	rt-PA i.v. i.a.	rt-PA i.a.	rt-PA i.v. i.a.	Uk i.a.
Collateral circulation	2	2	3	3	1	2	3	4	1
Reperfusion	3	1	4	4	2	3	2	1	0
Clinical course during treatment	=	=	=	++	−	+	=	+	=
Edema	2	3	3	1	1	1	1	0	3
Hemorrh. complic.	0	0	0	HT 2	HT 1	HT 1	0	0	0
Outcome after 1 month	0	0	0	80	0	50	40	80	0

Occluded artery	Carotid artery							
Chronolog. case no.	2	4	8	14	15	21	25	27
Age	60	70	47	55	52	37	71	63
Sex	m	m	f	f	m	f	f	m
Embolic occlusion	?		x	x	x		?	
Athero-thrombot. occl.	?	x				x	?	x
Delay of treatment: hrs	5	5	4	3	4	5	3	4
Thrombolytic method	rt-PA i.v.	rt-PA i.v.	Uk i.a.	rt-PA i.v. i.a.	rt-PA i.a.	rt-PA i.v. i.a.	rt-PA i.v. i.a.	rt-PA i.v.
Collateral circulation	3	1	4	3	3	4	2	2
Reperfusion	2	0	1	2	4	3	3	4
Clinical course during treatment	=	−	=	+	+	=	+	+
Edema	2	3	1	2	1	2	3	0
Hemorrh. complic.	0	0	HT 2	0	HT 1	0	HT 2	0
Outcome after 1 month	40	0	40	60	50	60	0	40

Occluded artery	Middle cerebral artery										
Chronolog. case no.	3	5	6	7	11	12	18	20	24	26	28
Age	63	69	50	38	51	67	54	51	45	65	60
Sex	m	f	f	f	m	f	m	m	f	f	f
Embolic occlusion	x	x	x		x	x	x	x	x	x	x
Athero-thrombot. occl.				x							
Delay of treatment: hrs	5	6	5	?48	6	5	6	4	5	4	4
Thrombolytic method	rt-PA i.v.	rt-PA i.v.	rt-PA i.v.	rt-PA i.a.	rt PA i.a.	Uk i.a.	rt-PA i.v. i.a.	rt-PA i.v.	rt-PA i.v. i.a.	rt-PA i.v.	rt-PA i.v.
Collateral circulation	4	3	4	1	3	4	4	3	3	2	2
Reperfusion	5	5	5	0	4	3	4	4	1	1	5
Clinical course during treatment	++	++	+	=	++	−−	=	+	=	=	++
Edema	1	1	1	3	1	2	1	2	1	0	1
Hemorrh. complic.	0	0	HT 2	0	0	PH 2	PH 2	HT 2	0	0	0
Outcome after 1 month	80	80	90	0	90	0	50	90	60	30	90

Hemorrhagic transformation of parts of the infarcted tissue was observed in 8 patients, but worsened the clinical course only in 1 case. We did not find any statistically significant association between hemorrhagic transformation and outcome ($G = 0.11$, $p = 0.58$).

There was a significant inverse association between patient age and outcome ($G = 0.34$, $p = 0.043$). However, age did not show any influence on the degree of reperfusion and was only weakly dissociated (weak inverse association: $G = 0.35$, $p = 0.055$) with collateral circulation. There was no influence of sex on collateral flow, reperfusion or outcome. The degree of reperfusion as well as the extent of collateral circulation was highly associated with outcome ($G = 0.56$, $p = 0.001$ and $G = 0.56$, $p = 0.003$, respectively). Taking into account survivors only, the correlation of reperfusion to outcome held its high level of significance ($G = 0.59$, $p = 0.004$), but there was no more significant association between collateral flow and outcome ($G = 0.23$, $p = 0.174$).

The combined effects of reperfusion and collateral flow on outcome were examined using multiple correlation methods [$r_{(rep. \times col.).out}$ = multiple correlation coefficient]. This correlation was highly significant ($r = 0.668$, $p = 0.001$), and exceeded all other investigated relationships. These findings support the general opinion about the role of collateral arteries, which are considered to be an essential prerequisite that reperfusion (spontaneously or not) will work to salvage penumbra tissue. Reperfusion was weakly dissociated with a higher tendency toward massive brain edema in our patients ($G = 0.32$, $p = 0.057$). Only a weak association was found between the degree of reperfusion and all hemorrhagic events (hemorrhagic infarction [HI] and parenchymatous hematoma [PH]) ($G = 0.34$, $p = 0.085$). Reperfusion and hemorrhagic infarction was not associated in our cases. The lapse of time between the first symptoms of ischemia and the start of treatment ("delay of treatment") did not influence significantly the outcome of the patients ($G = 0.09$, $p = 0.312$). There

Table 6.

Age	Outcome	Sign.	$p = 0.043$ (inverse)
Age	Reperfusion	No sign.	$p = 0.379$
Age	Collateral circ.	No sign.	$p = 0.55$ (inverse)
Reperfusion	Outcome	Sign.	$p = 0.001$
Collateral Circulation	Outcome	Sign.	$p = 0.003$
Reperfusion × collateral circulation	Outcome	Sign.	$p = 0.001$
Reperfusion	Brain edema	No sign.	$p = 0.057$ (inverse)
Reperfusion	Hemorrhagic event (PH + HT)	No sign.	$p = 0.085$
Reperfusion	Hemorrhagic transformation (HT)	No sign.	$p = 0.12$
Collateral circulation	Brain edema	No sign.	$p = 0.057$ (inverse)
Collateral circulation	Hemorrhagic transformation (HT)	No sign.	$p = 0.052$
Hemorrhagic transformation (HT)	Outcome	No sign.	$p = 0.58$
Delay of treatment	Outcome	No sign.	$p = 0.312$

Sign., significant correlation; No sign., no significant correlation; inverse refers to the test of an inverse association

was no association between delay and hemorrhagic events also. Within our patients there was only little difference in the delay of treatment. However, a larger number of patients would possibly reveal effects of little differences in the delay of treatment on clinical outcome. Table 6 shows a summary of our statistical analyses.

Conclusion

Though some correlations and associations between measured variables are highly significant, their predictive value for outcome seems to be relatively low. For example: even the highly significant correlation of reperfusion and collateral flow to outcome cannot obscure the fact that the two gross hemorrhages we observed occurred in such cases, which were well collateralized and rapidly recanalized under rt-PA treatment. This uncertainty of prediction may be due to our small sample size also. To date there are no conclusive results of large trials available. Therefore, whether or not a patient should undergo thrombolytic treatment remains to be an individual decision in every single case, weighing potential risks and benefits.

References

1. Burr EJ (1960) The distribution of Kendall's score for a pair of tied ranks. Biometrika 47:151–171
2. Goodman-Kruskal (1954) Measures of association for cross clarification 1. J Am Statist Assoc 49:732–764
3. Goodman-Kruskal (1959) Measures of association for cross classification 2. J Am Statist Assoc 54:123–163
4. Goodman-Kruskal (1963) Measures of association for cross clarification 3. J Am Statist Assoc 58:310–364
5. Goodman-Kruskal (1972) Measures of association for cross clarification 4. J Am Statist Assoc 67:415–421
6. Hacke W, Hirschberg M (1990) Thrombolytic therapy in acute ischemic stroke: An update. Stroke International 1:17–20
7. Kendall MG (1962) Rank correlation methods. Griffin, London

Factors Related to Intracranial Hematoma Formation in Patients Receiving t-PA for Acute Ischemic Stroke

D.E. Levy[1], T. Brott[2], E.C. Haley, Jr.[3], and J.R. Marler[4]

Tissue plasminogen activator (rt-PA) is used widely for acute myocardial infarction (MI) in the United States and is currently undergoing clinical trial in acute, ischemic stroke. Both theory and practice have raised concerns about intracranial bleeding induced by rt-PA, so that in the United States, rt-PA is contraindicated in MI patients with a "history of a cerebrovascular accident." An open-label, Phase I study sponsored by the NIH recently assessed the safety and efficacy of single-chain rt-PA. The trial required hyper-acute treatment, initially within 90 min and subsequently in a 91- to 180-min time window [6]; results of these trials have been published and suggest that rt-PA is relatively safe and may be clinically effective. Nonetheless, complicating intracerebral hematomas did occur, 3 in the 0- to 90-min group of 74 patients and 2 in the 90- to 180- min group of 20 patients. Analysis of the 74 0- to 90-min patients suggested that the risk of intracerebral hematoma increased with increasing rt-PA dose [3], but with merely 3 patients, only limited analyses were possible. Although total numbers are still small, the existence of 5 hematoma patients now permits a more detailed effort to identify risk factors associated with hemorrhage.

Subjects and Methods

Patients with acute, ischemic stroke were recruited from February, 1987 through September, 1989. To be eligible, patients 18 to 80 years old were to have a diagnosis of acute cerebral ischemia producing a serious measurable deficit, with established onset within 90 min of treatment (180 min after November, 1988). Exclusion criteria included any evidence of parenchymal or subarachnoid hemorrhage on a pretreatment computerized tomographic (CT)

From the Departments of Neurology at the Medical Centers of
[1] Cornell University Medical College, New York, NY,
[2] University of Cincinnati, Cincinnati, OH, and
[3] University of Virginia, Charlottesville, VA, and from the
[4] National Institute of Neurological Disorders and Stroke, Bethesda, MD, USA

G.J. del Zoppo, E. Mori, W. Hacke (Eds.)
Thrombolytic Therapy in Acute Ischemic Stroke II

scan of the head or coagulation variables or interventions likely to create an excessive risk of bleeding. Patients already anticoagulated with coumadin or heparin were excluded, but those on aspirin were not. Hypertensive patients were also excluded for a pretreatment blood pressure (BP) above 200 mm Hg systolic or 120 mm Hg diastolic, which was later changed during the study to 133 mm Hg mean.

Single-chain, recombinant t-PA (rt-PA, alteplase; Genentech, South San Francisco, CA) was administered intravenously in accordance with a defined dose-escalation schedule. The dose tiers (I–VI) were calculated on either a body weight (kg) or body surface area (m^2) basis, with maximum per-patient doses that ranged from 25 mg to 90 mg. Some patients subsequently received intravenous heparin.

The primary end-points and analytic techniques have already been described [3, 6]. As a safety end-point, intracerebral hematoma was distinguished from hemorrhagic conversion by contemporaneous neurological worsening or new mass effect on CT. Standard univariate and multivariate techniques were used for analysis; corrections for multiple comparisons were not made. None of the following results should be considered to establish causality but should be taken only as indications of factors possibly associated with intracerebral hematoma.

Results

Multiple analyses of most of the individual variables vs intracerebral hematoma failed to indicate anything other than a random association. Among these variables were prior use of aspirin, subsequent use of heparin, age, sex, a prior history of diabetes, hypertension, or cardiac arrhythmia, interval from stroke onset to treatment, initial aggregate stroke scale score, initial "cardinal sign" (the clinical abnormality most indicative of the patient's neurological deficit), and 3-h fibrinogen level. Two variables did show an association: baseline blood pressure and rt-PA dose.

In terms of blood pressure, hematoma was related to both diastolic and mean blood pressure, but not to systolic blood pressure. An intracranial hematoma developed in 4 of 22 patients (18%) with an initial diastolic BP of at least 100 mm Hg but in only 1 of the remaining 72 patients (1%; $p<0.01$) with initially lower diastolic blood pressure.

The relationship between rt-PA dose and intracerebral hematoma, however, is more complex. Patients in dosage tiers designed to deliver at least 0.95 mg/kg (IV-X, V, and VI) had a significantly increased risk of hematoma formation (4/32, 12%) compared to those at lower tiers (1/62, 2%, $p<0.05$), but the per-patient dose of rt-PA in mg was not related to the development of hematomas. The relationship of hematoma to dose per kg body weight was significant ($p<0.05$), whereas that to dose per square meter of surface area was not. To further clarify the discrepancy between the nonsignificance of per-patient dose and the significance of dose per kg, the relationship to body weight was assessed and found to be marginally significant ($p<0.10$), with lighter patients more likely to develop hematomas than heavier ones. Prior aspirin use was marginally associated ($p<0.10$) with bleeding.

Discussion

Although the relatively small number of patients with intracerebral hematoma in our two trials is encouraging, their relative scarcity complicated identification of factors for bleeding. As noted, two factors were consistently related to hematoma formation: rt-PA dose (particularly when represented as dose tier and as dose in mg/kg body weight) and initial blood pressure (particularly diastolic blood pressure).

Published experience of rt-PA in MI patients largely supports our findings. We never achieved a rt-PA dose of 150 mg in our trial, and possibly as a result, the relationship of bleeding to dose was somewhat less clear cut than in the larger experience with MI reported by the TIMI Operations Committee [12]: 1.6% of 1014 patients who received 150 mg rt-PA experienced intracranial bleeding, vs only 0.6% of 1452 patients given 100 mg. The possible risk in stroke patients of rt-PA doses approaching 100 mg is supported by the recent report of von Kummer and Hacke [13] that fatal parenchymal hemorrhage occurred in 3 of 32 patients (9%) given 100 mg of rt-PA within 6 h of acute stroke, a frequency somewhat higher than ours of 5/94 (5%). Physicians tempted to treat stroke patients with rt-PA should be very cautious in approaching doses of rt-PA currently used for MI patients since our experience suggests that a dose of 90–100 mg might be risky.

A possible relationship of bleeding to hypertension has been demonstrated by Anderson and colleagues [1] with streptokinase and rt-PA and is cited in review by Sloan and Price [10]. Our data support this concern. While a relationship of intracranial hemorrhage with high baseline blood pressure is not surprising, precise blood pressure criteria to be used in guiding thrombolytic therapy are not yet established. Issues that will require attention include effectiveness of antihypertensive therapy given in conjunction with rt-PA and the possible influence of blood pressure lability on the risk of bleeding.

Like Kase and coworkers [7], we found no relationship of bleeding to hypofibrinogenemia, an observation indirectly supported by the lack of any symptomatic intracranial bleeding in 132 stroke patients recently randomized to placebo and the fibrinogenolytic agent, ancrod [11]. Although Kase and coworkers report a possible association of bleeding to activated partial thromboplastin time (aPTT) [7], a variable we did not uniformly measure, we were unable to find any association with the use of heparin after rt-PA. We also found no association with age, as suggested by Sloan and Price [10] and shown by Maggioni and colleagues [8], although the fragile intracranial vessels of amyloid angiopathy [9], a condition of the elderly, could provide a mechanism for age-related bleeding. Our data suggest a greater bleeding risk in lighter patients; while Bovill [2] and Califf [4] and their respective colleagues made similar observations for MI patients, their failure to adjust rt-PA dose to body weight means that lighter patients might simply have had a greater dose effect. Finally, although our data suggest a greater risk of intracerebral hemorrhage with longer intervals to treatment, our results are not significant, in contrast to those reported by del Zoppo and colleagues [5], where intracerebral hematoma and hemorrhagic infarction are grouped and the interval to treatment in patients with either type of hemorrhage (6.1 ± 1.5 h) to those without hemorrhage (5.3 ± 1.7 h) was compared.

As various groups accumulate more experience with rt-PA (and other thrombolytics) in acute stroke, more definitive contraindications and warnings should emerge. The frequency of intracranial hemorrhage has, to date, been relatively small, but hints of circumstances that might promote bleeding are emerging and will require careful attention both experimentally and clinically.

References

1. Anderson JL, Karagounis L, Allen A, Bradford MJ, Menlove RL, Pryor TA (1991) Older age and elevated blood pressure are risk factors for intracerebral hemorrhage after thrombolysis. Am J Cardiol 68:166–170
2. Bovill EG, Terrin ML, Stump DC, et al (1991) Hemorrhagic events during therapy with recombinant tissue-type plasminogen activator, heparin, and aspirin for acute myocardial infarction: Results of the Thrombolysis in Myocardial Infarction (TIMI), Phase II Trial. Ann Intern Med 115:256–265
3. Brott TG, Haley EC, Levy DE, et al (1992) Urgent therapy for stroke. Part I. Pilot study of tissue plaminogen activator administered within 90 minutes. Stroke 23:632–640
4. Califf RM, Topol EJ, George BS, et al (1988) Hemorrhagic complications associated with the use of intravenous tissue plasminogen activator in treatment of acute myocardial infarction. Am J Med 85:353–360
5. del Zoppo GJ, Poeck K, Pessin MS, and 16 coauthors of the rt-PA Acute Stroke Study Group (1992) Recombinant tissue plasminogen activator in acute thrombotic and embolic stroke. Ann Neurol 32:78–86
6. Haley EC, Levy DE, Brott TG, et al (1992) Urgent therapy for stroke. Part II. Pilot study of plasminogen administered 91–180 minutes from onset. Stroke 23:641–645
7. Kase CS, Pessin MS, Zivin JA, et al (1992) Intracranial hemorrhage after coronary thrombolysis with tissue plasminogen activator. Am J Med 92:384– 390
8. Maggioni AP, Franzosi MG, Farina ML, et al (1991) Cerebrovascular events after myocardial infarction: Analysis of the GISSI trial. Br Med J 302: 1428–1431
9. Ramsey DA, Penswick JL, Robertson DM (1990) Fatal strepkinase-induced intracerebral hemorrhage in cerebral amyloid angiopathy. Can J Neurol Sci 17:336–341
10. Sloan MA, Price TR (1991) Intracranial hemorrhage following thrombolytic therapy for acute myocardial infarction. Semin Neurol 11:385–399
11. The Ancrod in Stroke Investigators (1992) Ancrod in acute ischemic stroke (Abstract). Stroke 23:162
12. TIMI Operations Committee, Braunwald E, Knatterud GL, et al (1987) Update from the thrombolysis in myocardial infarction trial (Letter). J Am Coll Cardiol 10:970
13. von Kummer R, Hacke W (1992) Safety and efficacy of intravenous tissue plasminogen activator and heparin in acute middle cerebral artery. Stroke 23:646–652

Transcranial Doppler Sonographic (TCD) Monitoring of Basilar Artery Thrombolysis

M.A. Williams[1,2], A.Y. Razumovsky[1], M.N. Diringer[2,5], L.H. Monsein[3], G.M. Debrun[3], R. Nick Bryan[3], and D.F. Hanley[2,4]

Acute basilar artery thrombosis is an often fatal disease which may be reversed by intra-arterial thrombolytic therapy. Important parameters for improving outcome include early identification of vessel occlusion, treatment before the onset of coma or tetraparesis, and successful recanalization of the affected arteries [1]. Transcranial Doppler sonography (TCD) has been used to monitor recanalization of the middle cerebral artery during intra-arterial thrombolysis [2]. We report our experience using TCD to identify vertebrobasilar occlusion and monitor vessel patency in 4 consecutive patients during and after intra-arterial thrombolysis of the basilar artery (BA).

Subjects and Methods

All patients were admitted via the emergency room or were already inpatients at Johns Hopkins Hospital. They or their families provided informed consent, and were given the option to be treated with intravenous anticoagulation or thrombolysis. Intra-arterial thrombolysis was performed with urokinase administered via a microcatheter placed as proximal to the thrombus as possible. This was begun within 12 h of identification of symptoms in all cases except one, in which the first attempt failed. TCD was performed via the transtemporal and suboccipital windows with a Medasonics Transpect instrument with a 2 MHz probe.

Case Studies

Patient 1. This 77-year-old man developed diplopia, left facial pain and weakness, and disequilibrium in the hospital one week after a distal pancreatectomy for carcinoma. TCD done 4 h later showed linear blood flow velocity (LBFV)

Departments of [1]Neurology, [2]Anesthesiology/Critical Care Medicine, [3]Neuroradiology and [4]Neurosurgery Johns Hopkins Medical Institutions, Baltimore, MD, USA, and [5]Department of Neurology, Washington University-St. Louis, St. Louis, MO, USA

G.J. del Zoppo, E. Mori, W. Hacke (Eds.)
Thrombolytic Therapy in Acute Ischemic Stroke II

of 13 cm/s with a delayed systolic upstroke in the BA; low amplitude, reverberating blood flow in the right vertebral artery (VA); and normal LBFV in the left VA. Angiography demonstrated occlusion in the mid-BA and proximal right VA, and a patent but atretic left VA. Thrombolysis was started 8 to 10 h after his initial symptoms. A total of 1.25 million units of urokinase recanalized the right VA, but the BA remained occluded distal to the superior cerebellar arteries. Subsequent TCD also confirmed flow through both VAs and absence of flow in the BA. The patient did not recover consciousness or brain stem reflexes and later died.

Patient 2. This 47-year-old man presented to the emergency room with somnolence, left facial weakness, diminished cough and gag reflexes, and left hemiparesis. MRI demonstrated small infarctions in the pons and both occipital poles. Angiography showed occlusion of the BA distal to the posterior inferior cerebellar arteries (PICA), delayed right VA flow, a small left VA, and an occluded proximal right internal carotid artery. Thrombolysis was started 10 to 12 h after symptoms began. The BA thrombus was lysed with 750000 units of urokinase and the vessel was recanalized, but a severe stenosis persisted. Subsequent TCD showed BA LBFV of 30 cm/s. He was clinically stable, but one week later new brain stem deficits developed. TCD indicated BA occlusion which was confirmed by angiography. Repeat intra-arterial thrombolysis was performed with 750 000 units of urokinase, but the basilar artery could not be reopened. This patient was later declared brain dead.

Patient 3. This 51-year-old man presented to the emergency room with dizziness, slurred speech, and unsteady gait. The BA was occluded distal to the anterior inferior cerebellar artery. Thrombolysis was not started until 28 to 30 h after onset of symptoms because of technical difficulty, but recanalization was attained with 750000 units of urokinase. One hour later, the BA LBFV was 8 cm/s and increased to 22 cm/s 6 days later. The patient was orally anticoagulated and later discharged to home with dysarthria and mild right hemiparesis, but was functionally independent.

Patient 4. This 49-year-old woman who was orally anticoagulated for chronic atrial fibrillation and a prosthetic aortic valve suddenly fell to the floor, unconscious, at home. In the emergency room she had sluggishly reactive pupils, no spontaneous or reflex eye movements, diminished corneal reflexes, and mixed extensor and flexor posturing. CT scan showed no hemorrhage, and TCD revealed low amplitude, reverberating signals in the right VA, LBFV of 13 cm/s in the BA, and 28 cm/s in the left VA. Angiography demonstrated occlusion of the right VA from the origin, and the entire BA to the top. The left VA was patent to the posterior inferior cerebellar artery (PICA), and the top of the BA and the posterior cerebral arteries filled via the posterior communicating arteries. Thrombolysis was begun 8 h after symptom onset. Using a total of 1.25 million units of urokinase, the right VA and BA were recanalized. TCD 6 h later revealed no audible signal in the right VA, and LBFV of 32 cm/s in the

BA and 35 cm/s in the left VA. This patient never regained consciousness and died within 36 h of presentation.

Discussion

BA occlusion often presents with a stuttering, progressing course. Anatomic correlation of vessel patency with neurological signs is necessary to properly identify patients with BA occlusion who may be candidates for thrombolytic therapy. Cerebral angiography shows the degree and location of BA occlusion and must be done to perform intra-arterial thrombolysis, but it is not a practical monitoring technique. Vertebrobasilar occlusion may be classified as single-sector, multi-sector, or top-of-the-basilar. Nadeau and colleagues [3] studied 57 patients with vertebrobasilar stroke not treated with thrombolysis, and found the highest mortality in the multi- sector group, with 7 of 11 patients dying within 60 days. Three of those 7 patients had stroke progression within 3 weeks of presentation. All of our patients had clinical and angiographic evidence of multi-sector vertebrobasilar system thrombosis and were at risk for death or re- occlusion.

In this small cohort, TCD demonstrated changes in vertebral artery or basilar artery LBFV which corresponded to changes in the neurological examination and angiography. In one case, TCD indicated re-occlusion of the BA, prompting repeat angiography and thrombolytic therapy. We conclude that TCD is an effective monitoring tool that correlates with angiographic findings and clinical symptoms. Its use should be considered during intra-arterial thrombolytic therapy for acute basilar artery occlusion and during the recovery period when re-occlusion is likely.

References

1. Hacke W, Zeumer H, Ferbert A, Bruckmann H, del Zoppo GJ (1988) Intra-arterial thrombolytic therapy improves outcome in patients with acute vertebrobasilar occlusive disease. Stroke 19:1216–1222
2. Karnik K, Stelzer P, Slany J (1992) Transcranial Doppler sonography monitoring of local intra-arterial thrombolysis in acute occlusion of the middle cerebral artery. Stroke 23:284–287
3. Nadeau S, Jordan J, Mishra S (1992) Clinical presentation as a guide to early prognosis in vertebrobasilar stroke. Stroke 23:165–170

HMPAO SPECT Measures Reperfusion After Thrombolytic Therapy in Acute Stroke

A.E. Baird[1,4], G.A. Donnan[1,4], M.C. Austin[2], G.J. Fitt[3], and W.J. McKay[2]

The introduction of thrombolytic therapy is potentially a major advance in the management of patients with acute stroke. Important applications of Single Photon Emission Computed Tomography (SPECT) may be the early identification of the site (and possibly severity) of cerebral ischemia, and the measurement of reperfusion after thrombolytic therapy. We are using hexamethylpropyleneamine oxime (HMPAO) SPECT to measure cerebral perfusion before and after streptokinase administration in patients entered into the Australian Streptokinase (ASK [1]) Trial. We are aiming to measure the degree of cerebral reperfusion within the first 48 h of ischemic stroke, and to correlate this with thrombolytic administration and functional outcome.

Subjects and Methods

Study Period. May, 1991–April, 1992.

CT Scans. At presentation and after 7 days.

Streptokinase. Intravenously (1.5×10^6 units) within 4 h of stroke onset, and intra-arterially (250000 units) between 4 and 24 h. Controls were patients excluded from thrombolytic therapy [1].

^{99m}Tc-HMPAO. Injected prior to streptokinase administration and at 24 h. Reperfusion was defined as a return of perfusion to within 12% of the homologous region in the contralateral cerebral hemisphere [2], and $\geqslant$30% in area. Hyperemia was defined as a perfusion level of $\geqslant$26%. Tissue salvage was defined as normal CT topography (after 1 week) occurring in a region which had

Drs. Baird and Donnan are supported by the National Health and Medical Research Council of Australia
Departments of [1]Neurology, [2]Nuclear Medicine and [3]Radiology, Austin Hospital Melbourne, Vicotria and [4]University of Melbourne, Melbourne, Victoria, Australia

G.J. del Zoppo, E. Mori, W. Hacke (Eds.)
Thrombolytic Therapy in Acute Ischemic Stroke II

previously reperfused. Fourteen patients with normal perfusion scans were not included in the analysis of reperfusion [1].

Outcome. Functional outcome at 3 months (Barthel index).

Results

Thirty-eight patients were studied (20 male, 18 female), mean age 71.3 ± 1.9 years. Sixteen patients were treated with streptokinase, with 22 controls. Fifteen patients were studied within 4 h of stroke onset (10 streptokinase), and 23 patients were studied between 4 and 24 h (6 streptokinase). The distribution of events was: middle cerebral artery (MCA) territory, 26; subcortical, 9; brain stem, 2; and uncertain, 1.

Reperfusion. Reperfusion was identified in 15 of 24 patients, always in the MCA territory. In the majority it was partial (12 of 15), often involving one of the MCA branches. Hyperemia was identified in three cases. Six of 10 patients treated with streptokinase (60%) had reperfusion, compared with 9 of 14 (64%) controls. Seven of 11 patients studied within 4 h of onset had reperfusion (4 of 7 streptokinase, 3 of 4 controls), compared with 8 of 13 patients studied between 4 and 24 h (2 of 3 streptokinase, 6 of 10 controls).

Tissue Salvage. Eleven of the above 15 patients had normal CT topography (after 7 days) in the vascular territory which reperfused. In 3 other patients, infarction occurred in a portion of the reperfused zone. Partial voluming from border zone perfusion may have masked underlying hypoperfusion in two of these cases. One patient died before a late CT was performed.

Functional Outcome. Two patients were excluded because of stroke recurrence during follow-up. Four of 8 patients with no reperfusion died, compared with 1 of 14 in the reperfusion group, and none in the normal perfusion group (Fisher's Exact test, $p < 0.01$). Median Barthel scores at 3 months were: normal perfusion studies, 100; reperfusion, 90; and no reperfusion, 35 (Mann-Whitney U-test, $p < 0.05$ when no reperfusion group compared with normal perfusion group).

Discussion

Reperfusion usually occurred in one of the MCA branches, and most likely corresponded to embolic migration/lysis during the first 24 to 48 h of cerebral ischemia. Total reperfusion occurred in 3 of 15 cases (20%), previously reported at 25% within 48 h. The levels of 60% – 64% partial reperfusion were higher than seen previously (8 of 24 cases of MCA occlusion studied within 4 days).

Reperfusion rates were expected to be higher in the 4 to 24 h group, although rates were similar in both groups; it is impossible to be certain when reperfusion occurred in the 24-h period between ^{99m}Tc-HMPAO injections. Patient numbers are too small to comment on the efficacy of thrombolysis.

The good outcome of patients with normal scans is most likely related to the presence of subcortical ischemia (lacunar infarcts in the majority), which have a better prognosis than cortical infarcts, and to early reperfusion in two cases of MCA ischemia. Patients with reperfusion were mostly functionally independent, although the majority still had regions of infarction, but smaller than the nonreperfused group, where the high death and dependency rate related to large MCA territory infarcts.

We have reservations about interpreting reperfusion and performing semiquantitative analysis, because the retention of ^{99m}Tc-HMPAO in both intact and ischemic brain is incompletely understood. In cerebral ischemia, more knowledge is needed about HMPAO uptake in relation to blood flow, as well as HMPAO retention in relation to glutathione and cellular organelle binding in ischemic tissue. At present, HMPAO SPECT must be regarded as measuring tissue perfusion, and not viability or metabolism. The results presented here are preliminary only.

References

1. Steering Committee Australian Streptokinase Study (1991) The Australian Streptokinase Study Protocol and Operations Manual
2. Podreka I, Suess E, Goldenberg G, et al (1987) Initial experience with technetium-99m-HMPAO brain SPECT. J Nucl Med 28:171–177

A Cell Culture Model of Reperfusion Injury: Neutrophil-Mediated Brain Endothelial Cytotoxicity

D.C. Hess[1,2], X. Chen[3], A. Griezkiewicz[2], and J. Catravas[3]

With the advent of thrombolytic therapy for acute ischemic stroke it may soon be possible to rapidly restore blood flow to an ischemic area of the brain. However, reperfusion may carry its own attendant risk of further tissue injury. There is an increasing body of evidence which suggests that neutrophils play an important role in mediating tissue damage during acute ischemic stroke [1, 2, 4, 5]. Moreover, there are suggestions that neutrophils may be at least partially responsible for the "no reflow" phenomenon [3].

Neutrophil–endothelial cell interactions may account for the tissue injury found during reperfusion. Three potential mechanisms by which neutrophils may enhance injury include: 1) cytotoxic effects upon the microvasculature with development of cerebral edema and hemorrhage; 2) neutrophil plugging of the microvasculature with impediment to further flow; and 3) direct cytotoxic effect on neurons and glia. This latter mechanism would require margination and passage through the endothelium.

In order to test the hypothesis that neutrophils may abnormally adhere to or injure cerebral endothelial cells during reperfusion, we developed a cell culture model of reperfusion injury in which cultured human microvascular brain endothelial cells were exposed to severe hypoxia followed by reoxygenation.

Subjects and Methods

Endothelial Cells. Human brain microvascular endothelial cells were isolated from temporal cortex specimens from patients undergoing ablative surgery for epilepsy. After removal of the meninges, the tissue was minced and homogenized. The homogenate then underwent dextran centrifugation to pellet the microvessels. Next the pellet was passed through successive nylon mesh screens. After overnight digestion with collagenase-dispase, the cells were allowed to attach to a fibronectin-coated plate. Contaminating cells (pericytes) were re-

Department of [1]Neurology, V.A. Medical Center, Augusta, GA, and Department of [2]Neurology and Medicine, Department of [3]Pharmacology, Medical College of Georgia, Augusta, GA, USA

G.J. del Zoppo, E. Mori, W. Hacke (Eds.)
Thrombolytic Therapy in Acute Ischemic Stroke II

moved by treatment with pancreatin. Endothelial cells were identified by morphologic features, immunofluorescence (*Ulex europeus*), and ACE activity by radiometric assay. Endothelial cells were grown in 75 cm^2 flasks in M199 with 10% fetal calf serum (FCS) with penicillin and streptomycin.

Neutrophils. Venous blood was obtained from healthy donors and neutrophils were isolated by density gradient centrifugation (Cardinal Associates, Santa Fe, NM). Cells were counted with a hemocytometer and concentrated to 2×10^6/ml in M199.

Cytotoxicity Studies. Endothelial cells from the first through fourth passage were grown to confluence in 24-well plates. The cells were incubated overnight with ^{51}chromium in 10% FCS in M199 (Gibco, Gaithersburg, MD). After washing and removal of unincorporated radioactivity, the monolayers were covered with 250 µl of M199 and placed in either an anaerobic chamber with $0_2 < 1\%$ (Forma Scientific, Marrietta, OH) or in a CO_2 incubator with 21% O_2 (Forma). After specified times of 1 to 24 h the plates were removed and neutrophils in M199 (1×10^6/well) or M199 alone were added. At set time periods of 1, 2, 4, and 20 h, 100 µl aliquots of media from the wells was removed and released chromium measured in a gamma counter. The remaining unreleased ^{51}chromium was measured by lysing and solubilizing the remaining cells with 1 ml of 1% Triton and measured in a gamma counter. The percent cytotoxicity in each well was calculated by the formula: cpm supernatant/(cpm lysate + cpm supernatant) × 100.

Adherence Studies. Endothelial cells were grown to confluence in 24-well plates and exposed to either anaerobic conditions or conditions or normoxia for 1 to 3 h. Neutrophils were labeled with ^{51}chromium and added upon reoxygenation (1×10^6/well). At set time periods the supernatant was aspirated, the wells washed once with M199 and these fractions pooled and counted in a gamma counter. The remaining endothelial cells and adherent neutrophils were lysed with 1% Triton and the radioactivity of this lysate measured in a gamma counter. The percent adherence was calculated by the formula: cpm lysate/(cpm supernatant + cpm wash + cpm lysate) × 100.

In other experiments, neutrophils labeled with ^{51}chromium were coincubated with endothelial cells in an anaerobic chamber for 2 h and then reoxygenated for a period of 1 h. As a control, labeled neutrophils and endothelial cells were coincubated for 3 h under conditions of normoxia.

Results

The addition of neutrophils upon reoxygenation significantly increased endothelial cytotoxicity. [1 h: 18.4% ± 1.5% (neutrophils) vs 12.7% ± 0.6% (no neutrophils), $p = 0.007$; 2 h: 22.2% ± 2.2% (neutrophils) vs 13.4% ± 0.7% (no neutrophils), $p = 0.003$; 4 h: 23.2% ± 1.9% (neutrophils) vs 14.4% ± 0.6% (no neutrophils), $p = 0.001$; 20 h: 48.6% ± 2.2% (neutrophils) vs 29.5% ± 1.0% (no neutrophils), $p = 0.001$, Student *t*-test, mean % of 6 wells + standard error of the mean.] No significant enhancement of endothelial cytotoxicity was found when neutrophils were added to endothelial cells exposed to conditions of normoxia. There was also no significant difference in cytotoxicity between endothelial cells exposed for up to 6 h of severe hypoxia and those exposed to normoxia. When endothelial cells were pretreated with allopurinol (10 μm) prior to exposure to severe hypoxia, the neutrophil-mediated cytotoxicity was significantly attenuated ($p < 0.05$). Moreover, similar attenuation was found when the cells were pretreated with 15 μm dimethylthiourea. No significant inhibition was found with pretreatment with indomethacin.

There was increased adherence of neutrophils to endothelial cells exposed to severe hypoxia (3 h) followed by reoxygenation compared to endothelial cells exposed to normoxia. This increased adherence was found at 1, 2 and 4 h after reoxygenation. [1 h: 23.3% ± 0.6% (severe hypoxia) vs 16.9% ± 0.7% (normoxia), $p = 0.0001$; 2 h: 32.1% ± 0.8% (severe hypoxia) vs 18.4% ± 0.9% (normoxia), $p = 0.0001$; 3 h: 38.0% ± 2.3% (severe hypoxia) vs 29.7% ± 1.3% (normoxia), $p = 0.0113$.]

When neutrophils and endothelial cells were both exposed to severe hypoxia for 2 h followed by 1 h of reoxygenation there was significantly greater difference than neutrophils coincubated with endothelial cells under conditions of normoxia (53.8% ± 2.6% [hypoxia] vs 27.1% ± 2.4% [normoxia], $p = 0.0001$).

Discussion

These observations demonstrate that under conditions of severe hypoxia followed by reoxygenation there is increased adherence of neutrophils to cerebral microvascular endothelial cells. Under our experimental conditions, neutrophil-mediated cytotoxicity occurred during reoxygenation. This cytotoxicity could be attenuated with allopurinol and dimethylthiourea. These latter findings suggest that oxygen-free radicals are involved in the pathogenesis of the cytotoxicity. A more specific role may be assigned to the xanthine dehydrogenase–xanthine oxidase system as at a dose of 10 μM, allopurinol is an inhibitor of xanthine oxidase but does not act as a free radical scavenger.

Further work is needed to define the mechanism of the increased neutrophil adherence under conditions of hypoxia and reoxygenation. It is known that neutrophil-endothelial cell interactions involve adhesive proteins expressed by both cells. Hypoxia-reoxygenation may cause an up-regulation of endothelial adhesive proteins or lead to the release of a chemotactic factor by endothelial cells.

References

1. Bednar MM, Raymond S, McAuliffe T, Lodge PA, Gross CE (1991) The role of neutrophils and platelets in a rabbit model of thromboembolic stroke. Stroke 22:44–50
2. Clark WM, Madden KP, Rothlein R, Zivin JA (1991) Reduction of central nervous system ischemic injury in rabbits using leukocyte adhesion antibody treatment. Stroke 22:877–883
3. del Zoppo GJ, Schmid-Schönbein GW, Mori E, Copeland BR, Chang C-M (1991) Polymorphonuclear leukocytes occlude capillaries following middle cerebral artery occlusion and reperfusion in baboons. Stroke 22:1276–1283
4. Dutka AJ, Kochanek PM, Hallenback JM (1989) Influence of granulocytopenia on canine ischemia induced by air embolism. Stroke 20:390–395
5. Hallenbeck JM, Dutka AJ, Tanishima T, et al (1986) Polymorphonuclear leukocyte accumulation in brain regions with low blood flow during the early postischemic period. Stroke 17:246–253

Modification of Brain Ischemia Due to Embolic Stroke by Tissue-Type Plasminogen Activator With and Without Heparin in a Rabbit Model

L. P. Carter, A. N. Guthkelch, J. Orozco, and O. Temeltas

This communication presents the results of an assessment of the ability of tissue-type plasminogen activator (t-PA), with and without heparinization, to modify the volume of ischemic brain tissue resulting from the introduction into the anterior cerebral circulation of the rabbit model of an embolus of standard size composed of white thrombus [5].

Subjects and Methods

The model comprised a group of 2–3 kg adult New Zealand white rabbits of either sex. In each animal, an arterial thrombus was created by scarifying the intima of the central pinnal artery under ketamine anesthesia. Two to three days later, under acetylpromazine/xylazine anesthesia, the thrombus was harvested. A portion of thrombus exactly 7 mm in length and 5 mm in diameter was cut, suspended in buffered saline and injected in retrograde fashion into the surgically exposed right internal carotid artery via the external carotid artery. Following embolization animals were randomized to receive either 2 mg/kg recombinant t-PA (alteplase; Genetech, South San Francisco, CA), or 200 U/kg/h heparin, or both of these together, by intravenous injection at intervals of 1, 2, or 4 h after embolization. Each subset contained 5 animals. Additional subsets of 5 animals received intravenous saline alone after an interval of 1 h or 4 h after embolization. Full details of our technique and of the results for 1-h and 2-h intervals have been published elsewhere [1].

Four hours after treatment had commenced, the animals were sacrificed with an overdose of barbiturates and their brains were rapidly removed and placed in 2,3,5-triphenyltetrazolium chloride (TTC) at 38 °C for 35 min. They were then photographed, immersed in ice-cold saline for a few minutes and cut into 2 mm thick sections. The sections were again treated with TTC and photographed so as to reveal the extent of ischemic tissue. This was then measured with a planimeter, and the volumes calculated using an appropriate computer

Department of Surgery (Section of Neurosurgery), University of Arizona Health Sciences Center, Tucson, AZ, USA

G. J. del Zoppo, E. Mori, W. Hacke (Eds.)
Thrombolytic Therapy in Acute Ischemic Stroke II

program for conic section models. Later, histologic preparations were made and examined by an independent observer to verify that the extent of ischemic change was about the same as the pale areas revealed by TTC staining. Note was also taken of the presence or absence of visible emboli in the middle cerebral artery and its branches. It was immediately clear that in the animals treated 1 or 2 h after embolization, the volumes of ischemic brain were smaller than in animals not so treated.

Results

The results were examined statistically. Because the data showed standard deviations from the group means which were roughly in proportion to the magnitude of these, it was deemed appropriate, after consultation with the Biostatistical Service of the University of Arizona College of Medicine, to express the results in relation to the logarithms of the volumes of ischemic brain. Statistical procedures included analysis of variance, which showed that only the interval elapsing before beginning treatment and the administration of t-PA made any significant difference to these volumes. Linear regression analysis showed that there was a significant increase in the volume of ischemic brain as t-PA administration was delayed to 2 and then to 4 h after embolization.

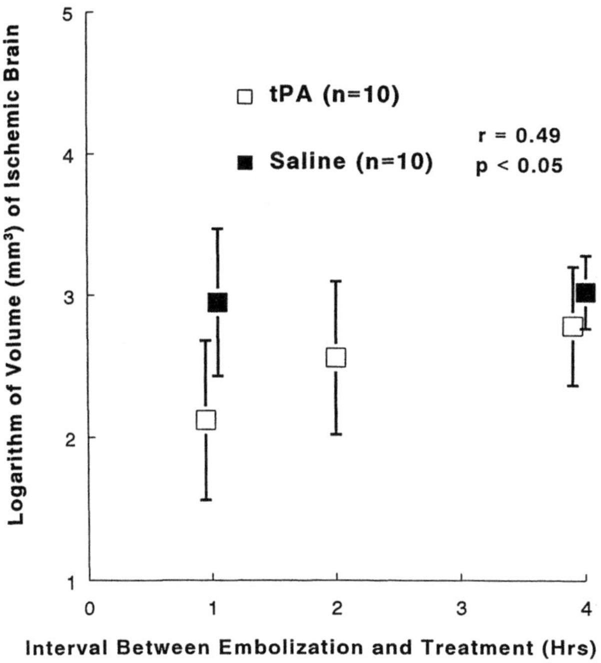

Fig. 1. Inflluence of tPA and interval before administration on volume of ischemic brain

At 4 h this was not significantly different from that observed in saline-treated controls (Fig. 1). On the other hand, the addition of heparin to t-PA made no difference to ischemic volumes and there was no difference between the volumes in the control series and those of animals receiving heparin alone at the intervals after embolization already specified.

In a small number of animals, a nuclear magnetic resonance scan was obtained prior to sacrifice. In those that had not received t-PA, ischemic changes were noted within 3 h of embolization.

Comment

These results are in conformity with a growing body of studies suggesting that the critical time within which, to be effective, thrombolytic treatment must be commenced after a stroke is of the order of 3 h [2–4]. While this study does not exclude the possibility that administration of an anticoagulant in combination with thrombolysis may, in the long term, increase the likelihood of hemorrhagic transformation of an infarct, over the short term there is no evidence of this. We shall soon be commencing a further series in which cerebral protective agents will be administered in combination with thrombolytics, to see whether such agents afford the brain any extra protection against ischemic change in conditions of acute embolism.

References

1. Carter LP, Guthkelch AN, Orozco J, Temeltas O (1992) Influence of tissue plasminogen activator and heparin on cerebral ischemia in a rabbit model. Stroke 23:883–888
2. Kaplan B, Brint S, Tanabe J, Jacewicz M, Wang X-J, Pulsinelli W (1991) Temporal thresholds for neocortical infarction in rats subjected to reversible focal cerebral ischemia. Stroke 22:1032–1039
3. Levine SR, Brott TG (1992) Thrombolytic therapy in cerebrovascular disorder. Prog Cardiovasc Dis 34:235–262
4. Okada Y, Sadoshima S, Nakane H, Utsunomiya H, Fujishima M (1992) Early computed tomographic findings for thrombolytic therapy in patients with acute brain embolism. Stroke 23:20–23
5. Rigamonte D, Uede T, Johnson PC, et al (1989) A new model of cerebral embolic ischemia using autologous arterial thrombus. Barrow Neurol Inst Q 5(4):2–7

Reduction of Infarct Volume and Mortality by Thrombolysis with rt-PA in an Embolic Stroke Model

T. Sereghy[1], K. Overgaard[1], G. Boysen[1], H. Pedersen[2], and N.H. Diemer[3]

The efficacy of thrombolysis with recombinant tissue plasminogen activator after embolization with microemboli was tested in a stroke model.

Subjects and Methods

Sprague-Dawley rats weighing 300–400 g were anesthetized with diazepam, fluanison, fentanyl, and atropine. The body temperature was kept between 37 ° and 38 °C. Blood pressure, p_aO_2, p_aCO_2, and pH were monitored through femoral arterial line.

Preparation of the Emboli. A 1-ml syringe with 28-gauge needle was filled with 50 µl of saline containing 2.5 units of thrombin. Then, 150 µl ($n = 33$) or 200 µl ($n = 17$) blood was drawn into another syringe of the same type. The two syringes were interconnected from tip to tip with a PP10 tube, and the suspension was moved alternatingly 70 times from one syringe to the other.

Carotid Operation. The right external carotid artery was cannulated and the pterygopalatine, thyroid, and occipital arteries were ligated. Clotting in the catheter was avoided by continuous flow of heparinized (5 IU/ml) saline through the line.

Embolization and CBF Measurement. The preformed embolus suspension was injected into the carotid catheter during 30 s. Just prior to and after embolization, CBF was measured using an intracarotid ^{133}Xenon bolus injection method.

Angiography. Immediately after and 2 h after embolization, angiography was performed via the carotid catheter by bolus injection of 0.2 ml heparinized

[1]Neurovascular Research Laboratory, Department of Neurology, [2]Department of Neuroradiology, University Hospital of Copenhagen, Rigshospitalet, and [3]Cerebral Ischemia Research Group, Institute of Neuropathology, University of Copenhagen, Copenhagen, Denmark

G.J. del Zoppo, E. Mori, W. Hacke (Eds.)
Thrombolytic Therapy in Acute Ischemic Stroke II

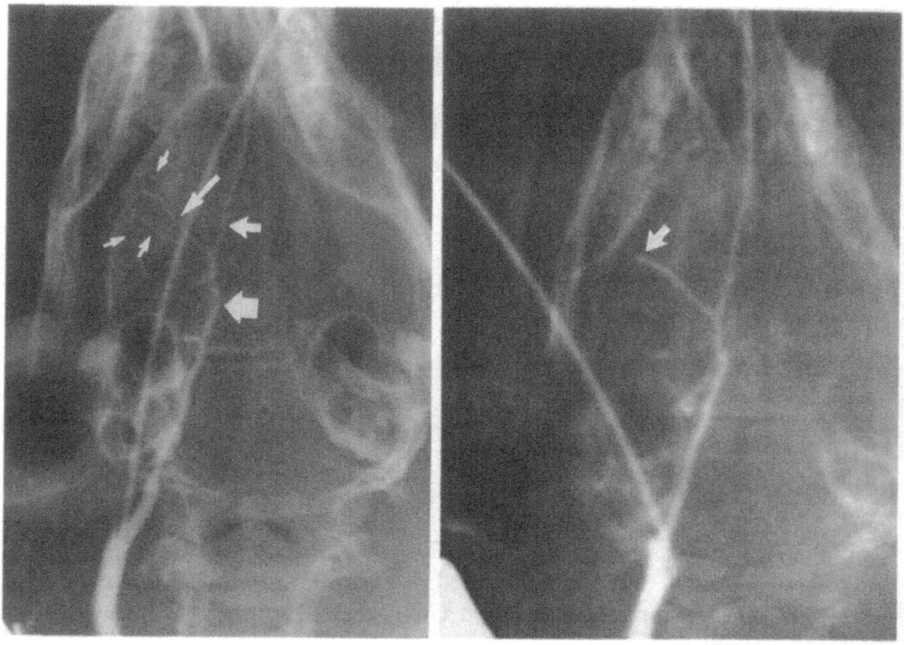
A B

Fig. 1. Angiography. **A** Normal filling of arteries supplying the brain; angiographic score value 0. The following arteries are identified: Internal carotid artery (*large thick arrow*), anterior cerebral artery (*small thick arrow*), middle cerebral artery (MCA) (large thin arrow), MCA-branches (*small thin arrows*). **B** Occlusion (*arrow*) of main-stem MCA; angiographic score value 2

(5 U/ml) iohexol. The angiograms were evaluated blindly by a neuroradiologist according to the score: 0 = patent arteries, 1 = middle cerebral artery (MCA) branch occlusion, 2 = MCA stem occlusion (Fig. 1), 3 = internal carotid artery occlusion.

rt-PA Administration. Eight animals embolized with 200 µl embolus suspension received rt-PA (alteplase), 3 mg/kg. Eight animals embolized with 200 µl embolus suspension and 8 animals embolized with 250 µl embolus suspension received rt-PA, 10 mg/kg. Intravenous infusion started 15 min after embolization and was administered during 30 (3 mg/kg dose) or 45 (10 mg/kg dose) min. Control animals received an equal amount of saline.

After the second angiography, all vessels were ligated, the wounds closed, and the anesthesia was reverted with naloxone. After recovering from anesthesia, the neurological status was evaluated, 0: normal rat, 3: maximum clinical damage.

Measurement of Infarct Size. Four to six days after the operation, the animals were again clinically examined and euthanized by cardiac perfusion-fixation with formalin solution. The brains were removed, postfixed, dehydrated, embedded in paraffin, sectioned and stained with hematoxylin-eosin. Using a Leica plus image analyzer, the hemisphere and infarct volumes were measured blindly.

Results

No differences were found in any parameters between the groups of animals treated with 3 mg/kg and 10 mg/kg rt-PA. The groups were therefore pooled.

Microscopy of Emboli. The emboli were heterogenous in size and shape, although the majority were elongated, irregularly outlined, less than 0.2 mm in cross-sectional diameter and resembled arterial "white" thrombi, rich in fibrin and platelets. The main results are displayed in Table 1.

CBF Reduction. Animals embolized with larger volumes of embolus suspension had larger CBF reduction after embolization ($p = 0.0025$).

Recanalization. Only slight spontaneous recanalization appeared in control animals, but significant recanalization was achieved by the thrombolytic therapy assessed by comparing the pre- and posttreatment angiograms of each animal ($p = 0.0005$ in 21 treated animals) as well as by comparison of the posttreatment angiograms of all thrombolysed and all control animals ($p = 0.036$, Mann-Whitney tests).

Clinical Effect. Recovering from anesthesia, the damaged animals were lethargic, showing asymmetrical posture, flexion of the forelimb contralateral to embolization, circling, tilting of the head, and pallor of the eyeball. The treatment increased the survival rate, from 0.48 in all controls to 0.96 in all treated animals ($p = 0.0004$, Fisher's test). The treated animals had better clinical recovery than controls, comparing the presacrifice Bederson scores ($p < 0.00005$, Mann-Whitney test), even when animals dying before sacrifice were not included in this calculation.

Reduction of Infarct Volume and Edema. Neuropathological examination showed infarctions affecting preferentially the MCA area (Fig. 2). Almost all infarcts were clearly demarcated with a border zone of only 5 to 10 cells in width, and sporadic neurons with eosinophilic cytoplasm. The treatment reduced the infarct size (Table 1), such that upon comparing all 23 treated animals with all 27 control animals, the significance reached $p = 0.0002$. Treatment reduced edema formation when we compared 23 treated animals (median embolized hemisphere volume of 265 mm^3) with 26 controls (median of 399 mm^3) ($p = 0.0001$, Mann-Whitney tests).

Correlation Between Angiographic Findings and Infarct Volume. Twenty-eight animals, which, on the second angiography, had patent arteries or only MCA

Table 1. Main results

Volume of emboli (µl)	Treatment with rt-PA	Number of animals	Survival		CBF reduction (%)	Angiography			Clinical score			Infarct volume	
			Rate	p		immediately after embolization	two hours after embolization	p	postop.	day 5	p	% of hemisphere volume	p
200	No	18	12 67%	0.15	71.5 (62.8 – 84.8)	2.0 (0.4 – 3.0)	1.0 (0.4 – 2.3)	0.14	3	3	0.0001	43.7 (8.8 – 68.7)	0.016
200	Yes	15	14 (93%)		70.0 (59.5 – 82.0)	3.0 (1.3 – 3.0)	0.0 (0.0 – 2.0)	0.003	3	0.9		11.3 (1.4 – 30.4)	
250	No	9	1 (11%)	0.0007	81.5 (66.3 – 90.0)	2.0 (2.0 – 2.6)	2.0 (1.0 – 2.5)	n.s.	3	3	n.s.	66.0 (57.5 – 68.9)	0.0006
250	Yes	8	8 100%		86.0 (81.0 – 97.0)	2.5 (2.0 – 3.0)	0.5 (0.0 – 2.5)	0.125	3	1.3		27.5 (12.6 – 50.0)	

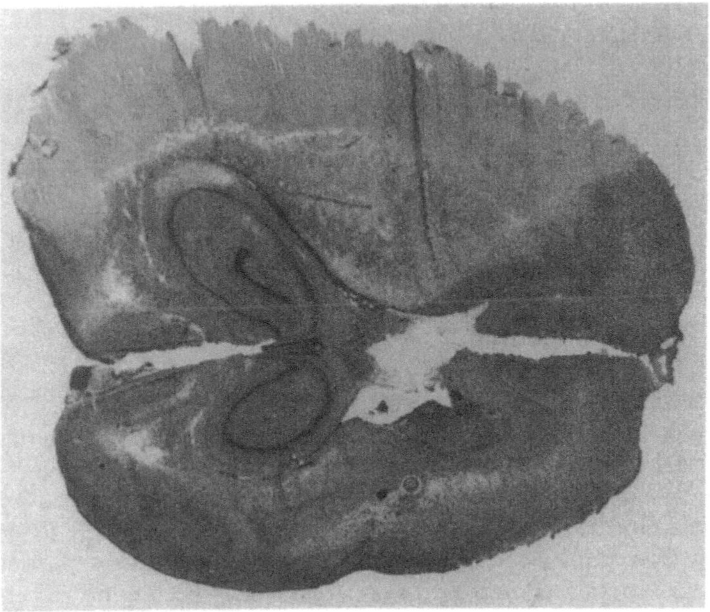

Fig. 2. Brain damage. Microphotograph of horizontal brain section with middle cerebral artery and posterior cerebral artery area infarction. Hematoxylineosin stain, original magnification 8

branch occlusion, developed smaller infarcts than 19 animals with more severe occlusions ($p = 0.0099$). Eight thrombolytic treated animals, embolized with 200 µl suspension, recanalized completely; infarct volume of those animals (median 2.8%) was smaller than infarct volume of the 7 nonreperfused (median 29%) in the same group ($p = 0.04$, both Mann-Whitney tests).

Correlation Between Clinical Findings and Infarct Volume. There was a strong correlation between the presacrifice clinical score and the infarct volume of the 35 surviving animals ($p = 0.0096$), and among survivors in the treated groups ($p = 0.003$). The body weight reduction (median 10.2%) correlated with the infarct volume ($p = 0.0027$, all Spearman tests).

Conclusion

Thrombolytic therapy reduced infarct size and mortality in this stroke model.

Discussion Summary: Open Communications

Chaired by E. Feldmann[1] and A. J. Furlan[2]

Discussion for Papers Presented by Drs. Wardlaw, Alberts, and Welch

Dr. Feldmann opened the discussion with a question to Dr. Welch: "The data [in the current NIH trial] reflect aggregate recruitment on a center-by-center basis. Are all centers ahead of schedule?" Dr. Welch replied that, "All the centers are up with the expected schedules. The one not up to schedule is no longer part of the study. Everybody is recruiting and some more than others, particularly those who are experienced in the process. It has really been quite successful."

Regarding the delays to treatment with fibrinolytic agents, Dr. Feldmann asked Dr. Alberts whether the timing of the presentation was affected by whom the patient initially contacted or by the stroke subtype? Dr. Alberts indicated that, "We found that those patients with intracerebral hemorrhage or cardioembolic strokes came in much sooner than patients with thrombotic strokes or small vessel lacunar strokes. Patients with hemorrhage or large ischemic strokes have dramatic deficits that are very difficult to ignore. I do not have any data about where the patients came from, but we have the impression that those patients who saw their local physician were much more delayed than those who consulted an ambulance service or came directly into the emergency room. A very common scenario was that a patient would go to an outlying hospital with a focal deficit and the physician would notice that their blood pressure was elevated. They would administer sublingual nifedipine to lower blood pressure and send them home. The patient would come to our hospital 6 or 12 h later with a more severe deficit, although their blood pressure was well-controlled. It was a sad but very common scenario. We have gone through tremendous local and regional educational efforts to try to improve the situation."

Dr. Brott added that, "Dr. Barson, who is now at Michigan, analyzed the NIH pilot study data and found that a call to the local doctor was a significant

[1] Department of Neurology, Rhode Island Hospital, Providence, RI, USA
[2] Department of Neurology, Cleveland Clinic Foundation, Cleveland, OH, USA

G. J. del Zoppo, E. Mori, W. Hacke (Eds.)
Thrombolytic Therapy in Acute Ischemic Stroke II

factor in slowing patient admission to the study. But before we come down too hard on the local doctor, I am a local doctor, too, and my patients who are ready to die do not call me either. They call 911 and that is quite appropriate. So there is a major distortion of that variable and it has to do with the severity of illness." Dr. Alberts agreed: "I also think patient presentation has to do with the area you work in. If you are working in a large metropolitan area with community hospitals and fairly sophisticated emergency room staff, you could set up a much more productive referral network. Duke University is in a small urban area with very small, rural outlying hospitals. We have to rely heavily on the helicopter to go back and forth to these local hospitals because we routinely transport patients from more than 100 miles away. It is a challenge to do that quickly."

Dr. Furlan commented, "I think we are hearing some very novel ideas on how to enhance patient recruitment, particularly from the NIH group. Demming, whom you may or may not know, is noted for his 14 points, the Bible of total quality management. Now we need a 15th point. Get the patient treated within 90 min. I would like to ask Dr. Welch a final question. There are 32 emergency rooms involved in the process management [you described]. Did you come up with 32 processes or was your strategy to move toward a standardized process that would be followed by all of these emergency rooms?" Dr. Welch responded, "There are different processes. The standard process is the flow charting. We walk through it, involving everybody. That is the equalizer and probably the only way to do it. I do not know one emergency room that works the same as another."

Discussion for Papers Presented by Drs. Freitag, Brucker and Brott

Dr. Furlan opened by asking Dr. Brott whether "... delay in treatment was a factor responsible for hematoma in your material?" Dr. Brott stated: "No,... but I would like to mention that we had a clustering of 'times.' While we had two time groups of 0–90 and 90–180 min, in the 0–90 group better than 85% of the patients were treated between the 85th and 90th minute, and in the 3-h group obviously our numbers were very low. [Therefore,]... we could not answer the question you posed."

From the audience a physician asked Dr. Brucker: "Imagine that you are deciding whether to use an intra-arterial or systemic approach. Could you comment on the variables that make you decide in some patients to use the intra-arterial route and in others to use the intravenous route?" Dr. Brucker responded that, "We begin the angiogram with the suspected vessel and if we find it occluded we start intravenous treatment. Then, we complete the angiography to document the collateral flow. We then again catheterize the occluded vessel to bring the catheter tip as close to the thrombus as possible, perhaps even entering the thrombus. We then initiate intra-arterial thrombolysis."

To Dr. Brott, Dr. Donnan noted that in the (ASK) streptokinase pilot study, the (parenchymatous) hematomas occurred in cases of massive middle cerebral artery infarction in patients with atrial fibrillation. "Can you comment on the size of the infarct with reference to the likelihood of forming a hematoma?" In reply, Dr. Brott stated that, "We have not analyzed the relationship of infarct volume by CT measurement at one week with the prior development of hematoma. However, the stroke scale score is some index of the size of the infarct and on that basis we did not see a relationship. One of our 5 hematomas occurred in a patient with a small vessel occlusion in the internal capsule. That patient had a cerebellar hematoma that obviously occurred at a site distant from the infarction. One of the problems with trying to learn about hematomas is that our numbers are so extraordinarily small and our patients are so heterogeneous."

Dr. Feldmann raised two questions for Dr. Brott. First, "Was the elevation in blood pressure that you detected in patients with rt-PA-related hemorrhage treated?" Dr. Brott replied, "I just took care of three of the patients. In one instance, the blood pressure was treated just prior to identification of the hemorrhage. In only one case was the blood pressure extraordinarily elevated. As you might have noticed, the pressures we found were not particularly high. One of the problems with the blood pressure and the possible relationship to hemorrhage is that the study does have blood pressure exclusion criteria. [Therefore,] we have a skewed sample with regard to blood pressure." Dr. Feldmann, in follow-up: "You did not have a control group. Would you speculate as to whether the five patients with symptomatic hemorrhage, out of 94 treated patients, reflect what you believe is an excess over the natural history of post-infarction hemorrhage?" Dr. Brott noted that, "Each of these hemorrhages developed within several hours of the cessation of thrombolytic therapy, so each was identified clinically and radiographically within about 8 h of the occurrence of stroke symptoms. We have not previously had the opportunity to identify such patients in the previous 10 years in our institution, so I have never seen a post-infarction hemorrhage within the first 6 h in the absence of anticoagulation. However, in our Bridging Study, I can say that one of the two hematomas that developed very early was in the placebo group."

Discussion for Papers Presented by Drs. Williams, Donnan, and Boysen

Following this group of papers, a physician from the audience asked Dr. Donnan what was about the time delay in terms of initiating treatment engendered by performing SPECT prior to thrombolytic therapy. Dr. Donnan, in reply stated, "In our series of 23 patients, it was 180 min on average. It did not delay the treatment to inject the tracer. We injected the tracer and scanned after treatment was given. That is the great beauty of SPECT scanning. You are able to inject the tracer and you still have about 4 h before you take the patient down for scanning."

The physician continued, "I know the numbers are only small but you have two treatment groups. The first group was treated between 0 and 4 h and then the next group between 4 and 24 h. Was there any difference in the percentage of patients who achieved reperfusion between those two groups?" Dr. Donnan replied, "There was not any difference. The numbers are very small, but it did not seem to matter when the scans were done as to whether reperfusion was documented."

Another physician in the audience stated, "One thing I missed in the discussion is any measurement of metabolic response of the brain to this type of treatment. Other than the neurological examination we are hearing about reperfusion rates, but I am not seeing anything about coupling those with the metabolic activity which is really what we want to salvage. An EEG may give us this information."

Dr. Donnan noted that the best indication of metabolic activity "... is that the patient is improving and is walking out of your department. I do not think that an EEG is going to help us. Very often, you may see a patient who has a clear-cut infarct on the CT scan and the EEG will be normal."

Discussion for Papers Presented by Drs. Hess, Carter, and Overgaard

Dr. Gordon raised a question for Drs. Overgaard and Carter regarding thrombus composition in their repetitive models. Because discussions have suggested that thrombolytic therapy might work best "on red clots, maybe on cardioembolic clots, rather than the clots that form in the arteries," it is apparent there is no agreement. "Dr. Carter's model is clearly a white or pale clot model formed in the artery, and Dr. Overgaard's clot model was also arterial, and yet both found some efficacy. I am a little confused by this, being not a hematologist, just a simple neurologist." Dr. Carter answered, "I am not a hematologist either, but I think that it was the suggestion of our pathologist that if we wanted a realistic model to study [the clinical condition], then we needed to use an arterial thrombus. rt-PA seemed to be effective, at least at 1 and 2 h after the embolization occurred. I think that subtyping on the basis of clot type or stroke type is very difficult to do clinically. It is almost easier to do the subtyping after the fact than before the fact. I do not think we can eliminate any patient whatsoever based on the etiology of the thrombus from these thrombolytic trials." Dr. Overgaard added that a technical difficulty with the rat model was that thrombi from whole blood would fragment easily, producing little or no damage in more than half the rats.

Dr. Furlan directed a question to Dr. Hess: "I was interested to see that indomethacin did not seem to offer any protective effect in your culture models. I believe there is some evidence from Hallenbeck and others that indomethacin seems beneficial in postischemic hypoperfusion. Can you comment on that in terms of the findings in your study?" Dr. Hess responded, "We have not tested indomethacin's effect on adherence, so it could play a role in adherence. In the cytotoxicity studies it did not show an effect, so [it does not protect against] cytotoxicity."

Dr. Grotta noted that re-occlusion had not been addressed during the Symposium. "I wonder whether in either of these animal models if the animals were left alive for any length of time before sacrifice re- occlusion would occur. I would also throw the question open to the TCD'ers and angiographers, and anybody, how frequently re-occlusion is occurring after thrombolytic therapy when not coupled with anticoagulation?" Dr. Carter indicated that in his study it was likely that the presence of heparin would have prevented re-occlusion if it occurred. Subjects receiving heparin "... were no different than those treated with rt-PA or the controls." Furthermore, it was very difficult to find thrombi when they were looked for. "They would usually be fragmented and presumably lodged in smaller vessels." In clinical situations, Dr. Furlan added, "Re-occlusion probably hinges on the preexisting stenosis. I think that was emphasized in the basilar artery cases." Here, due to the atheromatous base, re-occlusion may be a significant problem.

Finally, the issue of species differences in response to pharmacologic thrombolysis was brought forward. Dr. Zivin suggested to Dr. Overgaard that "... rat clots are not a very good substrate for human t-PA," and questioned why his experiments were performed with thrombi from a rat source. Dr. Overgaard replied that human source thrombi were not used for practical reasons. "We felt that we needed more security in our laboratory if we had to use human clots, and why use them if it was not necessary? In fact, t-PA works on rat blood and on rat plasminogen. This has been shown by Cotton and coworkers." Dr. Zivin: "It is only about 10% as effective." Dr. Overgaard: "Yes, we now use 20 mg/kg [alteplase] which is close to what is used in humans. Our problem was that we felt that we had to take care of HIV if we used human material, so it is a matter of practical approach in our laboratory."

In closing, Dr. Furlan stated: "I have one other comment on re-occlusion and I don't know if Dr. Zeumer or anyone else in the audience can comment. We have had a single case of high grade basilar stenosis that reperfused, but left a tight residual stenosis. We attempted balloon angioplasty. In fact, the stenosis was so tight the balloon could not be passed. Has anyone else in the audience had experience with balloon angioplasty following intra-arterial thrombolytic therapy or other similar techniques?" Dr. Monroe: "Yes, in fact, in a patient much like that described, a cardiologist was able to get a guidewire, a very soft platinum guidewire, through the region of stenosis. But re-opening the very tight stenosis with a balloon combined with urokinase led to a large area of hemorrhagic infarction throughout the brain stem. So, it is a really tough problem."

Clinical Trial Development

Clinical Trials Sponsored by Companies *Versus* the NIH

J.P. Mohr[1] and D.E. Levy[2]

This subject receives less attention in the literature than do the many other topics covered in the Symposium. Instead of buttressing the contents of this article by reference to the medical literature, the authors have decided to offer their own views based on personal experience. This experience includes the following: both have held full-time academic positions, from which they have sought and been funded both by the NIH and various drug companies; one is now a member of a drug company research firm, the other is a consultant to a company; both have participated in clinical trials assessing surgical versus FDA-approved medical therapy, medical therapy between two FDA-approved agents, and medical therapy for agents not yet approved by the FDA for any indications or for the indication for which a given trial has been organized; and, both have participated in trials funded by the NIH alone, drug company alone, or a mixture of the two. Each of these experiences has provided some insights into the similarities and differences between the various forms of sponsored research. Similarities exceed differences, and in recent years similarities are growing.

Perhaps most important, both the NIH and pharmaceutical companies formulate their research questions similarly and attempt to recruit the best investigators for their trials. Clinical NIH-sponsored research is generally directed at a clinical problem (e.g., therapy for acute ischemic stroke) while company-sponsored trials have the extra element of wishing to test one of their own compounds as the treatment for such a problem, aimed ultimately at seeking approval for such use by the Food and Drug Administration (FDA). Although pharmaceutical companies are believed generally to be motivated by desire for profit, they will be successful in generating profit only if they develop drugs that benefit mankind. Thus, they are driven ultimately by the same goals of helping people that motivate investigators receiving Federal funds.

This difference in purpose, however, is the crucial point on which the two sources of funding differ. For recipients of NIH funds, the timetable of funding cycles is critically important, whereas for pharmaceutical companies, the life of the patent is vital. Companies have great concerns that the patent might

[1] The Neurological Institute, Columbia-Presbyterian Medical Center, New York, NY, USA
[2] CNS Research, Knoll Pharmaceuticals, Whippany, NJ, USA

G.J. del Zoppo, E. Mori, W. Hacke (Eds.)
Thrombolytic Therapy in Acute Ischemic Stroke II

run out before the clinical trials are completed, the drug approved, and some of the investment recouped.

Further, companies remain alert to the possibility that safety concerns raised during a trial for a new indication of a drug already approved by (or submitted for approval to) the FDA for another indication could adversely affect the latter indication; and more than one trial has been still-born over this concern. For different reasons for concern over FDA review, companies usually prefer their agent to be tested against placebo. The coexistence of other concomitant treatment, it is sometimes believed, might complicate interpretation were the FDA to rule that benefit from the trial was from a combination of the tested drug and concomitant management (such as volume expansion therapy).

One other difference is that company-sponsored research scrupulously records all patient changes that might be interpreted as drug-induced "adverse events." This preoccupation with safety tends to make company-sponsored trials more cautious regarding inclusion and exclusion criteria, with the result that NIH-sponsored trials are often more generous in patient inclusion and company-sponsored trials far more limited, often requiring a larger number of centers and a longer time period for completion.

The issue of FDA approval also plays a huge role in the conduct of the trial. NIH-sponsored work is generally judged by peer review and reaches the physician and general public through scientific publications. For company-sponsored research, the principal target is the FDA, and publication in scientific journals, while important evidence the work has passed muster by peer review, is a separate issue. Achieving acceptance of the data by the FDA is an over-riding concern to companies, who go to great lengths to show that the only issue being tested is the utility of their agent in a given setting. Consequently, innovations in placebo-controlled trial design, data collection, and analysis tend to be suppressed in favor of forms, protocols, scales and analyses which have heavy precedent. As already mentioned, there is also great concern for the documentation of every detail of side effects, which are generally checked by a host of field personnel hired by the company to ensure completeness of the data set for outcomes which could be considered adverse effects of the therapy.

Confidentiality is a minor but recognized additional difference between NIH- and company-sponsored trials. Periodic publication of progress and free discussion among participants is a common feature of NIH trials, although increasingly the presence of external monitoring committees and scrupulous blinding of participants means that preliminary results are not available. Company-sponsored research also increasingly utilizes external monitoring committees, but additional factors that limit early public exposure of results are the concern about the possible impact on financial markets, good and bad, and the worry that some preliminary release of information may somehow jeopardize FDA action.

Perhaps it is concern for commercial impact which also influences the conduct of the trial, but NIH-sponsored trials tend not to suffer from issues of credibility, as they are typically run from university-based research units. Company-sponsored research tends to be the more credible when it is conducted at "arm's length" by a contractor, university-based or not, and when external monitoring committees are established.

Company-sponsored programs can cause additional problems, moreover, because of the need to negotiate the legal agreements, including "hold harmless" clauses, each time a new company or new trial is undertaken, which often result in long delays before implementation. The NIH also has standard language, at least for consent forms, but possibly because of presumed immutability of the government, investigators rarely try to change some of this dictated language.

Two additional trends are worth mentioning, one in funding, the other in staffing. Earlier, the funding mechanisms differed, with NIH sponsorship generally based on the "best effort" rules which provided for a grant to the local investigators, incorporating the necessary proportion of salary, supplies, and other costs (including indirect costs). University research offices followed federal rules for NIH-sponsored research, where indirect costs were based on the federal guidelines. Company-sponsored research more often had a much lower indirect cost, if any, and a per-patient flat-rate reimbursement (capitation) in contract form. The NIH has recently evolved toward this latter position as well, with payment in some trials, such as the Trial of Acute Stroke Therapy (a trial of the Organon heparinoid) now almost entirely based on case recruitment (Table 1).

However it is organized, most current clinical trials have local staffs consisting at a minimum a local investigator, usually an M.D. with an academic ap-

Table 1

Subject	Company	NIH
Focus	FDA drug approval	Therapy for a problem
Design	Active *vs* placebo	Active *vs* other active or placebo
Emphasis	Safety	Efficacy
Methods	Standardized, precedent-dependent	Sometimes innovative
Monitoring	Company field personnel and, increasingly, external monitoring committee	Trust and, increasingly, external monitoring committee
Results	Prepublication very unusual; concerns regarding both FDA and financial markets	Preliminary results may be disseminated; sometimes essential to maintain funding
Timetable	Governed by patent life	Governed by funding cycles
Credibility	Best if at arm's length and with external committee	Not so great a problem; may be a problem if result is unpopular
Reimbursement	Capitation (per case) and low indirect	Capitation or effort-based with high indirect
Other	Concern that safety issues could jeopardize other indications	

pointment, and a "patient care coordinator," usually an R.N. or L.P.N., qualified to act as the contact person for the patient, the central coordinating center for the trial, and as data clerk and keeper of records. Serious efforts in the past decade or so have developed this position into a profession, and many trialists prefer dealing with the coordinator as the surrogate investigator; the physician is left as the person responsible for finding patients, performing examinations and recording the clinical data, while the coordinator is responsible for most of the other details. This desired professional status has brought with it a steadily climbing income and has led more than one such professional to a supervisory position or to career moves to larger academic centers, rather like the traditional academic career path. The development of these professionals has strengthened clinical trial technology to a degree that their presence is an expected, even demanded, component of research teams. While a healthy development, it has had an unintended but clear negative effect on the training and development of the careers of clinical physician- investigators, who formerly often handled such tasks. Physician-investigators are sometimes now thought to be less qualified than the patient care coordinators and may even be thought to have salaries too high for what they do. For this and other reasons not covered in this presentation, it is not entirely clear who will comprise the next generation of clinical investigators.

Blindness and Thrombolysis

D. Stump and J. Breed

A major concern in clinical research is that of bias. Protocol design, data collection, analysis of results and presentation of data are all areas of potential bias. Trials shown to have been biased tend to lose their validity. Consequently, it is crucial to recognize when and where bias may occur and to guard against it. A significant research technique for minimizing bias is blinding, that is, keeping some or all participants in the protocol from knowing the treatment assignment, active agent or placebo. Bias may be either negative or, more likely, positive. There is often an assumption by the patient and investigator that the intervention will be helpful, and reporting of side effects and outcome measures may therefore not be accurate. The impact of bias on a study is particularly critical when the study is small and the end-points subjective [1, 2]. It is the purpose of this review to identify sources of bias and to suggest mechanisms of prevention. Potential sources include: the research subject, the physician-investigator, the research staff, the laboratory, the study medication, and the sponsor. The sponsor is assumed to be a pharmaceutical company.

An unavoidable source of bias is the patient himself. Most research patients participate in a protocol because they believe they will benefit from the intervention. When it is known that an active agent is being administered, a placebo effect may occur, resulting in a positive outcome. Consequently, trials are blinded. However, the research subject receiving an unknown (blinded) drug may exhibit subjective symptoms, for example, an allergic response to the test treatment, making it obvious that the active agent was administered. Objective responses, such as bleeding in a patient receiving thrombolytic therapy versus placebo, may also occur. While neither type of response is preventable, the practice of good medicine concurrently with the study protocol, as well as respect for the blind, is crucial.

Physician-investigators are in an excellent position for both the manifestations of bias as well as its prevention. They have a broad exposure to a protocol and are usually in contact with other participating investigators. In addition, physician-investigators may be on decision-making committees that have a maximal exposure to the data. Physician-investigators often have direct patient contact, and not only administer treatment but also evaluate patient responses.

Genentech, Inc., Clinical Research Department, South San Francisco, CA, USA

G. J. del Zoppo, E. Mori, W. Hacke (Eds.)
Thrombolytic Therapy in Acute Ischemic Stroke II

Outside the hospital setting, the physician-investigator is also in contact with the sponsor of the study. Communications with the company supplying the drug may include elements that would also lead towards bias on the part of the physician- investigator. The potential for bias in this group, therefore, is very strong.

Respecting the blind is the singularly most important mechanism available to physician-investigators for preventing bias. The intellectual challenge of determining the randomization scheme and/or blinding code is to be avoided. This can be done by keeping unblinding information secure and with limited access. Additionally, clearly defined end-points may be assessed by an independent observer. Use of Core Laboratories for selected end-point measures is a useful mechanism for accomplishing this goal. The need for limited to no access to Core Laboratory data that cause bias should also be respected by the physician-investigator.

Execution of research protocols usually involves several study staff members in addition to the physician-investigator. These individuals may have concomitant exposure to the patient, the study drug and the data, each of which can be a point for introduction of bias. While these three areas of exposure are requisite for any drug protocol to be carried out, some precautions can be taken to minimize bias. This is ideally accomplished by separation of the tasks of patient care, drug preparation and administration, and data collection so they are done by different staff members. While drug preparation in an acute setting may easily be assigned to a hospital pharmacist, it may be more difficult to assign drug administration and patient care to different staff members. Data collection may also be assigned to a specific individual who is not involved with direct patient care and evaluation of outcome measures.

In the setting of thrombolytic therapy, specific laboratory values, e.g., coagulation assays, can be predictive of the patient's treatment arm, placebo or active agent. This situation can be avoided by use of a Core Laboratory for such assays. Alternatively, assays done locally can be reported to a physician other than the physician-investigator. Filing of laboratory data in a protected file rather than placing results in the medical record can serve to maintain the blind. Standard procedures for computerized reporting of laboratory values, however, may make circumvention of the system more difficult than simply using a blinded Core Laboratory.

Corporate sponsors of clinical research protocols usually have several departments working together on protocol design and implementation. A study staff may consist of the following individuals or roles: medical monitor, clinical research associate, biostatistician, data manager and pharmacist. The company-sponsor may be the source of the randomization code. It will certainly be the supplier of study drug. It may also act as the data coordinating center and auditor of data for accuracy and completeness. Complicating the need for prevention of bias by the sponsor is the obligation for awareness and reporting of adverse events to the Food and Drug Administration (FDA). Adverse events may overlap with major end-points of the study, indirectly reflecting information about efficacy data.

A major mechanism for decreasing bias on the part of a company is control of access to specific types of information. For example, blinding codes generated by corporate biostatisticians should be done independently of the medical monitor, clinical research associate and data managers assigned to the project. Further, computer access to the program used to generate the blinding code should be strictly limited and protected by a secure password. Hard copies of the blinding code should be accessible only to the biostatistician generating the code and clinical drug personnel who are responsible for creation of appropriate labels for study drug and packaging materials. Additionally, any hard copies are kept locked.

Although preparation of clinical drug materials requires knowledge of the blinding information, thus inherently a potential source for bias, the Study Drug Coordinator has no access to study data nor any role in its collection or analysis. The study drug itself may be a source of bias if the treatment can be empirically determined. Therefore, in preparing study materials, it is incumbent upon the sponsor to provide placebo that appears identical to the active agent. When reconstitution of study drug is required, the process and end-product for both placebo and active agent need to be identical.

When the sponsor acts as the data collection center, medical monitors and clinical research associates necessarily have access to the data. This includes any laboratory results collected and reported on the data collection forms. Provision, however, can be made for use of a Core Laboratory as previously described. Additionally, Core Laboratory reports and files can be separated and reviewed by a clinical research associate whose involvement in the project is limited exclusively to Core Laboratory materials. This clinical research associate communicates directly with the Core Lab should there be a need for clarification or correction of data collection forms generated by the Core Laboratory. Clinical research associates and medical monitors remain blinded to the code prior to completion of data compilation. Furthermore, they do not participate in the primary, unblinded data analysis.

Both the data center and the biostatistical center remain blinded until termination of the study. Any predetermined interim analyses are done with treatment assignment remaining blinded.

Sponsors have alternative mechanisms available for limiting bias in clinical trials. Extramural agencies can be used for distribution of study drug, data coordination, data analysis and data reporting. Additionally, an independent group can be engaged to act as a Data and Safety Monitoring Board. A committee of this kind independently reviews the data from predetermined interim analyses. Based on data from these analyses, the Data and Safety Monitoring Board may recommend that a protocol either continue, be put on hold pending additional information, or be terminated.

The areas for bias in clinical research are myriad. Blinding that remains intact until completion of a study can minimize the occurrence of bias. Therefore, maintaining the blind should be a priority in all blinded studies. The key question when considering unblinding is whether knowledge of the actual treatment will alter subsequent medical intervention for an individual patient research subject. Unquestionably, if the answer is negative, the blind should remain intact.

References

1. Assenzo JR, Teal TW (1984) Clinical data management and statistical design in the clinical research process. In: Materon GM (ed) The clinical research process in the pharmaceutical industry. Marcel Decker, New York, p 153
2. Spilker B (1991) Guide to clinical trials. Raven Press, New York, p 15

Subject Index

Springer-Verlag and the Environment

We at Springer-Verlag firmly believe that an international science publisher has a special obligation to the environment, and our corporate policies consistently reflect this conviction.

We also expect our business partners – paper mills, printers, packaging manufacturers, etc. – to commit themselves to using environmentally friendly materials and production processes.

The paper in this book is made from low- or no-chlorine pulp and is acid free, in conformance with international standards for paper permanency.

GPSR Compliance

The European Union's (EU) General Product Safety Regulation (GPSR) is a set of rules that requires consumer products to be safe and our obligations to ensure this.

If you have any concerns about our products, you can contact us on ProductSafety@springernature.com

In case Publisher is established outside the EU, the EU authorized representative is:

Springer Nature Customer Service Center GmbH
Europaplatz 3
69115 Heidelberg, Germany

Batch number: 10704711

Printed by Printforce, the Netherlands